JOURNEY ACROSS
the Life Span

Human Development and Health Promotion

Birth is a beginning

And death a destination.

And life is a journey:

From childhood to maturity

And youth to age;

From innocence to awareness

And ignorance to knowing;

From foolishness to discretion

And then, perhaps, to wisdom;

From weakness to strength

Or strength to weakness

And often back again;

From health to sickness

And back, we pray, to health again;

From offense to forgiveness,

From loneliness to love,

From joy to gratitude,

From pain to compassion,

And grief to understanding

From fear to faith;

From defeat to defeat to defeat

Until, looking backward or ahead,

We see that victory lies

Not at some high place along the way,

But in having made the journey, stage by stage,

A sacred pilgrimage.

Birth is a beginning

And death a destination.

And life is a journey,

A sacred pilgrimage

To life everlasting.

With permission from The New Union Prayer Book. Central
Conference of American Rabbis: New York, 1978, p. 283

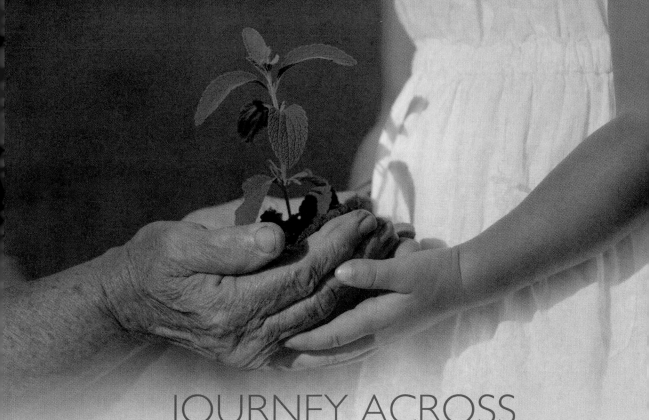

JOURNEY ACROSS
the Life Span

Human Development and Health Promotion

5TH EDITION

Elaine U. Polan, RNBC, MS, PhD
Retired Supervisor
Practical Nurse Program
Vocational Education and Extension Board
School of Practical Nursing
Uniondale, New York

Daphne R. Taylor, RN, MS
Retired Assistant Supervisor
Practical Nurse Program
Vocational Education and Extension Board
School of Practical Nursing
Uniondale, New York

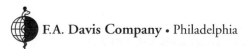 F.A. Davis Company • Philadelphia

F. A. Davis Company
1915 Arch Street
Philadelphia, PA 19103
www.fadavis.com

Printed in the United States of America

Last digit indicates print number: 10 9 8 7 6 5 4 3 2 1
Acquisitions Editor: Megan E. Klim
Developmental Editor: Rachel Miller
Director of Content Development: Darlene D. Pedersen
Content Project Manager: Echo K. Gerhart
Electronic Project Manager: Jaclyn Lux
Design & Illustration Manager: Carolyn O'Brien

As new scientific information becomes available through basic and clinical research, recommended treatments and drug therapies undergo changes. The author(s) and publisher have done everything possible to make this book accurate, up to date, and in accord with accepted standards at the time of publication. The author(s), editors, and publisher are not responsible for errors or omissions or for consequences from application of the book, and make no warranty, expressed or implied, in regard to the contents of the book. Any practice described in this book should be applied by the reader in accordance with professional standards of care used in regard to the unique circumstances that may apply in each situation. The reader is advised always to check product information (package inserts) for changes and new information regarding dose and contraindications before administering any drug. Caution is especially urged when using new or infrequently ordered drugs.

Library of Congress Control Number: 2014956160

Current trends indicate a need for changes in our health care system. The need is for a system that focuses on universal health care. This creates a need for emphasis on health promotion, maintenance, and restoration. In this new health delivery system, health care workers are expected to provide care to individuals in a variety of settings throughout their life span.

This textbook is designed to assist students in their study of the life cycle from conception to old age. Instead of having to read only certain sections of a core text or portions of a pediatric or maternity text, students can now see the complete presentation of growth and development across the life span. We hope this will be meaningful and will assist students in developing an appreciation for individuals in their struggle to maintain, promote, and restore health.

This edition has 14 chapters, each designed to make the book user-friendly. The last chapter deals with the topics of death, dying, and bereavement. The authors hope that readers will find comfort and guidance from this chapter when dealing with either personal or professional losses. A chapter outline, a list of learning objectives, and a list of key terms, which are considered important to the reader's understanding of the material, precede each chapter. Helpful Hints boxes, a special feature used in this text, are designed to draw the reader's attention to important facts. Other pedagogical features include tables, boxes, illustrations, and photographs. New with this edition are 10 Podcasts on the major chapters. These are for students to use at their convenience. By first reading the chapters and then listening to the Podcasts, students have a clearer understanding of the content. We hope that this new format will be enjoyable and educational.

At the conclusion of each chapter, a chapter summary highlights key points, followed by one or more Critical Thinking exercises to increase awareness and to challenge thinking. Multiple-choice questions at the end of each chapter help students test their content understanding. Suggested readings that enable students to further explore and research topics of interest and Web sites can be found on Davis Plus.

We wish to point out that the names of persons used in Critical Thinking exercises and in case studies are fictional and that any resemblance to names of actual persons is coincidental.

It is our hope that students will find this text easy to read and applicable to clinical practice and personal growth.

Elaine U. Polan, RNBC, MS, PhD
Daphne R. Taylor, RN, MS

Janice Ankenmann, RN, MSN, CCRN, FNP-C
Vocational Nursing Program Director
Napa Valley College
Napa, California

Linda M. Fleshman, MSN, HCNE, MST, RN
Director/Instructor
Mt. Hood Community College
Gresham, Oregon

Sharon Moore, RN, MSN-Ed
Practical Nursing Program Chair
Forsyth Technical Community College
Winston Salem, North Carolina

Robin Pearson, BSN
Nursing Instructor
North Florida Community College
Madison, Florida

Polly Reynolds, BSN, RN
Nursing Faculty
Galen College of Nursing
Louisville, Kentucky

Diane Roney, RN, BSN, MSN, **Certificate of Nursing Administration**
Professor; Program Director of the Practical Nursing Program
Eastern Gateway Community College, Jefferson Campus
Steubenville, Ohio

Acknowledgments

We, the authors, wish to extend special thanks to the following individuals without whom we could not have completed this task.

F.A. Davis and Acquisitions Editor Megan Klim, Project Editor Echo Gerhart, and Robert Craven III. We enjoyed working together again.

Last, we thank the many students whom we have taught over the years. Each of our students has enriched our lives and help inspire us. We hope that students will find this text helpful and enjoyable.

Contents

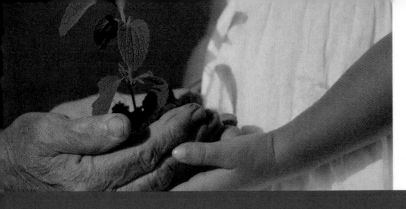

CHAPTER 1

Healthy Lifestyles

Key Words

anxiety

apathy

disease prevention

emotions

empowerment

equilibrium

fight-or-flight response

general adaptation
  syndrome

health

health promotion

health restoration

holistic

life expectancy

malnutrition

nutrition

regression

stress

substance abuse

wellness

Chapter Outline

Learning Objectives

At the end of this chapter, you should be able to:

- Describe the history of health.
- Describe the model for the nation's health as proposed by *Healthy People 2020*.
- Describe the concept of health.
- List five healthy lifestyle practices.
- State the role of the practical nurse in health promotion.
- List two factors that interfere with people's abilities to change their personal habits.

HISTORY OF HEALTH CARE

Early civilization was concerned with health and diseases. Illness was often attributed to natural and supernatural forces. Sometimes illness was thought to be the result of some evil wrongdoing. Diseases were often warded off by incantations, magic, or charms or with the use of herb concoctions. At times drastic measures were taken to rid the body of demons, such as beating, torturing, or starving the sick. Other cures relied on magic and folk remedies. Even primitive surgery existed before the advent of Greek medicine. In about the sixth century BC medical schools were established in Greece. Hippocrates was the first physician to believe that treatment should be based on the belief that nature has a strong healing component. Diet, exercise, and hygiene became important to treatment.

Throughout the Middle Ages medicine and religion were interwoven. Plagues and epidemics killed millions of people. Understanding of disease processes did not occur until the development of bacteriology, which took place in the 19th century. Louis Pasteur, Robert Koch, and Joseph Lister are some of the important scientists who made a significant impact contributing to the scientific understanding of health and disease during this time. During the 20th century a major cause of death was infectious diseases, but environmental improvements in sanitation, water, and food supply helped to further improve the quality of life. Between the years 1936 and 1954, the discovery and use of vaccines and antibiotics further reduced the number of deaths from infectious diseases.

Despite all the improvements toward limiting the incidence and numbers of deaths from infectious diseases, several diseases surfaced and reappeared in the 20th century. Diseases such as tuberculosis and measles have resurfaced, and new infectious diseases such as HIV, AIDS, Ebola virus, and drug-resistant strains of organisms (*Staphylococcus aureus, Streptococcus pneumonia*, and *Salmonella*) have become the current health challenges facing the population today.

Many other achievements have contributed to longevity and health. Improvements and advancements in maternal care have led to decreases in maternal and infant mortality rates. Better nutrition, better hygiene, and improved technology have also greatly reduced the risks to both mothers and infants during the first year of life. Still, the issue of access to health care for all remains a concern. Great numbers of childbearing women do not seek any medical care during pregnancy, increasing the risk for both themselves and their infants.

Other areas of improvement include recognition of the risks associated with tobacco use, genetic counseling, motor vehicle safety, and advances in diagnosis and treatment for heart disease and strokes. Improvements in the workplace regarding safety and job-related hazards have helped further reduce mortality rates. The mortality (death) rate today is lower than at any other time in history.

Healthy People

For three decades, the U.S. Department of Health and Human Services has published a 10-year agenda for improving the nation's health called *Healthy People. Healthy People* provides the scientific base for a 10-year projection that addresses national health care goals and objectives. The first volume published was *Healthy People 2000,* and the aim was to reduce health disparities among Americans.

Building on the objectives first identified, *Healthy People 2010* was published and continued its belief in a systematic approach to improving health. *Healthy People 2010* identified two major national health goals. The first goal was to increase the quality and years of a healthy life. **Life expectancy** is the average number of years a person is expected to live. Life expectancy has increased from 47.3 years at the beginning of the 20th century to nearly 77 years today. *Healthy People 2010* sought not only to extend life expectancy but also to improve the quality of life. The second goal was to eliminate the health disparities among persons that exist according to gender, race, ethnicity, education, income, disability, location, and sexual orientation. Regardless of differences, this initiative was dedicated to making certain that all persons in our nation have equal access to fulfilling their health care needs.

Healthy People 2020, launched in December 2010, continues the tradition with a 10-year agenda that promotes health and disease prevention services aimed at improving the health of all Americans. *Healthy People 2020* promotes collaboration across communities to disseminate health information needed to empower the individual to make decisions about his or her health. The outcome of these preventative health strategies is also continuously measured and evaluated.

The overarching goals of *Healthy People 2020* are to improve the quality of life of all Americans and keep them free of preventable diseases, disability, injury, and premature death. Equity in health care and the elimination of disparities among different groups will improve the health of all Americans. An emphasis must also be placed on a good quality of life and healthy behaviors at all stages of development across the life span for all individuals.

The health indicators spotlight the major health priorities for the nation. The Leading Health Indicators are listed in Box 1.1.

HEALTH CARE DELIVERY

The U.S. health care system in the 19th and early 20th centuries was dominated by physicians and hospitals. In these early times there was a close relationship between patient and doctor. Physicians set fees, billed, or collected payments. Often physicians adjusted fees based on the patient's ability to pay. For many years the American Medical Association (AMA) fought against having any third party interfere or come between the patient and physician regarding any medical matter.

In the early part of the 19th century some individuals had medical insurance from their trade union, fraternal order, or some commercial carrier. This sickness insurance, as it was first known, was simple coverage for lost time during sickness or injury. Years later this coverage was extended to include workers' dependents and others. Before World War I there was some impetus toward compulsory health insurance following the initiative taken by several European countries. "Industrial" policies were sold by Metropolitan Life and Prudential Life Insurance Companies. This early form of health insurance was low cost but provided for only a small

<table>
<tr><td>B O X</td></tr>
<tr><td>**1.1** **Leading Health Indicators**</td></tr>
</table>

- Access to health care
- Clinical preventive services
- Environmental quality
- Immunization
- Injury and violence
- Maternal, infant, and child health
- Mental health
- Oral health
- Overweight and obesity
- Physical activity
- Reproductive and sexual health
- Social determinants
- Substance abuse
- Tobacco use

lump sum at the time of death to cover final medical expenses and the cost of funeral and burial.

The Great Depression, which started in 1929, changed the financial security of hospitals and physicians. The AMA continued to protest the concept of health insurance, recommending that "persons save for the time of sickness." In 1935 the Social Security Act was passed by Congress. This act established federal aid to states for public health and assistance. The Social Security Act became the foundation for the growth of Medicare and Medicaid legislation in 1965. Many factors influence the financing of the health care system today, including providers, employers, purchasers, consumers, and politicians. Controlling the rising costs and making provisions for the estimated 48 million Americans who are underinsured or uninsured are the two most pressing concerns today.

The Affordable Care Act

The U.S. health care delivery system is one of the most complicated and expensive systems in the world. Despite its sophistication, this system has been unable to adequately address the need for universal coverage. On March 21, 2010, the first step in realizing health care reform took place with the passing of President Barack Obama's reform bill. The goal was to offer health insurance to the millions of Americans who are uninsured and improve the coverage of those who have insurance.

The main objectives of the Affordable Care Act (ACA) are to move away from a focus on illness and toward a focus on prevention and wellness, with the goal of creating a more equally accessible system for the population. The act also emphasizes improving the quality of care, improving patient care outcomes, accountability, and cost reduction.

The ACA will be phased in over several years. The major change is an expansion of Medicaid coverage, which will begin in 2014. Most of the population will then be covered by Medicaid and by the Children's Health Insurance Program (CHIP). The federal government will pay 100% of the cost for the delivery of care from 2014 to 2016 and 90% thereafter.

Some of the important provisions are as follows:

- Families are eligible for certain preventive health services at no cost.
- Insurance companies are no longer able to refuse health insurance to individuals with pre-existing health conditions.
- Uninsured children will be covered by their parents insurance until age 26.

- All companies with 50 or more employees must provide health insurance.
- State health care exchange programs will be created to allow consumers who are not covered by their employer or other types of entitlement programs to shop for health insurance coverage.

Types of Care Plans

Current health care delivery in the United States is provided by both public and private sector organizations. These organizations own and operate health care delivery facilities. Payment for care is traditionally through health care insurance, the majority of which is provided by the government and the rest by private businesses. The government agencies that pay for health care are Medicaid, Medicare, CHIP, and the Veterans Health administration (VHA). Other individuals pay private insurance companies, and 15% to 16% of Americans remain uninsured.

Traditionally, a person entered the health care setting and contracted directly with a health care provider. The provider was then paid a fee for service. In the 1970s, managed health care grew from the belief that costs could be contained by managing health care service delivery. Managed health care has become the dominant form of health care service in the United States today. Under this system a primary care provider (PCP) is assigned to provide basic health care services. The primary health care provider is a physician, nurse, or physician's assistant. The aim of this system is to reduce the numbers of hospital admissions, costly procedures, and referrals.

Health maintenance organizations (HMOs) became the managed care structures responsible for the financing, organization, and delegation of services for their members. The HMO provides a plan that has the provider assume some of the financial risks and uses primary providers as the gatekeepers.

Preferred provider organizations (PPOs) established a network of providers that deliver services to the private sector for a discounted fee. The patient assumes the financial burden rather than the provider. Those patients wishing to use providers outside the network can do so but will pay extra. For the PPO to make payment, the PPO must provide prior approval of visits to specialists or for hospitalization. Other plans are available that mimic features found in HMOs and in individual choice systems. In these plans, known as point-of-service (POS) plans, providers are paid a preset payment based on membership or a risk-based

system. Individuals may also choose their own provider at their own financial risk.

Official and voluntary public health agencies operate at the state, federal, and local levels. Health promotion, disease prevention, and education are key aspects of these agencies.

Comparison of U.S. and Canadian Health Care Systems

The health care systems of Canada and the United States are often compared. The two countries had somewhat similar systems until the 1970s, when Canada reformed its health care system into a group of socialized insurance plans that offered coverage to all Canadian citizens. This system is publicly funded and covers preventive medical treatment through primary care physicians, hospitals, dentists, and other providers.

Most Canadians qualify for coverage regardless of medical history, income, and standard of living. Statistics indicate that Canadians have a longer life expectancy and lower infant mortality rate than Americans. Many factors are believed to have contributed to these statistics, including different racial makeup, alcoholism, and obesity rates. Similarities also exist between the countries, including health care costs that are rising faster than the rate of inflation.

World Health Organization

The World Health Organization (WHO) is part of the United Nations and exists at the international level. It is concerned with worldwide health promotion, including disease prevention, early detection of disease, and treatment. The WHO also strives to improve access to health care in some local communities, as a lack of access impacts all aspects of a person's physical, mental, and social health. The organization coordinates global health care efforts against public health threats, such as the severe acute respiratory syndrome (SARS) and H1N1 (swine flu) outbreaks, and emergencies that require humanitarian aid. The WHO monitors global health care issues, such as the re-emergence of infectious diseases like tuberculosis and others, as increased international travel and commerce may contribute to the spread of such diseases.

THE CONCEPT OF HEALTH

Today's nurse must be knowledgeable about what constitutes health because one of the primary goals of nursing is to assist the individual in achieving the highest level of health. In 1947 the WHO defined **health** as "a state of complete physical, mental, and social well-being, not merely the absence of disease or infirmity." The authors here attempt to define for the reader a concept of health that is **holistic** in its approach. That is, we consider health to include not only physical aspects, but also psychological, social, cognitive, and environmental influences. Physical health is influenced by our genetic makeup, which includes all the characteristics that people inherit from their parents. These characteristics not only include physical features, but also may encompass genetic weaknesses or disease. Genetic inheritance is further explored in Chapter 6. Psychological health refers to how a person feels and expresses emotions. Social health, however, deals with everyday issues of economics, religion, and culture and the interactions of people living together. Cognitive health encompasses a person's ability to learn and develop. Environmental concerns include such issues as water and air quality, noise, and biochemical pollution.

Throughout this text we refer to specific developmental theorists to support the holistic view of growth and development. These theorists include Freud (psychoanalytic theory), Erikson (psychosocial theory), Piaget (cognitive theory), Maslow (human needs theory), and Kohlberg (moral theory). The holistic approach to health, which recognizes individuals as whole beings, promotes consideration of all aspects of a person's life. This approach helps the practical nurse to understand each person and attach significance, value, and meaning to each life. The holistic view further helps identify similarities and differences among people, allowing decision making from the person's own unique perspective. Positive nursing outcomes using the holistic approach emphasize patient independence and maximize potential.

Throughout this text we use the terms *health* and *wellness* synonymously. We believe that health, from the holistic perspective, is a balance of internal and external forces that leads to optimal functioning (Table 1.1). True health produces a state in which individuals are able to meet their needs and interact with their environments in a mutually beneficial manner. Healthy individuals exhibit effective coping patterns and experience a certain degree of comfort and pleasure in their activities. Health may be visualized on a scale or continuum (Fig. 1.1). One end of the continuum depicts optimal health or wellness, whereas the other end shows disease, total disability, or death. *Disease* refers to an imbalance between the internal and external forces. Individuals find that,

TABLE 1.1 A Holistic Model of Health	
Internal Forces	**External Forces**
Body systems	Culture
Mind	Community
Neurochemistry	Family
Heredity	Biosphere

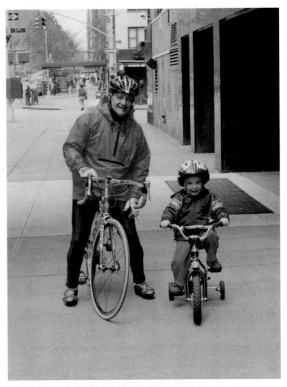

FIGURE 1.1 Exercise at all ages helps maintain health.

throughout the life cycle, health is not static but dynamic and can move backward and forward from a state of wellness to illness or disease.

Traditionally, health care has focused on an illness model, in which the primary role of the nurse is to relieve pain and suffering. Today, disease prevention is evolving as an area of nursing concern. This change places new demands on the practical nurse, emphasizing his or her role in patient education and health promotion throughout all stages of the life cycle.

PROMOTING, MAINTAINING, AND RESTORING HEALTH

Health promotion means health care directed toward the goal of increasing one's optimal level of wellness. Leading a healthy life means having full functional capacity at each stage of the life cycle, from infancy through old age (Fig. 1.2). Promotion of health can occur at any time and relates to individual lifestyles and personal choices. Health promotion allows people to enter into satisfying relationships at work and play. Health means being vital, productive, and creative and having the capacity to contribute to society.

The national aspirations for health promotion include three goals: healthy lives for more Americans, elimination of health care disparities among all ethnic and racial groups, and access to preventive services for everyone. The essential component of health promotion begins with the sharing of knowledge. The acquisition of knowledge then influences attitudes and leads to a change in behavior. Health promotion is most successful when placed in a supportive social environment. This environment first begins within the home and extends into the community. The community includes schools, churches, and businesses. Schools provide the location for the dissemination of health information among the young. More than 85% of American adults spend the greater part of the day in the workplace. The workplace, therefore, is another excellent site to

continue educating adults on health issues. Health promotion emphasizes nutrition, exercise, mental health, and avoidance of substance abuse. These health promotion issues are addressed throughout the text as they relate to specific age groups.

The practical nurse's first step in promoting health is assessing individuals and families for potential risks. Physical, social, and individual values must be considered essential components of the nursing assessment. Nurses can encourage patients to assume full responsibility for their behavior and to adopt a healthier lifestyle. Empowerment is a form of self-responsibility that encourages people to take charge of their own decision making. The practical nurse can play an important role in educating and guiding patients so that they have enough information to make critical decisions and be informed health consumers. Nurses must develop ways to help patients recognize their own needs, solve their own problems, and access resources that give them a sense of control over their own lives. Acts that empower patients place the nurse in the role of patient advocate. Nurses must be careful not to express their personal opinions, but rather to share enough information so that patients can make informed decisions. An example of the nurse's role as an empowering agent occurs when a patient newly diagnosed with cancer attempts to choose among the different treatment modalities offered by the physician. The nurse helps to assess the patient's knowledge level, communicates clear information, and supports the patient's decision concerning treatment. Throughout this text we discuss health-promoting activities that enable patients to maintain wellness, strive for their full potential, and enjoy a high quality of life.

The recent focus on health promotion and disease prevention has resulted in the introduction of alternative therapies as treatment modalities. Many of these therapies originated centuries ago in Eastern civilization. Today in the United States, these therapies are used along with Western scientific medical treatment. Managed care organizations may provide reimbursement for a few selected therapies. Nursing includes the practice of some of these therapies, such as therapeutic touch, acupuncture, and reflexology.

Disease Prevention

Disease prevention comprises three levels: primary, secondary, and tertiary (Table 1.2). Primary prevention occurs before there is any disease or dysfunction. The term *health promotion* may sometimes be used interchangeably with *primary prevention*.

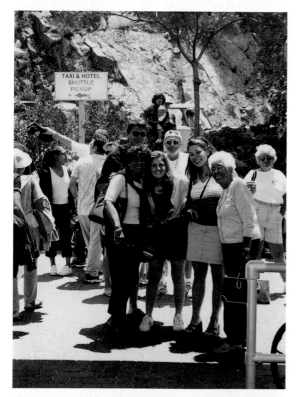

FIGURE 1.2 Health and wellness are promoted through an active lifestyle.

TABLE
1.2 Levels of Disease Prevention

Primary Prevention	Secondary Prevention	Tertiary Prevention
Immunization	Screening	Rehabilitation
Controlling risk factors	Treatment	Physical therapy, diet, exercise, stress reduction
HIV/AIDS education	Disease control	Pain control

An example of primary prevention includes patient education on basic hygiene, nutrition, and exercise. Other examples of primary prevention include immunizations against infectious diseases, avoidance of substance abuse, and regular dental examinations.

The most significant public health achievement in the past century is the reduction in the incidence of infectious diseases. Many factors have helped eradicate infectious diseases. Improvements in basic hygiene, food handling, and water treatment and the widespread use of vaccines have contributed to disease control. Antibiotics have further helped to successfully treat infectious diseases. Infants, older adults, minority groups, and health care workers are at increased risk for infectious diseases. All causative organisms, even those that are presently rare, may pose a potential threat of recurrence long after eradicating the illness. An example of this is the current reappearance of tuberculosis and smallpox. One major national goal is to effectively deliver immunizations to at least 90% of the preschool population. Special efforts should target minority populations, particularly African Americans and Hispanics, who, even today, receive fewer immunizations than the general population.

Many illnesses can be prevented worldwide by improving environmental quality. In recent years the United States has effectively moved to ensure clean water, safe food, and proper waste disposal, thus reducing the risk of infectious diseases. We still need to further improve air quality and develop new methods to eradicate other pollutants and environmental hazards. Environmental hazards today have taken on a new meaning since September 11, 2001. Concerns for the safety of air, water, food, and travel have evolved as a result of world terrorism. All persons are responsible for becoming informed and aware of their environment and its hazards.

Some people, such as older people, young children, pregnant women, and people with certain health conditions (such as asthma, diabetes, or heart disease), are at increased risk for serious complications from seasonal flu illness. The U.S. Centers for Disease Control and Prevention (CDC) currently recommends the influenza vaccination each year for the following groups (see the CDC website for up-to-date recommendations):

- Children aged 6 months and up; adults up to 24 years of age
- Pregnant women
- People 50 years of age and older
- People of any age with certain chronic medical conditions that put them at higher risk for influenza-related complications
- People who live in nursing homes and other long-term care facilities
- People who live with or care for those at high risk for complications from flu, including:
  - Health care workers and emergency medical services personnel
  - Household contacts of persons at high risk for complications from the flu
  - Household contacts and out-of-home caregivers of children younger than 6 months of age (these children are too young to be vaccinated)

Note: Current studies indicate the risk for flu infection among persons older than 65 years of age is less than the risk for persons in younger age groups.

In 2009, scientists discovered a new and very different flu virus called novel 2009-H1N1, sometimes referred to as swine flu, which caused many more people to get sicker than a regular flu would. It also caused more hospital stays and deaths than regular seasonal flu. It was first detected in people in the United States in April 2009, with the symptoms resembling those of seasonal flu. The H1N1 vaccine is now included in the influenza vaccine.

Personal injury is one of the leading causes of death in the United States. We must each identify and reduce our high-risk behaviors at home, on the job, and when we travel. The different health hazards that exist at each stage of the life cycle are outlined in later chapters.

Secondary prevention begins with diagnosis of disease or infectious processes. It focuses on the need for early diagnosis and treatment of disease to prevent permanent disability. Secondary prevention includes all interventions used to halt the progress of an already-existing disease state. It includes screening of all types (for example, breast self-examination or testing for hypertension and sickle-cell disease). In the latter stages of disease, secondary prevention often includes activities that prevent further disability. For example, the practical nurse may help the patient with diabetes prevent ulceration and loss of a limb by teaching and helping the patient to practice good foot care.

Tertiary prevention begins when a permanent disability occurs. Tertiary prevention is also referred to as **health restoration.** Health restoration begins once the disease process is stabilized. Nursing care is directed toward rehabilitation and restoring the person to an optimal level of functioning. The goal of tertiary prevention is to regain lost function and develop new, compensatory skills, possibly with the use of an assistive device such as a cane or hearing aid. Another goal is to help patients, including those with incurable diseases, attain the maximal level of health. To help patients achieve this objective, the nurse may collaborate with other health professionals, such as physical and occupational therapists. The nurse is also responsible for offering psychological support to patients and family members. The practical nurse can help an elderly patient who has had a stroke to achieve optimal functioning by first treating him or her with dignity and respect. Second, the nurse must provide individualized care that maximizes the person's strengths and minimizes weaknesses.

HEALTHY LIFESTYLES

In recent years it has become evident that many illnesses are preventable and that certain lifestyles greatly reduce the incidence of heart disease, stroke, and other diseases. There is a strong need to emphasize healthy behavior to reduce our current mortality rates. The overwhelming need is to learn to identify behaviors that place individuals at great risk for acquiring and possibly spreading disease. An individual's health also depends on his or her access to quality health care. An important goal on a national level is to expand health care opportunities and eliminate any disparities.

Health promotion campaigns should target nutrition, exercise, mental health, substance abuse, self-concept, and disease prevention (Box 1.2). Important to the success of any health promotion plan is the need to motivate and encourage patients to take responsibility for their own actions and health care practices. Involve the whole family in the needed

changes. The family must demonstrate healthy eating. Get children involved in meal planning and preparation.

Nutrition

Nutrition is a science that studies the body's need for foods, how foods are digested, and how food choices relate to health and disease. It is important throughout the life span, from conception to old age, to foster growth and maturation, and it is an important factor in promoting optimal health. Studies have shown that the five leading causes of death associated with poor dietary habits are coronary heart disease, cancer, stroke, non–insulin-dependent diabetes mellitus (type 2 diabetes), and coronary artery disease. **Malnutrition** is poor dietary practice that results from the lack of essential nutrients or the failure to use available foods. Malnutrition may involve undernutrition, including the symptoms of deficiency diseases, or overnutrition. This text focuses on dietary needs at each stage of growth and development

One of the goals of *Healthy People 2020* is to promote health and reduce disease by promoting the consumption of a healthy diet and maintaining a healthy body weight. An adequate diet provides sufficient energy and essential fatty and amino acids, vitamins, and minerals needed to support optimal growth and maintain and repair body tissues. It is not possible to design one diet for everyone because individual needs for nutrients vary greatly with age, sex, growth rate, and amount of physical activity, in addition to other factors, including social factors (Box 1.3). Because most nutrients are widely distributed in a variety of foods, it is possible to design a healthy diet or meal plan that satisfies an individual's personal and cultural preferences and lifestyle needs.

This means selecting a variety of foods from the five food groups as listed in the MyPyramid and MyPlate charts, while limiting intake of saturated fats, sugar, and alcohol. MyPlate, introduced in

B O X
1.3   Social Factors That Influence Diet

- Attitude
- Economic and price structuring
- Food and agricultural policy
- Food assistance programs
- Knowledge
- Skills
- Social support
- Societal and cultural factors
- Tobacco or drug usage

2011, builds on the basic MyPyramid. These guidelines are developed to help Americans make better food choices and understand that caloric intake must match energy output. See Figure 1.3 for the MyPlate chart.

Some of the conditions that are related to an unhealthy diet are obesity, malnutrition, iron deficiency anemia, heart disease, hypertension, type 2 diabetes, osteoporosis, oral disease, constipation, diverticular disease, and some cancers. Food provides the nutrients necessary to maintain health. These nutrients include protein, carbohydrates, fats, vitamins, minerals, and water (Box 1.4).

Causes of Obesity

Researchers believe that individuals can have a genetic predisposition for obesity. Other factors that can contribute to obesity are medications, fast foods, and a sedentary lifestyle, which might include more than 2 hours a day watching TV. See individual

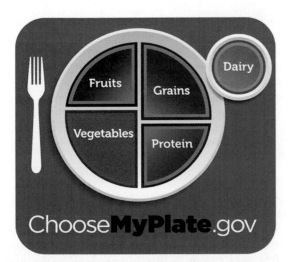

FIGURE 1.3 The MyPlate chart clearly outlines a balanced meal and diet. The MyPlate icon and the ChooseMyPlate.gov web page are from the U.S. Department of Agriculture.

B O X
1.4   Nutrients

Proteins
Proteins are broken down in the body into amino acids, which are the building blocks needed for repairing the body's cells and tissue. Sources of protein include meat, fish, eggs, legumes, milk, cheese, and nuts.

Carbohydrates
Carbohydrates are starches and dietary fiber that provide fuel for energy in the body. Carbohydrates are needed for brain, muscle, and heart function. They are divided into simple and complex forms: Simple carbohydrates are simple sugars found in fruits, while complex carbohydrates come from grains. Other sources for carbohydrates are breads, cereals, and vegetables. The fiber from carbohydrates is very important in lowering blood cholesterol levels.

Fats
Fats, also called lipids, cushion and provide insulation for the vital organs in the body. Fats also aid in the absorption of vitamins. They are divided into saturated or unsaturated: Saturated fats are those oils that are solid at room temperature, and unsaturated fats are oils that are liquid at room temperature. Unsaturated fats are the best types of fats to eat and cook with. Saturated fats raise the body's cholesterol levels. Sources of fats include meats, vegetables, and milk.

Vitamins
Vitamins are inorganic compounds that assist in building body tissues and are important in all chemical reactions in the body. They are found in a wide range of foods. Vitamin K is made by bacteria in the bowel.

Minerals
Minerals are inorganic substances that come from the earth and are important in body function. Calcium intake aids in the conversion of foods to energy; strengthens bones, teeth, and muscles; and aids in blood clotting. Iron is needed to make hemoglobin to carry oxygen to tissues. Minerals are found in a wide range of foods.

Water
Water aids in the regulation of body temperature, lubricates and cushions joints, protects the spinal cord, and eliminates waste from the body via urine, perspiration, and bowel movements.

chapters for further information on obesity and ways to counteract this growing health issue in different age groups.

Exercise

Regular exercise improves muscle strength and endurance, increases lung capacity, decreases tension and stress, and helps maintain adequate cardiovascular functioning. Studies have confirmed that regular exercise is useful in preventing heart disease, osteoporosis, diabetes, and other illnesses. The optimal benefits of exercise are seen when physical fitness is maintained throughout the life span (Fig. 1.4). Table 1.3 lists the positive effects of exercise.

There are two important points to remember about exercise. First, before beginning an exercise program, the individual should check with a physician. Second, moderation is better than excessive practice. The obstacles that many individuals face when trying to incorporate regular exercise into their daily lifestyles include lack of time and no place to safely exercise. It is recommended that adults get at least 30 minutes of moderate physical exercise daily or on most days. Children should limit inactivity and get at least 60 minutes of physical activity daily. The need for exercise and its applicability to the stages of growth and development are explored in each chapter of the text.

Mental Health

Mental health is a fluctuating state in which the individual attempts to adjust to new situations, handle personal problems without undue stress, and still contribute to society in a meaningful manner. Mentally healthy individuals see themselves and others realistically. A person's state of mental health fluctuates from day to day but maintains a certain degree of continuity and consistency. Certain behaviors may be normal in moderation but unhealthy in excess. For example, washing one's hands as part of everyday hygienic practices is considered acceptable. However, repeated hand washing unrelated to any activity is seen as bizarre and mentally unhealthy. A factor that may affect one's mental health is stress. Stress may be defined as anything that upsets our psychological or physiological equilibrium, or balance. Responses to stress may be physiological, emotional, or intellectual.

All humans experience many emotions. What is interesting is that human emotions are not the same for everyone. One individual may respond differently to a situation than another individual. During the course of a day, individuals experience a large range of different emotions.

Emotions are best defined as a feeling state. Our emotions produce both physiological and psychological changes. The physiological changes associated with an emotion are the result of motor,

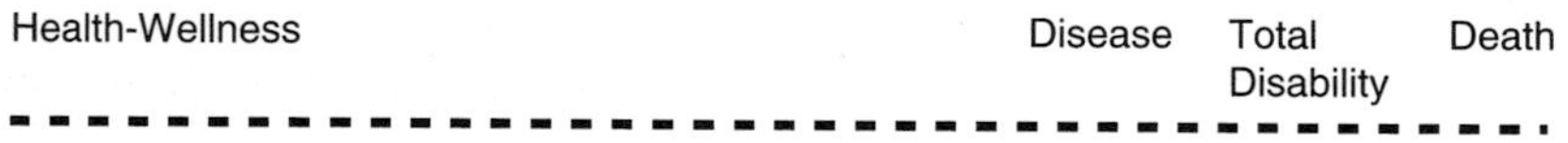

Health-Wellness		Disease	Total Disability	Death

FIGURE 1.4 The health-illness continuum.

TABLE
1.3   Positive Effects of Exercise

System	Effects
Cardiovascular system	Increases blood volume and oxygen content
	Increases blood supply to muscles and nerves
	Decreases serum triglycerides and cholesterol levels
	Reduces resting heart rate
	Increases heart muscle size
Respiratory system	Increases blood supply
	Increases exchange of oxygen and carbon dioxide
	Increases functional capacity
Neurological system	Reduces stress
	Improves mental health
	Decreases depression
Musculoskeletal system	Increases muscle mass
	Reduces body fat
	Increases muscle tone
	Improves posture

glandular, and visceral activity. Specific areas of the brain and the autonomic nervous system play a huge role in producing some of the physical changes one associates with an emotion. The areas of the brain known to play this role in a person's emotional response include the cerebral cortex and the limbic system. The cerebral cortex functions by receiving incoming sensory information. The limbic system of the brain comprises interconnected nuclei that affect memory and emotions. Conduction pathways in the brain produce many changes in the cardiac and smooth muscle contractions and in the secretion of some glands. Anger and fear produce an increased sympathetic activity. Increased heart rate, breathing, and intestinal tightening and cramping are just a few of the physiological reactions to certain emotions.

At birth, an infant's emotional experiences are simple and spontaneous. Most of their emotional responses are the result of their basic needs. For example, when the infant is hungry, his or her emotional response is likely to be crying with intense physical movements. Once satisfied, his or her response is one of pleasure and calm. With maturation and learning, emotional responses become more discriminating and individualized. See Figure 1.5.

Older children's and adults' emotions are expressed in a wide variety of responses with varying degrees of intensity. In fact, different stimuli produce different emotional responses in individuals. Common emotions include anger, jealousy, happiness, affection, fear, and anxiety. Emotional maturity exists when individuals are able to control their responses and can express their emotions in socially appropriate ways.

Some of the common physiological responses to stress include increased heart rate, respiratory rate, and blood pressure. Emotional responses to stress include irritability, restlessness, and a sense of discomfort. Intellectual responses to stress often include forgetfulness, preoccupation, and altered concentration.

Many years ago Hans Selye described three distinct stages of physiological response to stress, known as the general adaptation syndrome (GAS):

1. *Alarm stage:* Hormones from the adrenal cortex place the body in a state of readiness known as the fight-or-flight response.
2. *State of resistance:* The body attempts to adapt to the stressors.
3. *State of exhaustion:* After prolonged exposure to stress, the body's energy becomes depleted. This may result in disease or destruction.

Anxiety

Stress is a necessary part of life. It is unrealistic to expect to be able to eliminate all the stress from one's life, and it would not be healthy to do so. Stress triggers anxiety. Anxiety is the response to a stressful situation. Anxiety may be seen in four different levels: mild, moderate, severe, and panic. Mild anxiety is a part of normal, everyday life. Individuals experience some physical signs of mild anxiety such as restlessness, irritability, and mild discomfort. Mild anxiety sharpens one's perceptions and prepares the individual to act. Mild anxiety helps the student prepare for an exam. An example of mild anxiety can be demonstrated with the scenario of a young mother driving home with her children as it begins to snow and visibility is slightly hampered. The mother starts to feel tense and tells her kids that she has to concentrate on the road.

Moderate anxiety occurs with increasing discomfort. The individual's perceptions decrease. Persons experiencing moderate anxiety may focus only on certain aspects of what is happening. They tend to tune out what is considered less relevant. Learning can occur at this level of anxiety but not as effectively as at the mild level. Physical symptoms increase at this level, including heart palpitations, increased pulse and respirations, and mild gastric discomfort. The young mother is now experiencing greater difficulty driving through a heavier snowfall. She starts to feel gastric tightness, headache, and

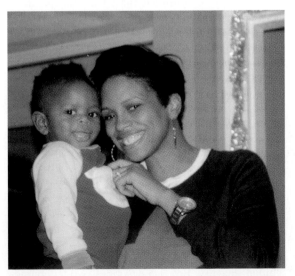

FIGURE 1.5 Infants' emotional experiences are instant and spontaneous.

marked irritability. She is unable to answer or talk to her kids as she recognizes the need to stay focused on her driving.

Severe anxiety decreases one's perceptions even further. The individual can focus only on one small detail of an event. Learning cannot take place at this heightened level of anxiety. Individuals may appear confused and complain of many physical symptoms. They experience a sense of doom and gloom. At this point the young mother has veered off the road and narrowly missed another car. She is in severe anxiety, and starts to cry and ignores her kids' responses.

The panic level is the most extreme form of anxiety. Individuals are unable to think clearly, reality is distorted, communication may be ineffective, and behavior is nonpurposeful. Physical symptoms are exaggerated. Our young mother has continued on her trip through very heavy snow and skids into another car. Although no one is hurt in either vehicle, the young mother is in a state of panic. When bystanders approach her, she is unable to describe what has happened and does not know how to proceed.

Stressors

Each of us perceives stressors differently, depending on our learned behavior, age, and personality (Fig. 1.6). For example, some individuals find air travel pleasurable, whereas others find it stressful. Stress may come from internal sources, such as

illness. It may also come from external sources, such as family, school, or peers. Stress can be acute or chronic.

Typical stressors in childhood include such events as birth of a sibling, death of a family member, onset of schooling, illness, and separation anxiety, to name a few. The practical nurse may witness stress or separation anxiety that a young child feels as a result of hospitalization. Separation anxiety may be seen in three phases: protest, despair, and detachment. Protest is evidenced by loud crying, restlessness, and dissatisfaction with substitute caregivers. Despair produces a sense of hopelessness and is seen as a quieter period. Detachment is a state of withdrawal and **apathy,** or lack of interest in one's surroundings. The nurse's awareness of these stages of separation helps both the child and the caregivers cope with and adapt to the stress. **Regression,** the return to an earlier stage of development, may be another childhood adaptation to stress. The stress of serious illness or hospitalization may cause the youngster to show regressive behaviors. The practical nurse can reassure the parent that bed-wetting after illness in a previously toilet-trained child is only temporary. After recovery from the illness, the child will return to the previous level of accomplishment.

Typical stressors during adolescence relate to an individual's search for identity. Decision making and the struggle for independence lead to family discord. Nurses can best assist adolescents in their struggles for independence by being supportive and encouraging decision making.

The main stressors of adults relate to their key relationships. According to the Social Readjustment Rating Scale (SRRS), death of a spouse, divorce, and separation are the events adults perceive as most stressful. During old age, life stressors include the loss of a spouse, retirement, and illness or loss of function. Nurses can help older adults cope effectively with stress by identifying and mobilizing their available support systems. For example, when an elderly patient is hospitalized, the family members need to be involved in the plan of care. Family involvement and frequent family contact help reduce stress for all involved persons. Another part of stress management is identifying what is perceived to be overly stressful. After identifying the stressor, a person must either reduce it or learn how to manage it in a healthy way. Healthy ways of adapting to stress include relaxation, exercise, humor, and guided imagery. Box 1.5 describes two techniques for reducing stress.

Responses to Stress

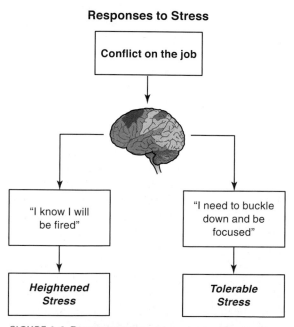

FIGURE 1.6 Responses to stress.

B O X
1.5 Stress-Reduction Techniques

Practice these techniques several times a day.

Relaxation Exercise
1. Assume a comfortable position.
2. Eliminate other distractions.
3. Close your eyes.
4. Regulate your breathing pattern and focus on inhaling and exhaling.
5. Progressively relax your muscles.
6. Refocus on your breathing, as needed.
7. Continue for 10 to 15 minutes.

Guided Imagery
1. Take a relaxed position.
2. Close your eyes.
3. Recall an image, event, or place that is pleasurable to you.
4. Focus your energy and thoughts on the image while relaxing your muscles from head to toe.
5. Concentrate on the image for 10 to 15 minutes.

Maladaptive Responses to Stress

Unhealthy or maladaptive responses to stress include denial, withdrawal, and acting-out behaviors. One example of denial is a surviving spouse who, after a prolonged period of mourning, is unable to change the deceased spouse's bedroom, leaving clothes and belongings in place as if the person were going to return. A detailed discussion on maladaptive responses to stress can be found in Chapter 5.

Substance abuse commonly refers to the abuse of drugs such as alcohol, nicotine, and caffeine, and legal and illegal pharmaceutical preparations. See Chapter 10 for further discussion of substance abuse. A substance abuser has more than a strong desire for the substance. Substance abuse is marked by gradual reduction in awareness, decline in self-esteem, and withdrawal from involvement. Recently, much attention has been given to educating the public about the effects of substance abuse. Tobacco use is one of the most important preventable causes of death in our society today. Recent research shows that every day 3,000 young persons start smoking. The connection between smoking and lung disease has been well documented for more than 40 years. Smoking also contributes to heart disease and fetal and neonatal abnormalities and deaths. Health promotion is aimed at encouraging cessation of smoking and avoiding exposure to secondary smoke. Because all behavior is influenced by role modeling, social education and individual responsibility are needed to further reduce the incidence of smoking in future generations.

Although moderate alcohol use may be beneficial in lowering blood cholesterol levels, alcohol abuse presents a serious health problem in our society. Alcohol abuse is not measured according to the specific amount consumed; rather, alcohol abuse occurs when the person cannot curtail the amount of alcohol he or she consumes or when alcohol interferes with the person's daily functioning. Alcohol use has been documented to begin at an early age. Recent studies have shown that many children ages 12 to 17 admit to drinking.

Long-term alcohol use has been linked to liver damage, heart disease, and an increased risk of neonatal disorders. Statistics indicate that alcohol contributes to serious social and health problems, including automobile accidents. Alcohol use is implicated in almost one-half of the deaths caused by motor vehicle crashes. It is also responsible for one-third of all homicides, drownings, and boating deaths.

Intravenous drug users and their sexual partners are at increased risk for AIDS and related sexually transmitted diseases (STDs). Drug treatment programs, counseling, education, and frequent testing reduce the many risks associated with drug use.

A Healthy Self-Concept

Knowing and practicing healthy behaviors and avoiding risky behaviors do not guarantee good health. Many factors influence an individual's health status, including family and community relationships, perception of various social pressures, and individual temperament. All of these factors cause each person to respond to the environment in a unique and sometimes unpredictable manner. Furthermore, perceptions of the environment, reactions to it, and individual needs are affected by a person's self-concept.

The relationship between the individual and the environment is reciprocal—that is, a person's self-concept is affected by the environment in which he or she lives. Self-concept also is affected by the individual's stage of development. Throughout this text we discuss the stages of development and how they might affect the individual's health and choices related to a healthy lifestyle.

Chapter 5 provides an explanation of several theories related to individual development: psychoanalytical, psychosocial, cognitive, moral, and others. Good health is more than a visit to the doctor. Healthy decisions, such as what we eat for lunch or the amount of exercise we get, can be made every day. Although many Americans are moving toward healthy living, others still need encouragement to practice healthy behaviors. Each person must set realistic goals that will reinforce positive behaviors. The first step is to make an inventory of healthy and unhealthy behaviors and develop a health assessment plan (Boxes 1.6 and 1.7).

ROLE OF THE NURSE IN HEALTH PROMOTION

As changes occur in the health care system, the role of the practical nurse also needs to change to meet the demands of the new health care delivery system. Practical nurses will need to work not only in traditional hospital settings, but also in the community.

B O X
1.6   Health Behavior Inventory

Before beginning any lifestyle change, it is important to assess your behavior. List below the healthy and unhealthy things that you do.

Healthy Behavior:

Unhealthy Behavior:

B O X
1.7   Personal Health Assessment Plan

In any health assessment it is important to first become aware of your personal quality of life. Complete the following statements and determine your personal health action plan.

1. Based on my readings, my personal health issues of most concern are:

2. My top-priority health issue is:

3. I can address the preceding issues by taking the following actions:

4. My goal is to:

Emphasis will be on prevention and health promotion. All levels of nurses will be accountable to both the employer and the client.

In the future, the practical nurse will have five roles and responsibilities:

1. *Caregiver:* Delivering health care services
2. *Teacher:* Educating the client, family, and community
3. *Advocate:* Helping clients choose between available options
4. *Collaborator:* Working as a member of a team, sharing and exchanging information
5. *Role model:* Practicing healthy lifestyle behaviors that will influence and reinforce clients' actions

SUMMARY

1. Early civilization was concerned with health and diseases.

2. Many improvements have contributed to today's increased life expectancy.

3. *Healthy People 2020* established two major goals for the nation: the first is aimed at increasing the quality and years of a healthy life, and the second is aimed at the elimination of health disparities.

4. Health is a balance of internal and external forces leading to optimal functioning.

5. Health promotion refers to health care directed toward increasing one's optimal level of wellness.

6. A change in lifestyle or personal habits is often necessary to promote maximal health.

7. Health maintenance focuses on prevention and the need for early diagnosis and treatment.

8. An important goal on a national level is to expand health care opportunities and eliminate disparities.

9. Health restoration begins after the disease process is stabilized. The goal is to either restore function or help the person compensate for losses.

10. Leading a healthy lifestyle includes paying attention to nutrition, exercise, mental health, substance abuse avoidance, and disease prevention.

11. Emotions are best defined as a feeling state. Our emotions will produce both physiological and psychological changes.

12. Factors that influence a person's health behavior include family, role models, social pressures, and self-concept.

13. Disease prevention is composed of three levels: primary, secondary, and tertiary.

14. The five roles for the practical nurse in health promotion are caregiver, teacher, advocate, collaborator, and role model.

CRITICAL THINKING

Exercise #1

Larry Woodhill, a 47-year-old bank manager, attends the wellness clinic offered by his organization. Larry weighs 230 pounds and is 5 feet, 8 inches tall. He has smoked two packs of cigarettes per week for the past 30 years. His recreational activities begin on Friday nights at the local bar, where Larry consumes five or six cans of beer. This activity is repeated on Saturday nights but not on Sundays. Through the wellness clinic, Larry embarks on an exercise program.

1. Without other major behavior changes, how do you evaluate the benefits of exercise for Larry?
2. Develop an approach to dietary counseling that may be beneficial for Larry.
3. What other healthy choices could Larry incorporate into his lifestyle?
4. Which of Larry's behaviors are considered high risk?

Exercise #2

A student begins classes after being out of school for several years. Prior to his first exam the student notes that he is becoming increasingly nervous and stressed. The night before his exam he stays up all night studying. On the morning of the exam he arrives feeling sick with stomach cramps and diarrhea. His muscles are tense, and he is jittery and sweaty.

1. What physiological responses is he experiencing?
2. Describe your own physiological responses to stress.
3. Describe what measures can be used to lower one's stress response in this situation.

MULTIPLE-CHOICE QUESTIONS

1. In early civilization, illness was often believed to be caused by:
   a. Bacteria and viruses
   b. Supernatural focus
   c. Internal imbalance
   d. External conflict

2. Knowledge of disease process occurred with the:
   a. Teachings of Hippocrates
   b. Use of herbal medicine
   c. Development of the U.S. Department of Health
   d. Advent of bacteriology

3. Which of the following statements best describes the Affordable Care Act?
   a. Medicare coverage will be available for all citizens.
   b. Expansion of Medicaid
   c. All health insurance companies will be owned and operated by the federal government.
   d. The major focus is providing inpatient care.

4. The health care worker is correct if she tells a client that *Healthy People 2020* provides a:
   a. Focus on world health issues
   b. Framework from which Canadian health care developed
   c. Scientific base for disease prevention and health promotion for all people in the United States
   d. National health insurance for low-income Americans

5. The objective of the managed care system is to:
   a. Decrease the number of hospitalizations
   b. Assign risk and quality to each case
   c. Increase the revenue for physicians
   d. Decrease the number of days spent in the hospital

6. Health can be defined as:
   a. Harmony between illness and wellness
   b. Balance between internal and external forces
   c. A state of mental thought process
   d. A state of physical functioning

7. The objective of health promotion is to:
   a. Hold the professional nurse responsible for the client's lifestyle practices
   b. Provide positive reinforcement to secure each healthy act
   c. Achieve an optimum level of wellness
   d. Decrease the person's tolerance level for stressful events

8. Empowerment is:
   a. The intensity of feelings generated by the client
   b. A needs-based behavior
   c. Client-centered decision making
   d. Open interaction between the client and the environment

9. Which of the following is a positive benefit of exercise?
   a. Decreased muscle mass
   b. Improved cardiac output
   c. Decreased blood supply
   d. Decreased nerve function

10. Mental health is best described as:
    a. Being problem-free
    b. Always consistent
    c. Ritualistic and excessive
    d. Realistic and adaptive

11. Physiological responses to moderate anxiety include:
    a. Improved mood
    b. Relaxed posture
    c. Slowed breathing
    d. Increased heart rate

12. Common responses to stressful situations may include which of the following? (Choose all that apply.)
    a. Decreased heart rate
    b. Smooth muscle contractions
    c. Glandular secretions
    d. Increased breathing
    e. Drowsiness

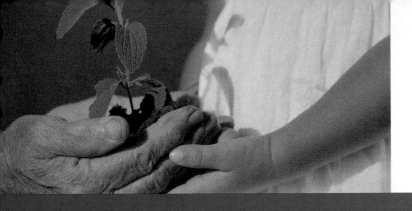

CHAPTER 2

Culture

Key Words

acculturation
beliefs
cultural awareness
cultural competence
cultural sensitivity
culture
diffusion
enculturation
ethnicity
folkways
globalization
individualism
language
laws
mores
norms
race
religion
sanctions
spirituality
symbols
technological innovation
transcultural nursing
values

Chapter Outline

Learning Objectives

At the end of this chapter, you should be able to:

- Define culture.
- Describe the difference between beliefs and values.
- State how culture is relevant to nursing practice.
- List and describe four common ethnic groups.
- Identify the basic components in a cultural assessment.

CULTURE, RACE, AND ETHNICITY

Each family has its own history, structure, and style of functioning. Within the framework of the larger society, groups of families are connected to each other by race, religion, and geographical proximity. Their shared beliefs, values, ideas, and religious doctrines—from their common culture—are handed down from generation to generation and adapted or changed to meet the current needs of the group. Culture refers to all of the learned patterns of behavior passed down through the generations that influence our thinking, decisions, and actions.

During recent years much attention has been given to cultural influences that affect health and health care (Fig. 2.1). The nurse can better understand patients' behavior and response to health care by understanding their histories and beliefs. Failure to develop cultural awareness may lead to misperceptions about patients' feelings and responses. These misunderstandings can increase the stress for both patient and caregiver. The definition of culture has been debated by anthropologists and sociologists since the 19th century. The points of agreement are that culture is not isolated but is universal to all society and populations despite variations in language. Similarities exist in all cultures including communication, social controls, family, marriage, education, and supernatural beliefs. To understand and study culture, researchers must first look at each culture's geographic location, population size, language, religion, economy, and political organization.

We believe that culture is broad and plays an important role in everything we do or think. Culture describes a social group within a society to which individuals belong and which gives meaning to their lives. It determines our own identity and forms the anchor for traditions, customs, and rituals. Culture determines how we view the world, how we practice religion, how we interact with each other, and how members understand their work roles and sexuality.

Modern social anthropology theorists consider culture as a set of standards set forth in these statements: Culture decides what is, what can be, what one feels about it, what to do about it, and how to go about doing it. The levels of culture can be described as follows:

- *National culture:* Learned patterns of behavior and values shared by a whole nation.
- *International culture:* Learned patterns of behavior shared across national borders because of migration and globalization.
- *Subcultures*: Subgroups within the dominant culture. Subcultures have common beliefs and interests. An example of a subculture would be health care workers as a group.

CHARACTERISTICS OF CULTURE

Social anthropologists have characterized culture as learned, shared, integrated or patterned, adaptive, and symbolic. See Table 2.1 for brief descriptions of these characteristics.

Learned

Culture is learned based on a human's unique capacity to learn symbols and signs. Culture is learned from birth because behaviors, values, beliefs, and traditions are passed down from one generation to the next through the acquisition of language. The ability to learn a language is based on our biological makeup, but the language we speak is what we learned within our cultural group. Culture is not genetically inherited, evidenced by the newborn baby born into a culture equipped only with basic instinctive reflexes such as sucking that help babies' survival. Newborn babies are not capable of caring for themselves and are totally dependent on their parents or guardians for food during the first few years of life. Newborn babies do not enter the world with a cultural template but learn culture through socialization within their respective groups. Newborn babies can learn the culture into which they are born through direct observation, using all their senses, as well as by being taught by members of

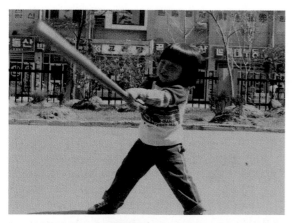

FIGURE 2.1 One's neighborhood supports cultural needs.

TABLE
2.1   Characteristics of Culture

Characteristic	Description
Learned	Culture is learned from birth as behaviors, values, beliefs, and traditions are passed down from one generation to the next through language.
Shared	Cultures share traditions, values, and beliefs. Shared values give cultures stability and security. Culture can be shared through interactions with members of the cultural group or by direct instruction.
Integrated or Patterned	Culture is integrated or patterned based on economics, social patterns, work ethics, and individualism.
Adaptive	Culture is a constantly adapting response to environmental and biological demands. Methods of change include diffusion, acculturation, technological innovation, and globalization.
Symbolic	Human culture uses symbols, especially language, gestures, and pictures, for communication among members.

their social group. Newborns learn their culture from their parents, siblings, and other children. In today's society culture is also learned through television shows such as *Sesame Street* and computer games. Cultural education and socialization occur in a more formal way in the school years. This process of learning is called enculturation. Enculturation means learning the culture through observation and instruction, thereby integrating oneself into the cultural group. Newborns will learn mealtimes, bedtime, types of foods, and manner of dress used by their culture. For example, in our culture we eat pigs and cows, while in other cultures this is forbidden and would be considered a violation of cultural or religious practices.

The cognitive level of an individual within the cultural group will determine his or her capacity for learning. For example, computers are widely used in our society, and the ability to be skilled in the use of the computers reflects the individual's level of education and motivation.

Culture is learned unconsciously because humans are able to think symbolically, meaning the object in reference need not be present. For example, we know the meaning of the U.S. flag without seeing it.

Shared

Culture is shared by members within that culture, and the most common practice shared by a cultural group is language. The language in a culture is shared by all members and is understood by all members of that group. Cultures also share the same ideas and ways of behaving, and the meaning of the behavior must be understood by individuals within that culture, thus providing a common experience and understanding. When a cultural behavior exists, that behavior is shared and must be practiced by more than one member in that cultural group. Cultures share traditions, values, and beliefs. Shared values give cultures stability and security. Culture can be shared through interactions with members of the cultural group or by direct instruction.

The degree of sharing within a cultural group varies because of the individuality of each member of the culture. Variations of behavior and traits can be seen within a culture based on age, gender, class, and religion. In North America, individuals share the feeling that they are special, and this fosters the common ideals of individualism. Individualism means that the individual's interests and needs are the primary focus.

Integrated or Patterned

Culture is integrated or patterned based on economics, social patterns, work ethics, and individualism. Forming the core of an individual's culture are the values, ideals, judgments, and symbols that are unique to each culture. All aspects must be integrated to comprise a whole culture. One anthropology theorist defined *patterned and integrated culture* as the following: elements or traits in a culture that are not a random collection of customs, but patterns that are mostly consistent with each other because they work together cognitively and emotionally help in adaptation. For example, child-rearing practices, expectations, and hopes for our offspring follow cultural patterns.

Adaptive

Culture is an adaptive response to environmental and biological demands. Humans must manipulate their environment to resolve problems of survival and reproduction. Humans are highly adaptive in comparison to other species. All cultures have demonstrated the abilities to develop tools to hunt for food initially and to adapt to climate changes, which have enabled the growth of cultural groups and populations.

Given time, all cultures adjust and respond to environmental crises. As new rules are embraced by a cultural group, old ones are dropped. Culture is not static but adaptive to a dynamic world. One of the changes society has experienced since the 1960s is the increased number of women in the workforce. Because of economic demands, many women are working full-time hours in North America and parts of Europe. According to the U.S. Census Bureau, in 1967 only 14.8% of women were in the workforce, and in 2009 that number had reached 43.2%.

Changes in a culture occur because of diffusion, which means borrowing cultural traits from another culture. Diffusion is responsible for the greatest amount of change seen within a culture. We adopt practices from other cultures that will enrich our culture without going through years of trial and error. Today cultures, societies, and nations are linked together in a mutually competitive way to ensure survival.

Change also occurs through acculturation, technological innovation, and globalization. **Acculturation** is when values and beliefs are exchanged as a result of continuous direct interactions between cultures. This occurs due to external pressures. An example of acculturation is when an individual immigrates to the United States and quickly adapts and believes in the U.S. right to free expression. Rapid changes in our society today are driven by **technological innovation.** Innovations developed to solve problems in society also create cultural change. For example, one of the first antibiotics discovered was penicillin, which has saved the lives of a large number of people throughout the world. Globalization is another cause of cultural changes. Globalization is change by a combination of diffusion, acculturation, migration patterns, and tourism. This change is commonly accepted in North America.

A culture can be maladaptive if it fails to change to meet the challenges of the group or goes through rapid changes that reduce the culture's chance of survival and would make that culture become extinct.

Symbolic

Culture is symbolic because the most fundamental aspect of a culture is the ability to develop symbols that allow for communication among its members. The most important symbols in human culture are the language, gestures, and pictures that people use to communicate with each other. Each symbol has a specific meaning within a culture and can be verbal or nonverbal. For example, an alphabet represents the sounds used within a language. Symbols are not timeless and can change as the culture evolves to maintain internal stability of the culture.

Symbols can be material or nonmaterial. Material symbols are objects made or built by the culture, such as clothes, art, or artifacts, that can identify how the culture was organized and how its people function and survive over time. An example of a material symbol in our culture is the stop sign. This red sign means a driver must stop and not proceed, and it is understood by everyone in our cultural group. Our culture also imposes penalties on individuals who violate the implied meaning of a stop sign. Nonmaterial symbols are ideas that have no physical characteristics and tell us about the culture's beliefs and values. Body language and other learned behaviors are examples of nonmaterial symbols.

CULTURAL ELEMENTS

Elements that make up all cultures are beliefs, values, norms, folkways, laws, mores, sanctions, race, and ethnicities.

Beliefs are the truths held by a culture's people. One's beliefs determine and influence how one deals with and views social problems and concerns. Beliefs affect our thinking and organizing ability. They also influence our behavior and concepts about health, illness, and death. Women's roles and child-rearing practices are also governed by cultural beliefs.

Values are deeply embedded feelings that determine what is considered good or bad, right or wrong. Cultural values give individuals direction and foundation for their decisions and actions. These values also provide a sense of stability and security. Absence of cultural values can lead to social problems. At an early age, children develop a sense of what is right or wrong and what behaviors are acceptable within their culture. Values can help to foster personal achievement. Conflicts may arise in an individual when his or her cultural values are challenged. For example, such conflict may occur when an individual moves out into the larger community and is then faced with the values of others. The individual must try to assimilate into the larger group without losing his or her own cultural beliefs and values.

Norms are socially accepted rules and practices that guide an individual's behavior and interactions within the culture. Norms also determine the role of each family member by age, gender, or ranking. Norms can be described in the following three ways:

- **Folkways** are the customs within the culture that determine how we greet each other. For example, in some cultures people greet each other with a handshake, whereas in other cultures they greet others with a kiss. These are not formally written laws, but a person's failure to extend the appropriate greeting may offend others in these cultural groups.
- **Laws** are written policies supported and enforced by the government. Breaking the law carries specific punishment. Violating a person's property and stealing are examples of breaking the law.
- **Mores** are moral beliefs that are strongly held by members of the culture. Failure to abide by these mores may lead to ostracism from the cultural group. Incest and child abuse are examples of these strong beliefs, or mores.
- **Sanctions** are the social remedies for violating any of the norms. These may be positive or negative. Positive sanctions may reward or honor an individual; negative sanctions exercise disapproval for violating the norm and may lead to imprisonment.

Symbols are expressed as language, gestures, or objects that people within a culture use to communicate with each other. Symbols can have different meanings among different cultures.

Race is defined as a group of people who share certain similar physical characteristics including skin color, hair texture, facial shape, and/or body shape or size. Race (and ethnicity) can determine our socioeconomic status. Race has also been defined as a social construct that categorizes people socially rather than biologically. Biological researchers once believed that race genetically isolated people. Recent research disputes this belief of racial isolation and supports a theory that there are no pure or distinct races because inbreeding and migration patterns throughout the ages have blended all people. These theorists ascribe differences such as skin color as the result of, or adaptation to, physical elements such as climate and sun. In regions with warm climates, dark skin tones are the result of an increase in pigmentation and melanin and help protect the skin from the sun's rays. In colder climates, less protection is needed; hence, skin is lighter in color. Racial categories emphasize physical characteristics rather than cultural differences.

Children are not born with prejudice; instead, they have a natural innocence and curiosity (Fig. 2.2). This curiosity leads them to become aware of differences in race and color as early as age 3. At this age children cannot fully understand the social concept of race—being either black or white—but they are able to describe themselves as pink, peach, brown, or chocolate colored. One researcher found that by age 6 many children have already developed some racial biases. To foster racial and ethnic tolerance in children, the issue of prejudice must be addressed at an early age. Negative stereotypes of race and ethnicity can be learned and reinforced from media depiction and from family members and friends. It is not unusual for well-meaning parents who are trying to teach their children to be color-blind to avoid

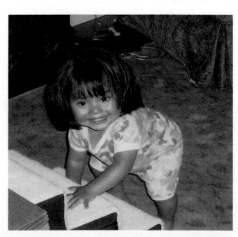

FIGURE 2.2 Children have a natural innocence and curiosity.

addressing the obvious differences children are able to see. Positive role modeling of racial and ethnic tolerance by parents is essential. Parents or caregivers must also include open, accurate, and positive discussions of color and race. Activities such as helping children track their cultural heritage can be enriching. A priority issue is helping children to understand that although people may look different and come from different countries, all of them feel, enjoy, and aspire to some of the same things. Box 2.1 gives some hints on fostering racial tolerance in children.

Ethnicity refers to stable cultural patterns shared by a group of families with the same historical roots. Ethnicity means that people have a shared cultural heritage and are from the same race and geographical area. They share the same language and other attributes peculiar to that group such as diet, customs, music and dance, family structure and roles, and religious beliefs or practices. These ethnic categories celebrate the diversity among racial groups. For example, people from the Caribbean have a diverse heritage consisting of African, Indian, French, Portuguese, English, and

Dutch ethnicities, to name a few. We are all born into a culture, race, and ethnic group. Although as individuals we are not totally defined by these categories, they are important elements in our lives.

CULTURE IN HEALTH CARE

Madeline Lenninger introduced the theory of transcultural nursing in the mid-1950s. Transcultural nursing is a formal area of study and practice focused on comparative human care and understanding the differences and similarities in beliefs, values, and practices among people. This theory uses a holistic care approach integrating concepts of humanistic caring philosophy grounded in scientific knowledge to deliver culturally congruent care. Culturally congruent care is care that incorporates the key values and beliefs of a culture. This was developed in response to changing demographics and globalization, or the movement of people from different cultures to different countries in the world. Major challenges in health care today include globalization and the new health care initiatives for cultural care. Other disciplines—such as medicine, social work, pharmacy, and physical therapy—now have become interested in providing culturally competent care to a rapidly growing multicultural population. The U.S. Census Bureau projection for 2020 is that one-third of the U.S. population will be composed of ethnic and racial minority groups. Presently, one-fifth of the U.S. population speaks a language other than English.

Because of the increasing cultural diversity of our nation, health care workers interact on a daily basis with patients from many cultural and ethnic groups. In response to our nation's increasing diversity, the emphasis must be on nurses and health care delivery systems that provide culturally competent care. Culturally competent care requires an understanding of culture, race and ethnicity, and diversity in minority groups.

The central purpose of transcultural nursing is to provide nurses with the education that was missing in nursing practice to promote and maintain the cultural care needs of the individual. This would benefit the individual and increase client satisfaction, promote an early recovery from disease, or support a meaningful death experience. Culturally congruent care is the ultimate goal of transcultural nursing.

In transcultural nursing theory, Lenninger viewed the patient as belonging to one world with many cultures and believed that nurses must be prepared to

---

B O X 2.1 Promoting Racial Sensitivity in Children

- Use positive role models.
- Answer questions factually.
- Have honest, open conversations.
- Do not deny differences in color of skin, hair type, or shape of eyes.
- Do not make children feel ashamed when they question race or color.
- Foster positive feelings toward individual heritage.
- Expose children to people of other races and cultures.
- Select dolls from different cultural and ethnic groups.
- Read your child stories depicting different cultural and ethnic groups.
- Read some of the following books together:
  - *The Hundred Dresses* by Eleanor Estes, Harvest Books, 1998
  - *The People Could Fly: American Black Folktales* by Virginia Hamilton, Random House, 2000
  - *Black Is Brown Is Tan* by Arnold Adoff, HarperCollins Juvenile Books, 1992
  - *Children from Australia to Zimbabwe: A Photographic Journey Around the World* by Maya Ajimera and Anna Rhesa Versola, Charlesbridge Publishing, 1997
  - *The Friendship* by Mildred D. Taylor, Penguin Group, 1998

care for anyone anywhere in the world. This world-view is a new way for nurses to learn about their clients' cultures and provide care that is culturally congruent and meaningful to the world's population. Without the knowledge of culture and a commitment to give culturally congruent care, nurses will be handicapped and culturally ignorant to care for people whose cultural values and beliefs are different from their own.

Culturally specific care is the art of using knowledge specific to the client's culture to determine the client's values and needs to plan and deliver care for a more positive outcome. For example, knowing that some clients from the Arab culture prefer same-sex caregivers and planning their care consistently will prevent unnecessary stress.

Health care workers must be careful not to become ethnocentric, believing that their culture, values, and patterns of behavior are superior to those of others. This type of belief breeds intolerance and insensitivity. Health care workers should practice cultural *relativism*, which means that the worker must learn and apply the other person's cultural standard to each situation. Furthermore, health care workers should respect and be open to new cultural experiences. Because we respect the individual's culture, we try not to stereotype and limit the person.

Cultural theorists believe that cultural challenges and health care disparities occur when health care providers do not understand the unique health values and beliefs of an individual's culture, race, or ethnic background. Traditionally, the health care system is organized in a paternalistic pattern, meaning male dominance of the greater society, and does not provide for the needs of women or minorities. To provide competent care, the health care system must be able to promote and maintain the health of all its patients. In this system the patient must be able to understand, interpret, and analyze health information that can complement his or her lifestyle. Individuals should be able to navigate the health care system, interact with health care providers, and advocate for their own rights. This will provide an outcome where client satisfaction, healing, and recovery take priority.

A culturally competent health care worker tries to understand the values, beliefs, traditions, and customs of diverse groups. The health care worker must understand each client's health problems, ethnic practices, language, literacy, and religious beliefs that will influence that client's attitudes and behavior. Health care workers should be able to appreciate the health practices of their patients without judgment, even if the practices go against their own beliefs. The care provided must be patient centered, taking into consideration a person's beliefs and priorities.

Cultural competence is a conscious process, which means the health care worker must apply knowledge and skills to enhance interaction with clients. **Cultural competence** is the ongoing and continuous self-evaluation and development of cultural skills, which can only be acquired by interacting with or learning about diverse cultural groups. This can be accomplished by health care workers while remaining true to their own cultural identities. To be culturally competent the health care worker is not required to have detailed knowledge about all cultures that exist, but he or she must have *cultural sensitivity* and *cultural awareness*. These two concepts are sometimes discussed as one and other times discussed separately.

Cultural awareness means understanding of culture, race, and ethnicity of diverse minority groups. This is not as easy as it sounds. You must enter the individual's world to learn about him or her. We must learn the history of the patient's ancestry and appreciate and celebrate cultural differences. Cultural awareness also means learning the cultural values and beliefs of the client and how he or she copes with difficulties and solve problems. Celebration of a culture can be seen in the food and clothing choices people make. This involves knowing their cultural expectations and needs from their point of view.

Cultural sensitivity recognizes that diversity exists and one needs to respect a person's uniqueness. It also means being correct in your language and interaction to avoid offending anyone's belief or practices. It is essential for nurses to understand differences in communication styles, use of space and time, and family roles so that they may provide competent nursing care. Being culturally sensitive when giving care provides the client with satisfaction and a quick recovery. The client can quickly become frustrated, resentful, and dissatisfied with nurses who are unable to provide culturally sensitive care. In this climate, healing can be compromised. Box 2.2 lists ways to express cultural sensitivity toward your patients.

CULTURAL GROUPS

Today the United States is no longer considered a "melting pot." Instead, we celebrate our diversity.

Our population is heterogeneous, consisting of many ethnic groups: European Americans, African Americans, Hispanics, Asians and Pacific Islanders, Native Americans, and others. Any generalization or stereotyping regarding these groups of people can be dangerous because exceptions exist within each one.

Hispanic Americans

Hispanic Americans are the largest ethnic minority and the most rapidly growing ethnic group in the United States. More than one-third of Hispanic Americans are children younger than 15 years of age. Hispanics are a diverse group made up of Puerto Ricans, Mexicans, Dominicans, Cubans, and people from South and Central America. The majority of Hispanics share a common cultural heritage in language, religion, and values.

In general, Hispanics believe in a large extended family headed by the man. Women have an active role in health and childbearing decisions. Children are valuable to the culture and cared for by all. Elders are respected and useful to aid in childrearing. Hispanics stand close to one another when communicating, frequently touching the other person, but this practice is usually with family members primarily and less with strangers. Direct eye contact is avoided because it can be interpreted as the "evil eye." Religion is a strong force in this culture, and the majority of Hispanics are Catholics who often blend their religious beliefs with those of their cultural tradition. An example would be the use of African drums in their mass service. Life is seen as a gift from God, and death is considered to be a natural part of the life cycle. Illness is believed to be caused by internal and external imbalances between hot and cold temperatures and the "evil eye."

A patient who is postpartum may believe that she will become ill if she is exposed to a cold draft. Good health is seen as a strong body able to perform a high level of physical work. Maintaining a constant environmental temperature is believed to prevent illness and maintain good health. Illness may be thought to result from natural causes or may be seen as God's punishment. The way in which a person views illness will also determine the person's response to pain and use of pain medication. Hispanics believe that when they are ill, they should try not to become a burden to others. Health indices for Hispanics are markedly poorer than for other groups.

Many Mexicans are migrant workers. Their living conditions, which are often overcrowded, increase the risk of accidents and the spread of viral and bacterial infections. Many live below the poverty level, which further affects their state of health and puts their children's health at increased risk.

The major barriers to health care for this group are language, beliefs, and economics. Many believe in home remedies and folk healing. Most Hispanics have Medicaid health insurance to access health care. Health care is provided by both the native healer and the doctor, although the use of native healers is declining. The native healer is called a *Lurandua,* and Hispanics have a strong belief in herbal medicine. Food and herbal remedies are selected based on the "hot-cold" belief for the treatment of illness. Medical doctors, when used, make most health care decisions for these patients.

Pregnancy is seen as a natural, normal, healthy process. A religious medal may be worn for protection, and prenatal care is often delayed. Birthing is carried out mainly by lay midwives called *parteras.* Emotional support for the laboring mother is given by either the mother or stepmother. Specific rituals are followed after birth to ensure the health of mother and child. Breastfeeding is a prevalent practice that does not begin for 3 to 4 days after birth, at the time when milk is considered ready. The first milk secreted is considered contaminated, possibly causing the baby to become ill. The mother must be kept warm to regain her strength, and bathing may be delayed for up to 14 days.

The most common diseases affecting the Hispanic community are diabetes, hypertension, obesity, AIDS, alcoholism, and lactose intolerance.

Native Americans

The fourth largest major ethnic group in the United States—Native Americans—comprises more than 200 different tribes. Each tribe has its own language.

Families form very strong bonds, and the tribes tend to be organized along matriarchal roles. Gender roles, however, are flexible within large extended families, with elders being highly respected.

Native Americans communicate in moderate tones; talking loudly is considered rude. Direct eye contact is unacceptable even between friends. Touch is acceptable between friends and family. There is no touching between strangers.

Health is seen as a harmony between nature and the universe. To maintain good health, life must be lived based on the native teachings handed down by the creator. These beliefs include enormous respect for everything on the earth. Illness is a result of an imbalance between the environment and supernatural forces. Illness may be prevented by using charms and prayers. To treat illness, evil spirits are exorcized, allowing the individual to return to oneness with the environment. When death occurs, the body must remain intact to enter the afterlife. Touching the dead calls for a cleansing ceremony. Native Americans believe in and use herbal remedies in rituals designed to cleanse the body of evil and poisons. There are as many native healing beliefs as there are tribes. Doctors and medical treatments are used along with the medicine man and his healing powers.

Pregnancy is seen as a natural, normal state of being if the woman remains stress free. Prenatal care is usually delayed until advanced pregnancy. Although the midwife is preferred in this culture, support can be provided during birthing by several family members—the husband, mother, or father. Postpartum bleeding is prevented by the use of herbal medicines. Breastfeeding is usually not started until milk is present a few days after birth. Traditional caring for babies means they are touched less frequently than they would be in other cultures.

The basic diet of a Native American is high in fats and lacks fruits. Heart disease, diabetes, alcoholism, accidents, and lactose intolerance are common contributors to ill health.

African Americans

The African American group is made up of people who came to the United States from Africa as part of the slave trade and of immigrants with a similar history who came from the Caribbean. Each African American belongs to a common race and a specific cultural group. The primary language is English, but many speak Spanish, French, and *patois* (Creole). A loud voice can be interpreted as either jest or anger. More emphasis is placed on nonverbal than verbal behavior. Direct eye contact in this culture can be considered a form of aggression.

Family organization is largely matriarchal with a dominant extended family. Many families include a stranger into the family circle. Elders are respected and contribute to the rearing and nurturing of children (Fig. 2.3).

Health is seen as a gift from God; illness is caused by exposure to cold, drafts, or air. The ingestion of poor-quality food and water can also contribute to illness. Illness also may be seen as an act of God or caused by witchcraft or voodoo. The length of life is deemed more important than the quality. Death is not seen as the end but as the passing to a better life based on how the person lived. Because of religious and spiritual beliefs, burial of an intact body is preferred to cremation. Burial is ceremonious and ritualistic; wakes may go on for several nights to after-burial celebrations with singing of religious songs. Grief is openly displayed and accepted.

The African American cultures have a basic distrust of the health care system. Medical doctors provide health care, as do spiritualists and voodoo doctors. Traditional medicines are used along with herbal remedies, candles, and balms.

Pregnancy is viewed as a natural, normal process of life. This view can lead to delayed prenatal care. Normal discomforts during pregnancy are usually relieved by cultural therapies. The pregnant woman is taught to avoid certain practices that are believed to lead to complications in the pregnancy, such as reaching up or having her picture taken. Support during birthing can be provided by women, especially the mother. Postpartum concerns include

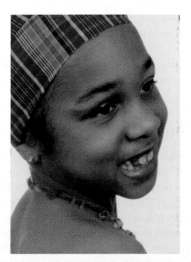

FIGURE 2.3 Cultural dress and beliefs are handed down to children.

exposure to cold or drafts. This concern may cause a delay after birth in the mother taking a shower or tub bath or washing her hair. Bottle feeding may be chosen over breastfeeding because of embarrassment. Solid foods tend to be introduced to the infant at an earlier age than in other cultures.

The death rate for both men and women as they age is related to exposure to hazardous materials in both home and work environments. Some can be exposed to chemical radiation, asbestos, and other pollutants in the work environment. Others live in overcrowded, substandard conditions. Common diseases affecting African Americans include hypertension, cancer, stroke, diabetes, and kidney and liver diseases.

European Americans

European Americans make up the largest cultural group in the United States. The predominant language is an English dialect, and any other language spoken represents the country of origin. Speech is usually loud, and eye contact is essential during communication but without staring. Touch is not an accepted method of communicating for most European Americans. Family life is equally matriarchal and patriarchal. Pregnancy focuses on care during and after for both mother and child. Birth preferences are most often vaginal deliveries, with elective cesarean sections in some cases.

Elders are loved but live outside of the family and have no input on child rearing. European Americans believe the individual is responsible for his or her health. It is believed that prayer and religious symbols can prevent illness. The search for healing and good health results in a reaching out and use of traditional and nontraditional methods that have succeeded in other cultures. Common diseases affecting European Americans include breast cancer and leukemia. Burial is based on religious influences. Open expression of grief is not accepted, and men should not outwardly grieve or cry.

Asian Americans

The Asian American group is made up of people from many different countries in the Pacific, including Korea, Japan, the Philippines, and China. Their languages are specific to the countries or origin, and one country may have many dialects. Communicating is done in quiet tones because loudness is considered disrespectful. It is considered disrespectful to look elders directly in their eyes. Touch is acceptable only between individuals of the same sex. It is taboo to openly express emotions—whether happy or sad. Households are divided along gender lines that are clearly patriarchal. Extended families within one household are common. The elders are protected within the family unit. Children are very important and must demonstrate respect for the family.

Health is seen as the balance between ying and yang—good and evil. Good health is seen as a gift from the ancestors. Cleanliness also is seen as a way to prevent illness. Eastern medicine predominantly uses meditation, acupuncture, and herbs.

In Asian American culture, it is believed that God determines who dies. The period of grief can be extended beyond 30 days after a death. It is appropriate for women to grieve, but grieving is highly unacceptable for men. Burial rituals vary among Asian American cultures, with some choosing burial and others cremation.

Pregnancy is viewed as a time of happiness and contentment for the woman. Discomforts of pregnancy are treated by omitting milk from the diet and maintaining a high level of activity to prevent a lazy baby and a difficult labor. Support during the birthing comes from the mother and other women. The father has a less active role than in Western cultures. Postpartum activity can be curtailed for 40 to 60 days while others tend to household tasks and help to care for the new child. Breastfeeding is encouraged but usually will start 3 days after the birth, when milk is present.

Asian Americans tend to suffer from lactose intolerance, hypertension, and, more recently, liver and stomach cancers.

Arab Americans

Arab Americans or Middle Eastern people come from countries such as Saudi Arabia, Egypt, Iran, Palestine, Turkey, Pakistan, and Syria. The primary language of Arab Americans is Arabic, but most have some mastery of English. Arab Americans communicate at close proximity. They tend to talk in loud voices with frequent and intense eye contact. Touch is permitted only with people of the same gender. Cultural laws specify that women wear clothing to cover their bodies from their wrists to their ankles, and their heads and faces. Many Arab Americans follow this rule of modesty, whereas others have assimilated into Western culture. Family organization is usually patriarchal with very clearly specified gender roles. Family loyalty and commitment are extremely important. Children, women, and older adults are protected within the family. Social functions and occasions are celebrated with food. There is strict adherence to diet and mealtimes, with periods of fasting during the holy month of Ramadan.

Several prayer and meditation sessions are interwoven into the Arab American's day. Illness is seen as a punishment for sin, and death is seen as God's will. At death, the body must be specially prepared, and the bed should be positioned to face Mecca. Arab Americans have a general belief in Western medicine along with prescription or nonprescription medicines. In sickness, men and women generally seek health care providers of the same sex.

During pregnancy, many of the cultural and religious practices continue. For instance, some women fast during pregnancy to be blessed with a son. Mothers-in-law act as role models and guide new mothers during pregnancy and delivery. During pregnancy and birthing, the woman must be attended by female doctors or nurses. Immediately after birth, some fathers read to the newborn baby from the holy book, the *Koran*, as a way of giving thanks to Allah. Breastfeeding is preferred by most Arab American women, and it can continue until the child is about 2 years old.

CULTURAL ASSESSMENT IN THE HEALTH CARE SETTING

To provide an optimal level of health care, the nurse should complete cultural assessments for all patients as they enter the health care environment. A cultural assessment should include determination of the patient's ethnic and racial origin, the patient's language of origin and language he or she is most comfortable using, the decision maker for the family, and if there is a preference in gender of the health care worker who will provide direct care. It is also important to understand how to use personal space in the communication process. The health care worker must be aware of the person's beliefs about medicine, pregnancy, and healing. Dietary laws and preferences need to be considered and respected. Box 2.3 contains an exercise to practice obtaining a cultural assessment.

B O X
2.3   Cultural Assessment Exercise

Sit with the oldest member of your family and trace your family history. Be sure to determine country of origin, cultural practices, food preferences, and dress protocol particular to your culture.

CULTURAL BARRIERS TO HEALTH CARE

The social, cultural, and ethnic differences between the client and the health care providers may contribute to many different attitudes and beliefs. These differences may either help support or conflict with the client's adherence to the medical plan of care. Common cultural barriers to health care include the following:

• Difficulties with English
• Lack of health insurance
• Knowledge deficit
• Reluctance to question the health provider
• Adherence to old cultural practices

Health care providers can minimize cultural and ethnic barriers by becoming culturally sensitive to clients' needs. To minimize language barriers, trained interpreters must be used along with translation sheets or devices. Food served should take into consideration common cultural preferences. For example, Chinese clients may prefer rice instead of potatoes. Health providers should acknowledge the importance of other cultural health practices. Nurses can encourage clients to ask questions regarding their treatment as a means of becoming empowered. Last, health care providers must be sensitive to the client's socioeconomic status and insurance coverage status.

SPIRITUALITY AND RELIGION

Religion is a specific system of beliefs and worship that is closely integrated with culture, ethnicity, and spirituality. Religion is an organized practice with rituals and symbols based on specific beliefs taken from the scriptures that provides a code of conduct for its members. Religion and spirituality are used interchangeably but are not the same. Religion is only one dimension of spirituality. Spirituality is concerned with how each individual finds a purpose and meaning to his or her life (Fig. 2.4 and Fig. 2.5). The outcome of spirituality is inner peace and a feeling of well-being with the world. Spirituality includes how one connects with nature or a supreme being.

Nurses who practice from a holistic perspective must make every effort to attend to patients' spiritual needs. This includes respecting patients' expressions of their spirituality. The nurse need not share the same spiritual ideals of his or her patients but must recognize them and allow freedom of expression.

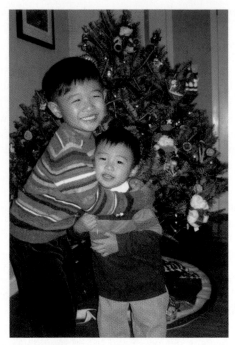

FIGURE 2.4 Holidays are special.

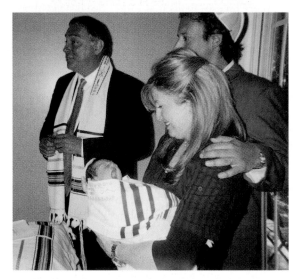

FIGURE 2.5 Religious practices are important in some families.

The nurse must be careful not to impose his or her own spiritual values on patients. The nurse should be able to identify a client in spiritual distress. This distress may be manifested in feelings of hopelessness, anger, depression, and withdrawal. Allowing the patient to get in touch with his or her spirituality is one way of providing emotional support. Spiritual and religious assessment must include the patient's preference for religious or spiritual practice and needs. Spiritual support is demonstrated in the nurse's ability to listen to the patient while being

nonjudgmental as the patient works through his or her spiritual issues. Some of the documented benefits of spiritual and religious expressions are a decrease in stress and relief from diseases such as hypertension, allergy, depression, and nausea. Patients known to engage in these practices may enjoy an increased life span, healthy self-concept, and improved mental health.

Religion also serves to satisfy several basic needs. Religion attempts to define the spiritual and give an explanation for otherwise incomprehensible events. Religion offers a sense of hope and the strength to endure. Religion guides individuals in the belief in a power greater than themselves.

Individuals are brought together through a common belief system without which they may share little else in common. Religion defines various rituals and rites of passage such as baptisms, confirmations, bar and bat mitzvahs, weddings, and funerals (Fig. 2.6). The partaking of rituals and the sharing of religious beliefs help assist persons in overcoming adversities, thereby contributing to their well-being. Religious affiliations may serve to reduce social isolation by bringing people together to worship. Friendships, community support, and other social networks are often outgrowths of religious affiliations.

Religion may encourage the community toward a healthy lifestyle and healthy behavior. Some religions promote health behaviors by supporting abstinence from smoking or alcohol usage. Most religions promote the family unit and the maintenance of marriage, family, and parenting. Religion also provides its followers with a moral guide that promotes well-being. One's religious faith or lack of it is most often

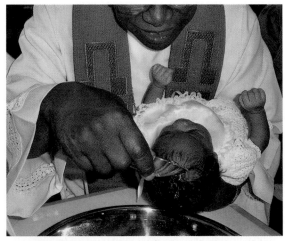

FIGURE 2.6 Baptism presents the infant into the teachings of the family's religion.

handed down by the family from generation to generation, linking the past and the future.

Several different Christian denominations are practiced in the United States: Protestants are the largest religious group and Catholics are the second largest. Protestants include subgroups such as Baptists, Episcopalians, Lutherans, Methodists, Presbyterians, and Seventh-Day Adventists. While Christianity remains the largest practiced religion in the United States, a minority of people practice other faiths, including Judaism, Buddhism, and Islam, and a growing percentage of individuals are unaffiliated with any organized religious group. Health care workers can best meet their patients' needs by exercising tolerance and understanding of the religious beliefs and practices influencing health and illness. Religious beliefs may offer people support during crises such as illness, family problems, or other stressors.

Box 2.4 offers an exercise to help you practice religious sensitivity.

B O X
2.4 **Religious Sensitivity Exercise**

The following questions should help to heighten your sensitivity to your own religious beliefs:

- Are you affiliated with any religious organization?
- How important is religion to your daily activities?
- What helps you renew your strength and hope?
- Is religion a source of comfort to you?
- What religious practices do you adhere to in your own life?
- How do you feel about other religions?

SUMMARY

1. Culture can be defined as socially acquired patterns of behavior that are learned and passed down through generations.

2. Culture is learned within the home and community. All groups have cultural beliefs and practices that they maintain. These cultural beliefs and patterns distinguish one cultural group from the other. The primary elements of culture are beliefs, values, norms, sanctions, symbols, race, and ethnicity.

3. Race is defined as a group of people sharing certain similar physical characteristics including skin color, hair texture, facial shape, and/or body shape or size. Race and ethnicity can further determine socioeconomic status.

4. Ethnicity refers to stable cultural patterns shared by a group of families with the same historical roots.

5. Ethnicity means that people have a shared cultural heritage and are from the same race and geographical area. They share the same language and other attributes peculiar to that group such as diet, customs, music and dance, family structure and roles, and religious beliefs or practices.

6. Cultural awareness means learning the history of the patient's ancestry and appreciating and celebrating cultural differences. Cultural awareness also means learning the cultural values and beliefs of clients and how they cope with difficulties and solve problems.

7. Cultural sensitivity means being correct in your language and interaction to avoid offending anyone's beliefs or practices.

8. Transcultural nursing involves understanding the differences and similarities in beliefs, values, and practices among people. This theory was developed to bring about client satisfaction, early recovery from illness, or a meaningful death experience.

9. Hispanic Americans are the most rapidly growing ethnic group in the United States. Hispanics are a diverse group made up of Puerto Ricans, Mexicans, Dominicans, Cubans, and people from South and Central America. The majority of Hispanics share a common cultural heritage in language, religion, and values.

10. Native Americans are the fourth largest major ethnic group in the United States and comprise more than 200 different tribes. Each tribe has its own language. Families form very strong bonds, and the tribes tend to be organized along matriarchal roles. However, gender roles are flexible within large extended families, and elders are highly respected.

11. African Americans include people who came from Africa as part of the slave trade and immigrants with a similar history who came from the Caribbean. Each African American belongs to a common race and a specific cultural group.

12. European Americans make up the largest cultural group in the United States. The predominant language is English. European Americans believe the individual is responsible for his or her health.

13. Asian Americans are made up of people from many different countries in the Pacific including Korea, Japan, the Philippines, and China. Health is seen as the balance between ying and yang—good and evil. Good health is believed to be a gift from the ancestors.

14. Arab Americans or Middle Eastern people come from countries such as Saudi Arabia, Egypt, Iran, Palestine, Turkey, Pakistan, and Syria. In general, they believe in Western medicine and prescription or nonprescription medicines.

15. Common cultural barriers to health care include difficulties with English, lack of health insurance, knowledge deficit, reluctance to question health providers, and adherence to old cultural practices.

16. To provide an optimal level of health care, cultural assessments should be completed for all patients as they enter the health care environment.

17. Religion is a specific system of beliefs and worship and is closely integrated with culture and ethnicity. Spirituality helps individuals find purpose and meaning to life, often through nature or a supreme being.

18. Health care workers can best meet their patients' needs by exercising tolerance and understanding of their religious beliefs and practices that influence health and illness.

Student Activity

Observe a person of a different cultural or ethnic background and list six beliefs that you have about this cultural group.

CRITICAL THINKING

Exercise #1

Juan Perez, age 70 and of Hispanic ancestry, is admitted to the nursing home with a history of heart failure. What elements would you include in a cultural history for Mr. Perez?

Exercise #2

An 18-year-old male of Arabic descent with a history of diabetes mellitus comes to the emergency room during a hypoglycemic reaction. He has little mastery of English. The nurse orders a snack for the patient. The kitchen sends a ham sandwich and milk. The LPN hears the client speaking rapidly and angrily in broken English but cannot clearly understand the content of the speech. She asks another member of the staff to interpret the patient's concerns. He expressed this food as a violation of his religious practice.

1. How was the patient violated?
2. What is the first action that the LPN should take?
3. What action should the nurse take before placing an order for food?
4. Is there anything that the diet kitchen could have done to prevent this outcome?
5. What knowledge deficit did the nurse show?

MULTIPLE-CHOICE QUESTIONS

1. Culture is learned because of which of the following?
   a. It is genetically inherited.
   b. Instinctive human reflexes
   c. Traditions passed down from one generation to the next
   d. The culture contains a smaller number of people.

2. The ability to learn one's culture within the cultural group is an example of:
   a. Sanction
   b. Mores
   c. Diffusion
   d. Enculturation

3. Nurses who respect the patient's cultural difference:
   a. Are less effective practitioners
   b. Deliver competent care
   c. Give low-level care
   d. Tend to stereotype patients

4. Culture includes one's:
   a. Age
   b. Handicap
   c. Disease
   d. Customs

5. Transcultural nursing theory states:
   a. One world, one culture
   b. One world, many cultures
   c. Socially relevant nursing
   d. Nursing of foreign people

6. Behavior that is correct within a culture is called a:
   a. More
   b. Value
   c. Sanction
   d. Symbol

7. The best way to provide culturally competent health care is to:
   a. Use only scientific knowledge to plan health care
   b. Involve patient and family in developing a plan of care
   c. Use only the medical information from the doctor
   d. Use folk laws and stories to guide your choices

8. Which of the following statements is true?
   a. Knowing a person's culture will help you understand his or her response to illness.
   b. Race is the sole predictor of disease and life expectancy.
   c. Elderly persons seek health care based on their cultural values.
   d. All cultures take responsibility for their members.

9. How an infant is treated after birth depends on the cultural background of his or her parents.
   a. True
   b. False

10. A client expresses a cultural belief that prayer and faith heal better than any medicine. The nurse assigned to care for this client can provide culturally competent care by:
    a. Challenging his belief
    b. Seeking to change his belief with education
    c. Attempting to use his family to persuade him
    d. Respecting his belief

11. The expected patient outcome when the nurse is culturally sensitive is:
    a. Frustration
    b. Recovery
    c. Dissatisfaction
    d. Resentfulness

12. The nurse is correct when completing a physical assessment on a newly admitted client if he or she includes elements of the client's culture such as: (Choose all that apply.)
    a. The client's connection to his or her supreme being
    b. Meaning of gender roles
    c. The use of touch
    d. Use of eye contact
    e. How the client derives meaning or purpose from life

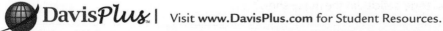

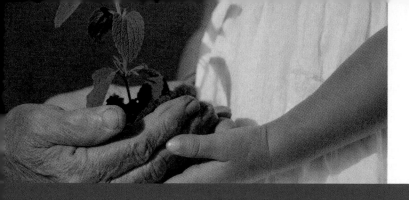

The Family

Learning Objectives

At the end of this chapter, you should be able to:

- Give the classic definition of the term *family*.
- Describe the eight family types.
- Name two groups that assist the family in socializing the child.
- List the four different stages of family development.
- Contrast the characteristics of functional and dysfunctional families.

The family unit is where the individual first learns to make decisions that will enable the promotion of health and well-being. Both children and adults are loved, protected, and taught within the family. Individuals learn about themselves, their relationships, and their behaviors within the family unit (Fig. 3.1). Each person in the family unit plays a role in the other members' health. Changes in the state of one member's health or illness may affect other family members. The nurse's understanding of the importance of the family helps to provide rationales and guidelines for clinical practice.

Health care workers must recognize the patient as a part of a family unit, not in isolation. This holistic approach to health care requires that the licensed practical nurse (LPN) be familiar with the meaning of today's family: its functions, types, stages, sizes, patterns, and cultural issues. Knowledge of culture and ethnicity will help the nurse to better understand how these issues affect a person's health actions and practices. In addition, it is important that nurses not only be aware of different family variations, but also be open and nonjudgmental in their approaches to patient care.

Until fairly recently, the basic family unit has usually been defined as two or more people related by blood, marriage, or adoption who live together. This definition of "family" is narrow in its scope and does not accommodate the many different living arrangements that are in place today. A more current definition of family might be "two or more people who have chosen to live together and share their interests, roles, and resources." Each family is unique in its style and makeup, but usually attachment and commitment are the features that bind people together.

FAMILY FUNCTIONS

The family is one of the most important and powerful groups that individuals belong to. Although each family is set up for a specific purpose, a common goal shared by all families is the growth and development of its members. The family progresses through distinct stages of development over time, but the ultimate goal of the family is the survival and personal fulfillment of each member. Every family has certain distinct strengths and weaknesses, but all families share certain basic characteristics.

All families have a basic purpose or function and a set of values and governing rules. Several functions help secure this goal. These functions are not exclusive to families, but in combination they are unique to the family institution. The basic functions of the family include physical maintenance, protection, nurturance, socialization and education, reproduction, and recreation. See Figure 3.2.

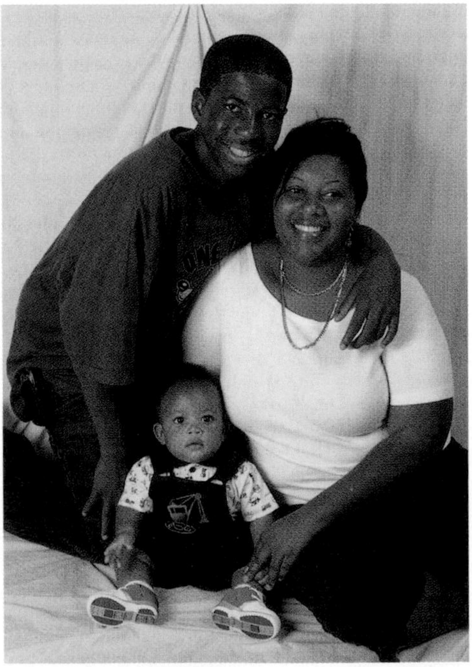

FIGURE 3.1 Each person in the family unit is important to the total well-being of the family.

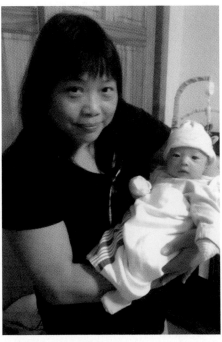

FIGURE 3.2 Nurturance provides love, care, and attention.

Physical Maintenance

The family must provide food, clothing, water, and shelter for each of its members. The ease and the manner in which a family can provide these necessities vary with each family and depend on the unit's economic success. Nearly one out of every eight American families lives below the federal poverty level. This low socioeconomic status results in a health disparity between the poor and higher-income families. Public assistance programs have been set up to help needy families meet basic family needs.

Protection

Each family member needs protection against inherited and acquired illnesses (internal forces) and injury (external forces). Protection may take different forms at different points of the life cycle. Before and during pregnancy, health screening and genetic counseling may offer individuals protection against certain diseases, including inherited diseases. After birth, immunization protects the infant and child against a number of illnesses. (The recommended immunization schedule is listed in Appendix B.) Diet, exercise, and health screening help protect adults from illness. Individuals in families are protected from external forces such as injury throughout all stages of growth and development. This protection is best accomplished through education, awareness training, and role modeling.

Families protect their children by using discipline. The words and actions of parents help shape the child's behavior.

Nurturance

The family provides nurturance—loving care and attention—to each of its members. In fact, it is the only group that offers almost unconditional acceptance, love, and emotional support for its members. Young infants need touching, cuddling, the sound of the caregiver's voice, and food if they are to thrive. As they grow, children also need to have limits set on their behavior. Without such discipline, a child feels unprotected and unloved. Adult family members need to nurture and care for each other because the need for love continues throughout the life cycle. If the family unit breaks down, other support systems must fill this need for nurturance. See Figure 3.3.

Family Loss and Breakdown

Illness or death of a family member may result in stress on the family unit. Untimely losses prevent

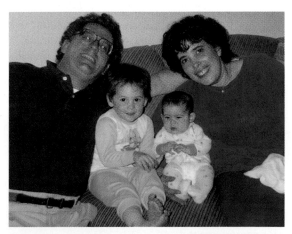

FIGURE 3.3 The family is the primary socializing agent for children.

individuals from having time to deal with crisis. Individuals left as survivors have no time to say goodbye or to express their feelings, and many survivors experience feelings of disbelief, anger, and even guilt.

Some experts classify deaths as premature, unexpected, and catastrophic. Premature deaths often are those of an infant or a child, often without warning. Unexpected deaths also occur without warning, frequently in seemingly healthy persons or in individuals who are not seriously ill. A death from a heart attack would be an example of an unexpected death. Catastrophic deaths are deaths that result from violent, destructive acts including murder, terrorist activity, or natural disasters.

Grief support means offering support to a person who has experienced a loss or death of a loved one. It is not an easy task for anyone. It is common to feel uncomfortable and ill prepared when talking to a grieving friend or family member. It is important to just be available to the person in need. Try not to "cheer up" the individual because each person needs time to feel and then to mobilize and proceed.

Parents should help their children understand the concept of death. This teaching is best done before a significant loss occurs and parents are grieving themselves. It is best to teach children about the "circle of life." Allowing a child to grieve for the small loss of a pet or an animal helps to accomplish such teaching. Children should be part of the lives of older family members and realistically be informed of their impending deaths. Introduce children to the concept of spirituality and the reality that we do not control death. Reinforce the memory of the loved one with openness and honesty. Counseling and grief support should be made available for anyone having difficulty coping with loss.

Divorce is another common example of family breakdown. Divorce presents a family unit with three challenges: moving forward, developing new ties, and redefining parenting roles. Divorce threatens the integrity of the family unit and, therefore, affects every member of the family. Parents need to be calm and keep their feelings under control so that they can

HELPFUL HINTS

Grief Support

Offer self and support.
Avoid clichés.
Recognize that time is needed for healing.
Be nonjudgmental.
Suggest professional help.

HELPFUL HINTS

Understanding Death

Children have different concepts of death at different ages. Their responses reflect their stages of emotional and cognitive development.

- Infants have no concept of death.
- Toddlers believe that death is temporary or reversible.
- Preschool children believe that their thoughts may cause death. This causes feelings of guilt and shame.
- School-age children understand the permanence of death but may associate it with misdeeds. They sometimes personify death as a monster or other evil thing.
- Adolescents have a mature understanding of death but may be subject to guilt and shame. This age group is least likely to accept death, especially if it happens to one of their peers.

talk openly with their children. The effect of divorce on a child depends on the child's personality, the nature of the custodial family, the involvement of the noncustodial parent, and the support systems and resources available. Children need to be able to express their feelings in an ongoing process. Many children of a divorce experience feelings of guilt and anger, often believing that they are the cause of the split. Children fear that one or both of their parents may abandon them. These feelings also give rise to anger. Unexpressed anger may cause children to act out or suffer depression. See Box 10.2 in Chapter 10 for common signs of depression.

Parents should be careful not to speak negatively about their former spouses in front of their children. It is important that children are not placed in the middle of feuding families. Parents should not send messages to one another via the children. Professional counseling may be necessary for all family members and should be instituted early to protect everyone's mental well-being. Expect resistance when new relationships begin. New partners mean that the child must cope with new relationships and new role assignments. Support, understanding, and open lines of communication are necessary during the adjustment period.

Socialization and Education

The family is the child's primary **socializing agent**. Children first learn how to interact with their social environment by observing how other family members act and respond (Fig. 3.4). It is within the family that the child first learns about the world and how to respond to it. The education of the child begins in the home. Other important socializing institutions—notably, school—may support and supplement the family unit, but educational success cannot be accomplished unless both family and school work together toward a common goal.

Today there is much debate about whether the schools can—or should—teach certain values and provide information about topics that have traditionally been considered part of the family's domain—for example, sex education and drug awareness. Other institutions and agents—the church, the media, or organizations such as the Boy Scouts and Girl Scouts—may support and supplement the family, but the family unit is still the primary socializing institution.

Reproduction

Reproduction is the means by which the family survives and passes its genes to succeeding generations. Reproduction is a bodily function that begins with puberty. However, it requires not only physical readiness, but also psychological preparedness and a lifetime of commitment.

Recreation

The family unit should be able to spend time together in pleasurable activity. Family time is one of the best indicators of healthy family functioning. It is important to the success and cohesiveness of the group that family members share fun time, work, and other roles. This creates a balance and opens the channels for communication. Family time has a positive effect on the child's emotional development,

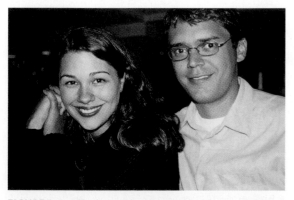

FIGURE 3.4 Affection and bonding begin at the couple stage.

behavior, and conflict resolution. In today's family, "free time" may be difficult when both parents work or a single parent must play multiple roles.

FAMILY TYPES

In today's world, there are a number of different family structures or types. The most common types include the nuclear or conjugal, the extended, the single-parent, the blended or reconstituted, the cohabitative, the communal, the foster or adoptive, and the same-sex family. For a summary of family types, see Table 3.1.

The Nuclear or Conjugal Family

The nuclear or conjugal family, also known as the traditional family, consists of a husband, a wife, and their children. Today statistics indicate that fewer than one-third of all families are of the nuclear type. Families consisting of two adults without children are referred to as a nuclear dyad. Marriage is the main binding force in both of these family types. In recent history, the nuclear family has become the model for other, more complex family types. Traditionally, the man was expected to be the breadwinner

TABLE 3.1   Family Types

Types	Members
Nuclear, conjugal, or dyad	Husband and wife, with or without children
Extended	Husband and wife, children, and grandparents or other family members
Single-parent	Mother or father and children
Blended or reconstituted	Mother or father, stepparent, and children
Cohabitative	Man, woman, and children
Communal	Individuals with their mates and children
Foster or adoptive	Parents or caregivers and children
Same-sex	Two women or two men, with or without children

and the woman was considered the caregiver and homemaker. In today's nuclear family, both parents are probably in the workforce and there is a sharing of roles. Fathers are more and more actively involved in raising their children. Someone other than the parents, or some outside agency, may provide child care while the parents are at work.

The Extended Family

The extended family type consists of the nuclear family plus grandparents, aunts, uncles, or cousins living together under the same roof. Children in this household have many role models from which to choose. In this family type there may be sharing of resources and roles. Elders living in the extended family can assist with child-rearing roles. This assistance may resolve their need for usefulness and increase their sense of belonging. An undesirable effect of the extended family occurs when the older person is undervalued and seen as a burden. It is important that nurses in all practice settings be able to assess and evaluate the coping abilities of extended families.

In recent years, extended families have become more commonplace as a result of certain outside forces—namely, increases in the cost of living, unemployment, longer life spans, and greater numbers of divorces and teenage parents. The extended family may provide a temporary respite from economic or social hardship; once recovery is achieved, family members may move out on their own. Often, however, the nuclear family may be set up in close proximity to parents and other relatives. In this case, the nuclear family has some of the feel of an extended family because of the regular, frequent contact among family members.

The Single-Parent Family

The single-parent family consists of an adult living with one or more children. In most cases, single parents are divorced, separated, or widowed. However, a growing number of adults are choosing this family type as an alternative lifestyle. Today, 60 to 70 percent of families are single-parent families. Most are headed by women, although recently more men are becoming single parents. A major challenge to this family type is that the single parent must assume the role of both caregiver and breadwinner. Single parents may look to their own families of origin for support and assistance. Other outside agencies or individuals may also assist this family type.

Divorce or separation may increase health risks for children. A recent study indicated that the children of divorced or separated parents had a one-third greater risk for developing health problems, including pneumonia, ear infections, and tonsillitis, than did children from intact families. The infant mortality rate has also been shown to vary based on marital status, race, and ethnicity. The infant mortality rate is the number of infant deaths occurring in the first year of life per 1,000 live births.

The Blended or Reconstituted Family

The blended or reconstituted family is created when one or both partners bring children from a previous marriage into the relationship. Divided loyalties and resentment toward the stepparent can create stresses, which may be compounded if one parent must pay support for a child living in another household. In addition, children have to adjust to multiple views, attitudes, and personalities. Conflicts frequently emerge over how to discipline the children. Open communication between family members is essential in resolving conflicts and uniting all the parties. After the initial adjustment period, the members may unite to form a new, congenial group. Coparenting is a family style that works in cases of divorce or separation. In this style, the parents continue to share parental responsibilities even though they have separated.

The Cohabitative Family

In the cohabitative family, a man and woman choose to live together without the legal bonds of matrimony,

---

HELPFUL   HINTS

Parenting Stepchildren

- Share and value history and memories through stories, pictures, and videos.
- Encourage respect for individual differences.
- Give everyone a place for belongings.
- Avoid taking sides and showing favoritism.
- Establish a united approach to child care.
- Avoid negative comments about the absent parent.
- Be sensitive to children's concerns about differences in their surnames.

Source: Lusk Lechlitner, S, Kerr, MJ, and Ronis, DL: Health-promoting lifestyles of blue-collar, skilled-trade, and white-collar workers. Nurs Res 44(1):20–24, 1995, with permission.

but in all other ways this type of family resembles the nuclear or blended family. This family type has gained popularity during the time before or between marriages. Many of these families include children from previous relationships. These relationships may be less stable and are subject to change at any time. Stability increases when couples remain together for a long time.

The Communal Family

The communal family consists of a group of people who have a common philosophy, value system, and goals and who choose to live together, sharing roles and resources. All the children become the collective responsibility of the adult family members. This family style became popular in the 1960s as a result of the political ferment of the period and disenchantment with society. It is difficult to track and document but still exists in rural areas.

The Foster or Adoptive Family

Foster families are those who take temporary responsibility for raising a child other than their own. Although these placements are temporary, they may extend over long periods depending on the stability of the birth family. This type of family faces a number of challenges. If the foster child is from a dysfunctional family, the child may experience behavioral problems as he or she attempts to cope in the new environment. The age of the child and the length of time that he or she has been in foster care will affect the child's ability to make the transition to the new setting. Foster parents assume legal responsibility for the child in their care.

The adoptive family permanently adds a child other than its own to its structure. This child has all the legal entitlements of a birth child. Adults who choose to adopt may do so because they want children but cannot or do not wish to give birth to a child. In the past, adoption records were not made public. Today many adoptees seek out their birth parents to better understand their identities and personal histories.

The Same-Sex Family

Same-sex families can also take the form of any of the preceding families except that they consist of two adults of the same sex living together and sharing common emotional bonds, resources, and parenting roles. Society's attitudes toward same-sex relationships have become somewhat more liberal in recent decades. The courts are increasingly willing to award child custody to parents with this alternative family style. Same-sex couples sometimes choose to adopt as a means of meeting their nurturing needs.

FAMILY STAGES

The following section contains brief descriptions of family stages. Not all families go through every stage. For example, a couple without children may still be considered a family. Other families may not survive into old age.

Couple Stage

Traditionally, a new family is launched when young, single adults decide to move away from their families of origin and start a unit by themselves. When two people form an affectionate bond and move in together, they become a couple (Fig. 3.5). This is the first stage of a new family, and emotionally it may be difficult as each person merges his or her original values and beliefs with those of the new partner. Many adjustments are necessary as each partner learns to accept the other's habits, preferences, and routines. Also, early in the couple stage, the couple will need to define roles and distribute and accept responsibilities. This is an important move. It allows the young person to try out the roles and values learned in his or her family of origin and test newly acquired skills and independence. This experience can be both exciting and threatening to the young adult. Throughout this testing period, the individual may remain tied to the family of origin. During stressful times, the young adult may rely heavily on the family of origin for financial and emotional support.

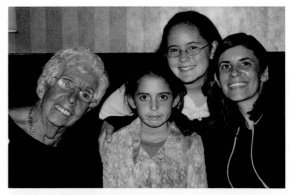

FIGURE 3.5 Grandchildren have strong bonds of affection toward their grandparents.

One of the objectives of this union is to establish a satisfying relationship built on mutual respect. Each party must be able to compromise and to recognize and accept the other person's point of view. Sometimes this means putting aside one's own needs and considering the needs of the other person.

Sometimes a couple decides to postpone marriage until their careers are started. Postponement may have certain advantages and disadvantages. These individuals may be more mature but also more set in their ways. Communication channels must be kept open to maintain a healthy, satisfying relationship. Intimacy must be valued but not to the exclusion of each partner's **autonomy,** or independence and sense of self. Pleasurable activities, humor, and relaxation should be integrated into the couple's daily living. It is important to the success of the marriage or relationship that the couple be separate from but still closely connected to their families of origin (Box 3.1).

Childbearing Stage

The arrival of a baby changes the family constellation dramatically. Both parents must have time to adjust to their new and expanded roles. Early preparation for parenthood can help decrease some of the anxiety and stress for the new parents.

When making decisions about child care, the mother and father should each consider the other's philosophy. Care and development of the child and parents are also enhanced by close interactions with

---

B O X
3.1
Maintaining a Healthy Relationship

- Clarify roles with families of origin while maintaining self-identity.
- Permit autonomy while reaching out to maintain intimacy.
- Value time for privacy.
- Recognize and seek support from outside agencies during periods of stress.
- Tighten family bonds in times of stress or crisis.
- Respect your partner's worth.
- Handle anger and conflicts with open communication.
- Maintain a sense of humor.
- Satisfy your mate's need for security and safety.
- Demonstrate caring while maintaining a romantic outlook.
- Be open and tolerant to your partner's point of view.
- Take time to have fun and share with each other.

---

grandparents and other relatives. Even with a close relationship to extended family members and with expansion of the family as other children are born, each family member must make new role adjustments without compromising his or her autonomy and sense of self. Parents and children alike can thus develop confidence and enhance their self-worth.

Delayed Parenting

The timing of parenthood varies now, as many couples are delaying parenting. This means different things to different individuals: Pregnancy may be delayed until career or financial goals are established, or it may mean waiting to start a family until the couple has had a chance to grow together. There are advantages and disadvantages to earlier and delayed parenting. Delaying parenting may result in having more established career goals, maturity, stable income, and valuable life experiences. Early parenting usually allows individuals to have more energy and fewer maternal health issues.

Grown-Child Stage

Once again the family must make adjustments to the new family unit when grown children leave home and start out on their own. For parents this scenario is sometimes described as the "empty-nest syndrome." The parents shift their focus from caring for the children to caring for each other once again. This can be a time for the development of new roles, interests, and accomplishments. Many adults return to school or begin new careers during this stage. This may be a very rewarding period, allowing each partner to fulfill lifetime goals. However, it may also be a period of stress and turmoil as some middle-aged adults reevaluate their goals, marriage, and priorities. For some individuals the earlier conflicts have been resolved, but for others they have contributed to the breakup of the marriage. Social expectations regarding economic stability and family and work satisfaction may place additional stresses on individuals during this stage of development.

Older-Family Stage

The transition into the elderly years generally begins with retirement of one or both spouses. Perceptions of retirement are often based on economic preparation and physical health. Many elderly families prefer to live separate from but within close proximity to their children. Older adults must often make several adjustments because of changing health, declining income, and reduced energy. Some older adults must also adjust to the death of a spouse and the resultant role changes that occur at this point in life. Older adults should be sure to include pleasurable recreational activities in their daily lives. Many continue to maintain rich, rewarding relationships with their children and grandchildren throughout their older years. These kinds of pleasurable activities help the older person maintain a high level of self-esteem.

Grandparenting Roles

Grandparenting may take on different styles, which can be described as formal, informal/spoiler, surrogate, wisdom provider, and distant figure. The formal grandparent allows the parents to discipline their children while maintaining a close interest in the children. The informal/spoiler style of grandparenting attempts to establish a close, somewhat indulgent relationship with grandchildren. The surrogate style is assumed by those grandparents who tend to do most of the child-rearing activities while parents are at work. Surrogate grandparents may be in the position to make many of the parenting decisions. The wisdom provider is a role bestowed by family beliefs and customs that imply that the older person is one of high esteem and regard. Family members look to the grandparent for knowledge and guidance. The distant grandparent role is one in which the grandparents have limited contact with their children and grandchildren. This role may be the result of living arrangements that prevent frequent visits, or it may be the result of earlier family conflicts. Grandchildren appear to have strong bonds of attachment and affection toward their grandparents (Fig. 3.6), and regardless of the style of grandparenting, the grandparents' role is important to children of all ages.

See Table 3.2 for a summary of family stages.

FAMILY SIZE, BIRTH ORDER, AND GENDER OF CHILDREN

Decisions about family size are important. Family planning—the spacing and numbering of children in the family—requires both maturity and responsibility. Effective family planning (or the avoidance of unwanted pregnancy) can improve overall infant health. It has been shown that women who plan their pregnancies tend to seek out earlier prenatal care than those who have unplanned pregnancies.

The family unit is not constant; it changes with the addition of each new member. Each child has a

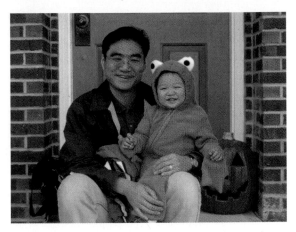

FIGURE 3.6 Adult males play an important role in parenting.

TABLE
3.2   Summary of Family Stages

Stage	Task
Couple stage	Establish bonds between individuals. Adjust to new routines. Define roles and responsibilities.
Childbearing stage	Integrate baby into the family unit. Adjust to new roles; extend relations to extended family. Explore and establish child care philosophy.
Grown-child stage	Adjust to new roles and empty nest. Focus on reestablishing marital relationship. Develop new roles, interests, and accomplishments.
Older-family stage	Adjust to retirement living. Adjust to decline in income. Adjust to changing health and reduced energy. Maintain rewarding relationships with children and grandchildren. Establish pleasurable activities to build self-esteem.

distinct place in the family. A child's birth order can provide some clues to his or her behavior because ordinal position affects the child's perception of and response to the world.

The *oldest child* has the parent's undivided attention for a period, creating a sense of **omnipotence,** or unlimited power or authority. The oldest child may always want things to go his or her way. This perception can lead to difficulties within the family and within the larger community. Parents often have very high expectations for a firstborn. This places great demands on the firstborn.

The *second child* (or middle children) never has the undivided attention of the parents in the same way as the first child. This child has a need to compete with the first child, always wanting to be as good as or better than the older sibling. This may motivate the second child to work harder to achieve. Or the child may give up and settle for less than he or she is capable of attaining. Parents may be more relaxed in their approach to child care.

The *youngest child,* the baby of the family, may gain attention and importance from this position, which can serve as either a positive or a negative influence on his or her development.

The *only child* has only adults for company and role models. How the child handles the presence and attention of adults varies with the individual.

Ordinal position alone cannot be used as a determinant of behavior. The size of the family and spacing of the children may also influence each child in his or her particular position.

The gender or sex of the child also may influence upbringing. It is unfair to make generalizations regarding the differences or similarities between girls and boys. Each family has its own cultural influences and expectations, which undoubtedly affect a child's perception of gender.

FAMILY PATTERNS

Family patterns can be classified as authoritarian, authoritative, permissive, or uninvolved, depending on how family members relate to each other.

In the *authoritarian* or *autocratic family,* parents usually make all decisions. Rules are made and enforced by the adults without input from the children. Parents demand and expect respect from their offspring. Parenting is rigid and punitive. Parents expect children to just "do it" their way without question. The *authoritative* or *democratic family* offers its members choices and encourages participation and individual responsibility. This family works on a philosophy of mutual respect. It is thought that children develop a greater sense of self-esteem and gradual autonomy in this style of family. Children become self-reliant, self-controlled achievers who work well with others. The family meeting is an

effective tool used to air and work out differences. The *permissive* or *laissez-faire family* offers its members complete freedom. Parents do not try to regulate or set limits on the family members. Children raised under this style of parenting often do not learn the rules that teach impulse control. Parents practicing the *uninvolved* parenting style show little or no commitment to parenting. They emphasize meeting their own needs first and foremost. These adults are emotionally unattached, often overwhelmed by stress, and indifferent to the child's developing autonomy. Children raised in this style may become impulsive and immature and often may act out of control.

Families may also be considered functional or dysfunctional. A **functional family** is one that fosters the growth and development of its members. Cohesion among family members also helps to promote emotional, physical, and social well-being. Meeting each family member's needs for love, belonging, and security helps to maintain the stability of the family. See Figure 3.7. The functional family readily admits new members into the circle without compromising the worth and individuality of its members. Healthy families can recognize and accept the differences among individual members and accommodate stressors from inside or outside the family. Common family stressors include financial problems, parenting concerns and conflicts, illness, death, divorce, lack of time, and unequal distribution of roles. Healthy families are not problem-free, but they are able to deal with their problems as a group or seek outside assistance to help them preserve their integrity.

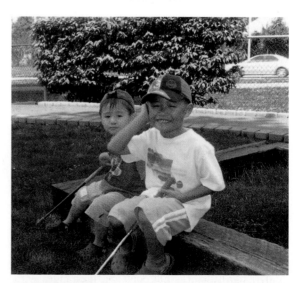

FIGURE 3.7 Recreation is important for a healthy family life.

The **dysfunctional family** is unable to offer its members a stable structure. As a result, family members may have poor interpersonal skills and lack the ability to deal with stress and conflict. A lack of proper discipline and consistency can lead to acting out or antisocial behaviors. Dysfunctional families have trouble reaching outside of the immediate family boundaries for help. Dysfunctional families often have less skilled parents who exhibit difficulties handling confrontation and stress. Things that start out as minor irritations become larger ones, causing family members to react emotionally and inappropriately. Pleasure and affection are rarely expressed. Factors that often contribute to creating an "at-risk" climate for families include unemployment, young maternal age, low income, lack of education, alcohol and drug usage, and lack of adequate social support.

Family members in these families are at risk for physical, sexual, and psychological abuse or neglect.

Although most families are warm and loving, a number of families may suffer from domestic violence, child abuse, and elder abuse. These cases are difficult to measure because they occur in the privacy of the home. Victims are ashamed and reluctant to report this abuse to the proper authorities. Family violence may affect any family.

Factors that may contribute to family violence include marital conflict, financial problems, social isolation, poor parenting skills, and alcohol and drug use. Two approaches for dealing with family violence are primary prevention, which is aimed at reducing the risks by teaching parenting skills, and secondary prevention, which focuses on rehabilitating families after abuse is identified.

SUMMARY

1. A current definition of family is two or more people who have chosen to live together and share their interests, roles, and resources. All families are bound together by attachment and commitment.

2. Each family is unique, but all families share the goals of survival and personal fulfillment of family members.

3. Basic functions of the family are physical maintenance of family members, protection, nurturance, socialization and education, reproduction, and recreation.

4. Families may go through distinct stages of development: the couple stage, the childbearing stage, the grown-child stage, and the older-family stage.

5. Birth order may influence the child's development.

6. Families may be classified as autocratic, authoritative, permissive, or uninvolved, depending on how family members relate to each other.

7. Family violence exists on all levels. Primary prevention is aimed at reducing the risk through teaching parenting skills. Secondary prevention is focused on rehabilitation after the abuse has occurred.

MULTIPLE-CHOICE QUESTIONS

1. Which of these descriptions provides a modern definition of a family?
   a. Two or more people who live together and share a bond of love and intimacy
   b. Two or more people who are related by blood, live together, and share the same values
   c. Two or more people who share common bonds
   d. Two or more people who are related by adoption and share the same ethnicity

2. Which characteristic do all families have?
   a. A specific purpose
   b. Specific roles for their members
   c. A specific number of members
   d. Specific behavioral regulations

3. Which goal is common to all families?
   a. Disciplined action
   b. Ritual acts within the group
   c. Monetary success
   d. Personal fulfillment of the members

4. Which of the following is a basic family function?
   a. Philosophical ideals
   b. Honesty
   c. Protection
   d. Creativity

5. One of the advantages of early parenting is:
   a. Established career goals
   b. Stable income
   c. More valuable life experiences
   d. More energy and fewer potential health problems

6. Which is a common family type?
   a. Open
   b. Closed
   c. Bonded
   d. Extended

7. Characteristics of functional families include:
   a. Freedom from problems
   b. The ability to prevent stressful situations
   c. The ability to foster growth and development
   d. The discouragement of role sharing

8. The primary socializing agent for children is:
   a. School
   b. Church
   c. Family
   d. Friends and peers

9. The nurse advocates for secondary prevention of family violence by providing:
   a. Incarceration
   b. Use of pharmacological agents
   c. Probation
   d. Rehabilitation and education

10. To clarify the roles of members within a family, it would be best for the nurse to ask:
    a. "When your father comes in drunk, what does your mother say?"
    b. "Who do you go to in the family when you need someone to talk to?"
    c. "Tell me how your mother feels about your father's illness."
    d. "What do you believe caused your illness?"

11. In the formal grandparenting role, discipline of the child is left to the parent.
    a. True
    b. False

12. The community health nurse is working with a family after one of its members experiences a major health crisis. The nurse records signs of a healthy family when:
    a. There is very little communication between the family members.
    b. She walks in on an angry disagreement between members.
    c. The family states they have plans to share caregiving.
    d. The recovering member states, "Can you help me? I can't stay here anymore."
    e. After each visit different members of the family question if everything is going well.

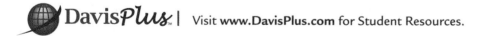

DavisPlus | Visit **www.DavisPlus.com** for Student Resources.

Student Activity   **Family Observation**

Select a family that you can observe closely for a brief period. While observing the interactions of the family members, try to answer the following questions:

1. What is the specific role of each family member?

2. What are three strengths unique to this family?

3. What are two outside support systems available to this family?

4. What stresses can be identified during this observation?

5. What three interventions might enhance this family's coping abilities?

CASE STUDY

A Preschooler's View of Death

The parents of 4-year-old Sara prepared her for the death of a seriously ill uncle. They spoke about illness and answered all of her questions honestly. When the uncle died, it seemed appropriate for the whole family to attend the wake. In preparation, the parents explained that Uncle George was going to heaven. Several days after attending the wake, Sara asked, "Do you think Uncle George got where he was going yet?" Questions like this one or others—such as "Will he be cold?" or "How does he breathe?"—indicate that the concept of death is too complex for young children to comprehend at the moment. It is important that parents recognize these questions as cues to the child's own concern about his or her safety and place within the family.

CASE STUDY

Problem-Solve

Claris and John come from low-income, working-class families in the Midwest. They are the first in their families to complete college and earn a degree. They were childhood sweethearts and married after graduating from college. They moved from the Midwest and settled in a major city in the East where John worked as a financial analyst, while Claris worked as a schoolteacher. They have three children, ages 14, 12, and 7. As John worked his way up the ladder in the company, they enjoyed the life of upper-middle-class Americans with a home in the suburbs, two cars, college funds for the kids, and funds in the money market. Now Claris stays at home and cares for the children.

The sudden economic recession caused John, who is now 44, to lose his job and his search for a new job was not going well. The couple's savings are depleted, and they have suffered major losses in the money market. Since being out of work, John has been experiencing episodes of depression. He has been admitted to the hospital with chest pains and diagnosed as having an inferior wall myocardial infarction.

In the step-down unit, the nurse is planning discharge teaching for John and has set up a meeting with Claris and John. During the interview John begins to cry and says it would be better for his family if he had died. Claris begins to cry too and expresses their inability to even find food for the children or pay the hospital bills. She also says they cannot meet their mortgage payment and may lose their home.

1. How should the nurse respond to validate this family concern?
2. What could the nurse do to help relieve the family stress?
3. Is this a good time for the nurse to continue discharge teaching?
4. What impact can the changes in the family health and financial status have on the children?

CRITICAL THINKING

Mavis Citro, 38 years old, was summoned to an interview with the school nurse because Reginald, her 9-year-old son, had had several altercations with his peers and teachers. During the interview the school nurse discovered that Ms. Citro and her first husband had divorced when Reginald was 5 years old. Two years later she began seeing another man, also divorced and custodial father of two older boys. After a yearlong courtship, the couple got married; shortly thereafter they bought a new home and moved out of the neighborhood. Almost immediately, Reginald, then age 8, started having conflicts with his stepfather and stepbrothers. These conflicts have been escalating lately.

1. What is Reginald's current family type called?
2. Give two reasons for the conflict between Reginald and his new stepfamily.
3. What can be done to establish harmony in the family?

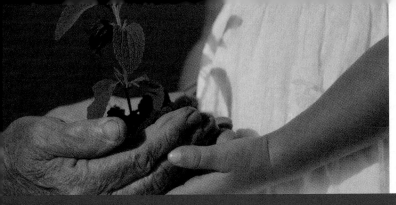

Communication

Learning Objectives

At the end of this chapter, you should be able to:

- Define communication.
- Describe the difference between verbal and nonverbal communication.
- Distinguish between social and therapeutic communication.
- List responses that block effective communication.
- Name techniques for effective communication.

Communication is an interaction between two or more persons—an exchange of information, ideas, feelings, or emotions. Communication is complex, dynamic, and ongoing. In the health care setting, communication serves as a vital link among patients, families, nurses, physicians, and other health care workers. The development of communication is a continuous process. Communication begins during infancy and is a necessary part of our existence. Communication and language acquisition will be further explored in the chapters that follow.

THE COMMUNICATION PROCESS

The communication process (Fig. 4.1) consists of five parts: message, sender, method, receiver, and feedback. The **message** is the expression of your thoughts and feelings in words, symbols, or body language. The **sender** delivers the message by initiating the conversation. Factors that determine how the message is developed are varied. These include the sender's knowledge base—his or her past experiences. The **method** used to convey the message is determined by the sender and can be words or symbols or a combination of both. The **receiver** is the person to whom the message is sent. The receiver must interpret and reconstruct the message. How the receiver interprets the message will be influenced by his or her age, knowledge, and past experience. Age, feelings, attitudes, and emotions also shape how the message is sent and received. **Feedback** is the response to the message. Feedback is necessary because it serves to verify that the message was received as intended.

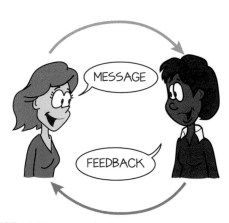

FIGURE 4.1 The communication process.

TYPES AND STYLES OF COMMUNICATION

There are two basic types of communication—verbal and nonverbal. **Verbal communication** transmits attitudes, thoughts, and feelings using spoken or written words. Much of the meaning of words depends on the person's understanding of the words, how the words are used, and the individual's emotional state. Culture may influence the meaning of words. **Nonverbal communication** is also referred to as *body language*. Individuals may choose to use body language to emphasize their thoughts or feelings, and they may use gestures without being aware of doing so. The nonverbal method of communication is partly learned and partly instinctive. It is the most accurate method of sending a message.

Eight Modes of Nonverbal Communication

The eight modes of nonverbal communication include the following:

1. **Physical appearance and dress.** The way a person appears may give information about his or her mental, physical, and emotional states. Dress may also indicate a person's work role, culture, or religion. For example, seeing a young man wearing a collar sends the message that he is a clergyperson. A person's choice of colors or adornments such as jewelry, lipstick, and perfume, or the lack thereof, may reveal additional information. Persons who are depressed rarely take interest in their appearance or wear makeup. A nurse whose appearance is professional communicates competence and pride, whereas a caregiver whose appearance is unkempt may communicate incompetence and a lack of care.
2. **Body movement and posture.** Body movement and posture can convey many different messages. The way in which individuals position their bodies when they sit, stand, or move communicates messages such as self-esteem and attitude.
   - A person whose posture is open sits relaxed, with hands and legs uncrossed, facing another individual. This *open* posture communicates warmth, caring, and willingness to communicate.
   - A *closed* posture is best demonstrated by a person who sits with arms and legs tightly crossed. This position generally communicates

coldness, disinterest, and nonacceptance. Other postures, such as standing over someone, may convey authority and control. A slumped posture with head and eyes cast downward can suggest low self-esteem. Anger or anxiety is implied by a tense posture.

3. **Facial expression.** Next to speech, facial expression is the primary source of human communication and is universal to all cultures. Facial expression communicates sadness, happiness, anger, fear, and surprise. Facial expression serves to complement or qualify feelings. Children can often tell if their mother is angry or upset just by looking at her facial expression.

4. **Gestures.** Moving body parts can indicate feelings. For example, one of the first things babies learn and understand is the simple gesture of waving good-bye or shaking their head for yes or no. Pain and anxiety can be communicated by the wringing of one's hands or pacing.

5. **Eye contact.** The eyes are referred to as the "windows to the soul." Eye contact can suggest a willingness to communicate. To show respect, some cultures avoid direct eye contact. Staring can cause anxiety and is usually used to register disapproval or power, whereas lack of eye contact can suggest shyness, embarrassment, or nervousness.

6. **Tone and volume of voice.** Tone and volume of voice can express enthusiasm, sadness, annoyance, or anger. Speaking in a low volume may give the impression of hesitancy or lack of interest. Speaking loudly can be used to overcome the listener's hearing impairment. However, it is best to use low- rather than high-pitched tones for most hearing impairments.

7. **Touch.** Touch is a powerful communication tool that elicits positive or negative reactions. Touch is basic and primitive. It begins in infancy and helps an infant feel comforted immediately after birth. Touch is one of the most important tools we use to convey human emotions. Kissing, hugging, and patting the hand or cheek are several ways of showing affection (Fig. 4.2).

It is important that touch be used appropriately in each situation. Hugging or touching can be an appropriate greeting for someone you know but inappropriate for a stranger. Sudden touching can be threatening. Inappropriate touch can be viewed as an invasion of privacy or as a sexual advance. Children should be taught at an early age what is appropriate or inappropriate touching.

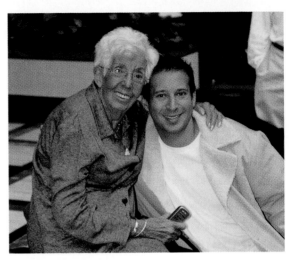

FIGURE 4.2 Touch conveys human emotions.

8. **Silence.** Silence conveys different messages depending on the accompanying gestures and body posture. Silence between individuals can provoke thought or anxiety. Silence can indicate acceptance, evasion, fear, uncertainty, anger, rebelliousness, or rejection. Some individuals think that they must always have something to say, making periods of silence uncomfortable. However, short periods of silence can be used to put thoughts and feelings into perspective.

Personality Types

Passive or Unassertive

Individuals with the passive or unassertive personality type are unable to share their feelings or needs with others. They have difficulty asking for help. They often feel hurt or angry and that others are taking advantage of them. They use apologetic words; have weak, soft voices; make little eye contact; and are often fidgety. They usually are compliant, ask for nothing, and get little attention. They usually sacrifice their rights to meet the needs of others.

Aggressive

An aggressive personality style is very destructive. These individuals use angry vocalization to dominate

---

H E L P F U L   H I N T S

Listening Is

- Sensing
- Interpreting
- Evaluating
- Responding

and harm other people. They may lack concern for others and often put their own needs first. They are demanding and manipulative.

Assertive

Persons who are assertive are empowered. They express confidence and are comfortable sharing their feelings. They use a firm voice with appropriate eye contact. They take responsibility for the consequences of their actions and behave in a manner to enhance self-respect. Assertive types encourage listening and reflect on the feelings of others.

Social Versus Therapeutic Communication Styles

Individuals can engage in two levels of communication in their interactions with others: interpersonal and intrapersonal. They may exist together or they may be used alone. *Intrapersonal* communication occurs when one is thinking to himself or herself. The purpose of these thoughts is to help control an emotional response. What a person is thinking affects how he or she will interact with others. Negative thoughts can result in negative interactions and may affect the individual's relationships. Positive thoughts can help make our responses more pleasant and optimistic. *Interpersonal* communication occurs between two or more individuals. Communication at this level varies with the type of relationship. In the nurse–patient setting the interpersonal communication is goal directed and purposeful, whereas between friends the communication is less purposeful.

These two styles of communication are known as social and therapeutic. **Social communication** is used in everyday life between family, friends, and coworkers. It serves the needs of participants (Fig. 4.3). It is sharing of thoughts, feelings, needs, and desires. Social communication is light and superficial. Therapeutic communication is the type used in professional nursing care, and it is discussed in detail in the next section.

THERAPEUTIC COMMUNICATION

Therapeutic communication is purposeful and goal oriented. It promotes trust and good rapport with others. It is open until the goals are reached. Health care professionals use this style of communication in their work interactions. Therapeutic communication is used between the physician and

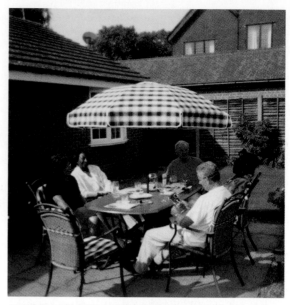

FIGURE 4.3 Social communication.

patient and among the nurse, patient, and/or family members.

Six Components of Therapeutic Communication

1. **Listening and observing.** Messages are sent in the cognitive or affective domains, or both. The cognitive domain is the message expressed in words. The affective domain expresses feelings through the tone of words. **Listening** can be active or passive and involves the interpretation of the spoken word. Listening also requires more than just hearing the words spoken. It requires that the listener consider both the verbal and nonverbal message. Distraction occurs when the listener is not concentrating. Active listening is outlined in Box 4.1.
2. **Warmth.** Warmth is a feeling of cordiality and acceptance that makes the person feel relaxed and secure.
3. **Genuineness.** Genuineness is being yourself—open and truthful. It is important to be honest

---

BOX 4.1   **Components of Active Listening**

- Sitting squarely facing the patient
- Using an open posture
- Leaning forward toward the patient
- Establishing eye contact
- Relaxing and concentrating

and say you do not know or are not sure of the answer. Being genuine means being caring.

4. **Attentiveness.** Attentiveness is concentrating on what the other person is saying to demonstrate that he or she has your full attention.

5. **Empathy.** Empathy shows that you understand a person's feelings and view the world as he or she does. Empathy is different from sympathy; in the latter, you adopt the other person's feelings. You lose your objectivity when you are sympathetic instead of empathic. Showing empathy allows you to stay in control of the interaction and act with confidence. This can be reassuring to the other party.

6. **Positive regard.** Positive regard is demonstrated by accepting the patient exactly as he or she is. This requires you to be nonjudgmental. The other person must be valued and respected. Positive regard may be another term for caring. It serves to make a person feel secure. Showing such acceptance does not mean you need to agree with the other person.

Functions of therapeutic communication are listed in Box 4.2.

Three Phases of Therapeutic Communication

Orientation Phase
In the orientation phase both the nurse and client will initially experience some anxiety. As a nurse, you can reduce this anxiety by introducing yourself and giving your title. This can be followed by a broad opening statement that helps set the tone and allows for an exchange of words. During the orientation phase, you learn about the individual and his or her initial concerns and needs. You listen to the patient and learn by observing. At the same time, the patient learns about you and your role, and a contract is established. The goal is to build trust. Trust is built slowly.

Working Phase
In the working phase the nurse determines the type of coping mechanisms that the client is using and what support systems exist. The nurse can then develop a plan of care and establish realistic goals. The plan of care is implemented to promote independence and optimal functioning. The client has a fundamental right to expect confidentiality from all members of the health care team. The client must be assured that the information shared will not go beyond the members of staff directly involved in his or her care. If this phase is successful, the client can share and explore thoughts and feelings and work toward a change in behavior or possible solution.

Termination Phase
The termination phase is the end of a relationship. Ideally it involves evaluating and synthesizing what has occurred and preparing for separation. At the termination phase, it is important to think and ask yourself, "Has the person been helped?"

FACTORS AFFECTING COMMUNICATION

Congruence

Congruence implies an agreement between the verbal and nonverbal language. It is important that the spoken word match the nonverbal communication. When congruence occurs, the message is clear to the receiver.

BOX 4.2 Functions of Therapeutic Communication

- Create an understanding with the individual to effect a change.
- Decrease anxiety by allowing others to talk about themselves and their feelings. Individuals cope with their feelings in different ways. Communication must be modified to meet each individual's needs.
- Provide information.
- Develop trust and show caring by answering questions honestly.

HELPFUL HINTS

Rules of Listening
- Do not talk while listening.
- Assume an open, relaxed posture.
- Focus on what the person is saying.
- Listen to understand rather than to respond.
- Secure a quiet environment, free of distraction.
- Show caring and understanding.
- Validate the other person's feelings.
- Do not criticize.
- Accept the person as he or she is.
- Be nonjudgmental.
- Ask open-ended questions.
- Rephrase questions to help verify the accuracy of the conversation.

Time and Setting

Time is very important in most Western cultures. Time is concerned with what precedes and follows an interaction. It is important not to promise that something will occur within an unrealistic time frame. Setting includes the physical environment in which communication takes place. Setting should be private and free from noise and distraction. Individuals should be comfortable in the setting used for meaningful conversation. Always ask for permission to have someone else present during an interview or private conversation.

Proxemics

Proxemics refers to how close a person can get to another individual before he or she begins to feel uncomfortable. Individuals need their own personal space. The amount of personal space varies with a person's age, sex, and culture.

Biases

Bias is a word used to describe a prejudice or a negative belief about someone or something. Most often these types of beliefs are not based on fact or evidence but rather on ignorance. To avoid biases you must know yourself and gain insight into your personal feelings. This process is called becoming self-aware. Achieving self-awareness is a lifelong process. Ask yourself what motivates your interest in helping others. Determine how you feel about other people's cultures. Learn to respect all cultures. Always try to look at things from the other person's cultural perspective. Box 4.3 offers suggestions for multicultural communication.

Physical Handicaps

Physical handicaps, such as problems with sight, hearing, or illness, can interfere with an individual's ability to properly communicate. When communicating with a patient who is visually impaired, tell the patient where you are and what you are doing before touching him or her. When communicating with an individual who is hearing impaired, it is best to speak slowly, face the person, and use sign language to emphasize the message.

BLOCKS TO COMMUNICATION

Blocks to communication are words or actions people use to obscure the messages they are sending.

BOX 4.3   Multicultural Communication

- Have the individual define his or her health care practices and beliefs.
- Respect cultural traditions and dignity of others.
- Listen to the language and words and provide a translator as needed.
- Avoid stereotyping.
- Recognize the individual as unique with individual needs.
- Help individuals make informed choices.
- Keep one's personal beliefs to oneself.
- Be open and aware.
- Identify the level of comprehension.
- Request feedback to gauge level of understanding.
- Give written handouts in the person's primary language.
- Remember, nonverbal communication may be understood by all.

Common blocks to communication include the following:

- *Belittling* is using a statement that dismisses or mocks a person's beliefs or fears. For example, a 3-year-old child says he is afraid of monsters. His mother responds by saying, "You're acting like a baby. There are no monsters." Or a patient says, "I won't leave here alive." The nurse responds, "That's ridiculous. You shouldn't even think that way."
- *Disagreeing* is giving a response that indicates you believe the other person is incorrect. When you disagree with someone, it causes the person to feel angry and become defensive. For example, a teenage girl tells her mother that her boyfriend is terrific. Her mother replies, "I think he's a loser. You can do better." Or a patient says, "Why am I here? Nothing is being done for me, and I'm not getting any better." The nurse responds, "You are getting better."
- *Agreeing* is using a statement to show that you believe what the person is saying is correct. This technique cuts off the conversation, making the other person's concern seem unimportant. For example, a person tells her neighbor that she is thinking of divorcing her husband. The neighbor replies, "I'd get rid of him too." Or the patient says, "I am afraid the doctor won't send me home tomorrow." The nurse responds, "I am sure you are correct. I doubt he will let you go home so soon."
- *Defending* is responding with a statement of justification or a counter-reply to a verbal attack.

For example, a teenage boy says he doesn't get as much allowance as his friends do. His father replies, "I do the best that I can." Or the patient says, "I had my call light on for 15 minutes." The nurse responds, "I am doing the best I can. You are not the only patient here."

- *Stereotyping* is offering an insincere statement. It is using clichés that keep the conversation superficial or never looking for any additional information or clarification. For example, a person says, "I know what is happening to you" or "All 2-year-old children are terrible." Or the patient says, "I am really worried about the children. I came to the hospital so quickly and didn't get to see them. They just won't understand. I wish I could talk to them." The nurse responds, "I know exactly what you are going through. I know what's happening to you."

- *Giving false reassurance* is offering a statement of reassurance without sincerity or justification. This technique causes the other person to feel unimportant and unworthy of your concern. Reassurance is most effective when it is valid and appropriate. For example, someone says, "Don't worry. Everything will be all right. You will feel better soon." Or the patient says, "What will I do if this is malignant?" The nurse responds, "Don't you worry. Everything will work out just fine."

- *Giving advice* is telling another person what you think they should do. By giving advice, you are implying that you know what is best for the individual, thereby making it more difficult for the person to know what is right for himself or herself. An example of giving advice is saying, "If I were you . . ." or "Why don't you . . ." or "I think you should . . .". Or the patient says, "I broke my arm when I fell off a skateboard." The nurse says, "At your age, I would suggest you give up skateboards."

- *Changing the subject* minimizes the significance of the speaker's feelings by introducing a new topic. This makes the other person feel that his or her concern is unimportant. For example, a patient says, "They are doing a biopsy tomorrow. I hope it isn't cancer." The nurse responds, "Are these pictures of your children? They are such a nice-looking family."

- *Asking closed-ended questions* should be avoided in therapeutic communication because they encourage a one-word answer of yes or no. This technique does not allow the individual to further explore concerns or feelings.

- *Asking "why" questions* often increases a person's uneasiness by demanding an immediate answer. Sometimes individuals will make up an answer to a "why" question to get off the hook. They simply tell you what they think you want to hear.

- *Probing* is questioning that seeks information beyond what is necessary. It can be very invasive and threatening.

TECHNIQUES USED TO ENHANCE COMMUNICATION

- *Giving information* helps the patient know who you are, what you are doing, and what you need from him or her. The information explains the purpose of the communication process and decreases the patient's anxiety.

- *Validating* is making a statement or question that attempts to verify your perception of the person's verbal and nonverbal message. In essence, you are determining whether the person's needs have been met. An example is saying, "Has the diarrhea stopped?"

- *Clarifying* is clearing up possible misunderstandings or seeking information necessary for your understanding. Clarification can help keep another person on the topic. The nurse should never pretend he or she understands what the patient is saying if the message is not clear. An example is asking, "Could you explain?" or saying, "I am not sure I understand." You might need to ask, "Who are 'they'?" A patient says, "There is no point in asking for pain medication." The nurse responds, "Are you saying no one gives you medication when you have pain, or do you mean the medication doesn't help your pain?"

- *Reflecting* is stating your perception of another person's message in the affective (feeling) domain. This puts the patient in control and promotes self-esteem by allowing him or her to get in touch with feelings and find solutions for problems. Reflecting on, repeating, or restating other people's words helps make them aware of the mood, affect, or feeling being expressed. Reflecting is also referred to as *flashback*. However, it is best to avoid negative comments or those that can reinforce guilt, hostility, or depression. For example, a patient says, "My sister won't help with our mother's care." The nurse responds, "You feel angry. Have you discussed this with her?"

- *Paraphrasing* or *restating* is using similar words for what the other person just said. This technique is used to determine whether you understand what the other person means. It can reflect part of or the whole theme that was originally expressed. For example, a patient says, "I was awake most of the night." The nurse replies, "You have trouble sleeping." Or the patient states, "I couldn't eat supper last night." The nurse responds, "You had difficulty eating."
- *Asking broad questions* is using open-ended questions. These questions are used to encourage individuals to share their feelings about a specific topic. An example is saying, "Would you like to tell me about it?" or "Is there something you would like to talk about?"
- *Using general leads* is giving one- and two-word responses to encourage the person to continue talking. Examples are, "Go on," "And then?" or "You were saying."
- *Stating or making an observation* helps to acknowledge and verbalize thoughts and feelings. This technique is similar to clarification. Examples are "You seem tense" or "You are trembling."
- *Offering self* when the patient will not talk or when the situation is highly emotional and words cannot adequately convey the message being transmitted is accomplished by listening in silence or touching. The nurse might sit with the patient. Other examples are saying, "I'd like to understand" or "I'll stay awhile if you'd like."
- *Focusing* is a way of directing the conversation to a specific topic when you are seeking more

information on a poorly defined topic. It requires total concentration on what the patient is saying without preoccupation or a wandering mind.
- *Using humor* that does not demean can serve to decrease anxiety, help a person face stress, increase a person's tolerance to pain, and build a trusting relationship. Laughter, the best medicine, also shows the nurse as human. Studies have shown that laughter can improve mood, decrease pain, lower blood pressure, and enhance the immune system.

HELPFUL HINTS

Interpersonal Skills

- Use good judgment in choosing humor. The same joke is not for everyone.
- Avoid cultural, ethnic, sexual, or religious jokes.
- Use humor sparingly until you know the person.

Tips for Good Communication Skills

- Approach the individual with a positive attitude.
- Minimize distraction and interruption.
- Face the person conversing with you.
- Position yourself at eye level.
- Lean forward as you listen.
- Use body language that shows interest, such as nodding.
- Rephrase as needed.
- Clarify to keep the focus.
- Use touch and silence as needed.

SUMMARY

1. Communication is an interaction between two or more persons. It is the exchange of information, ideas, feelings, or emotions.

2. The communication process consists of five parts including the message, sender, method, receiver, and feedback.

3. There are two basic types of communication—verbal and nonverbal.

4. There are eight modes of nonverbal communication:
   - Physical appearance and dress
   - Body movement and posture
   - Facial expression
   - Gestures
   - Eye contact
   - Tone and volume of voice
   - Touch
   - Silence

5. A person with a passive or an unassertive personality style is unable to share his or her feelings or needs with others.

6. The aggressive personality style is very destructive. These individuals use angry vocalization to dominate and harm other persons.

7. Assertive persons are empowered and are comfortable expressing their feelings.

8. There are two styles of communication—social and therapeutic.

9. There are six components of therapeutic communication:
- Listening and observing
- Warmth
- Genuineness
- Attentiveness
- Empathy
- Positive regard

10. The three phases of therapeutic communication are the orientation phase, the working phase, and the termination phase.

11. Several factors influence communication, including congruence, time and setting, proxemics, biases, and physical handicaps.

12. Blocks to communication are words and actions people use that tend to obscure their messages.

13. The techniques that are used to enhance communication include validating, clarifying, reflecting, paraphrasing or restating, asking broad questions, using general leads, stating or making an observation, offering self, focusing, and using humor.

CRITICAL THINKING

Therapeutic	**Nontherapeutic**
Using general leads	Giving advice
Focusing	Stereotyping
Reflecting	Belittling
Clarifying	Disagreeing

Using this list, identify which communication technique is being described:

"You're in love with that man?" _____

"Continue. I'm listening." _____

"You're saying that you are not happy about . . ." _____

"What about school is troubling you?" _____

"All women in their 40s feel that way." _____

"Perhaps you can describe how you felt when . . ." _____

"You better drop out of college before it's too late." _____

MULTIPLE-CHOICE QUESTIONS

1. When communicating with a patient from a different culture, the health care worker should:
- **a.** Limit the time spent with the patient
- **b.** Know that less emphasis should be placed nonverbal messages
- **c.** Keep personal beliefs to oneself
- **d.** Encourage the patient to change cultural practices and beliefs

2. One of the goals of communicating with a hospitalized patient is to:
- **a.** Help the patient make informed decisions
- **b.** Make medical decisions for the patient
- **c.** Act as a conduit for information between the patient and family
- **d.** Teach the coping methods and behavior expected of inpatients

3. Communication is the:
   a. Last step in the nursing process
   b. Most vital link between diagnosis and disease
   c. Exchange of information and ideas
   d. Basis for all thinking processes

4. A health care worker's professional appearance should communicate:
   a. Incompetence
   b. Lack of concern
   c. Knowledge
   d. Acceptance

5. Which of the following describes nonverbal behavior?
   a. Written word
   b. Spoken word
   c. Tone of voice
   d. Aggressive style

6. Periods of silence during the communication process allow the health care worker to:
   a. Redirect the client
   b. Observe nonverbal behavior
   c. Relieve the client's anxiety
   d. Minimize rejection

7. Assertive personality types are described as:
   a. Unable to share their feelings
   b. Making little eye contact
   c. Putting their own needs first
   d. Acting confident and being responsible for their actions

8. Gaining insight into your personal feelings is an example of:
   a. Empathy
   b. Bias
   c. Proxemics
   d. Self-awareness

9. You overhear Jane telling her mother that she is "afraid to ride over the bridge." Jane's mother responds, "Don't be silly. Let's go." This statement is an example of:
   a. Stereotyping
   b. Belittling
   c. Giving advice
   d. Giving false reassurance

10. You are the nurse assigned to a well-baby clinic. A mother comes with her 6-month-old infant for a well-baby checkup. The mother has been a resident in the United States for only a short time, and she speaks and understands very little English. The best action for you to take is to:
   a. Speak very slowly
   b. Attempt to use a foreign language dictionary
   c. Assume she understands if she does not ask any questions
   d. Arrange for a translator for the next visit

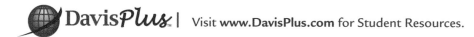

DavisPlus | Visit **www.DavisPlus.com** for Student Resources.

Student Activity   **Communication Observation**

Listen to and observe 10 minutes of an interchange between two adults speaking to one another at school, church, or work. Answer the following questions after your observation.

1. What verbal or nonverbal behavior, or both, did you observe?

2. Based on your observations, what feelings were expressed?

3. What inconsistencies did you observe between the verbal and nonverbal communication during the exchange?

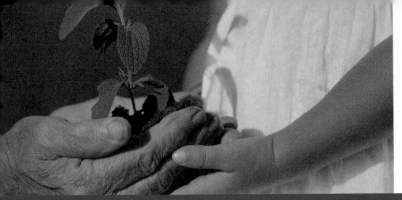

CHAPTER 5

Theories of Growth and Development

Key Words

accommodation

animistic

assimilation

autonomy

cephalocaudal

compensation

conscious

conversion

defense mechanisms

denial

development

displacement

ego

ego integrity

Electra complex

generativity

growth

heredity

id

identification

libido

maturation

Oedipus complex

personality

projection

proximodistal

puberty

rationalization

reaction formation

regression

Chapter Outline

Learning Objectives

At the end of this chapter, you should be able to:

- Describe the five common characteristics of growth and development.
- Name the two major influences on an individual's growth and development.
- Compare Freud's psychoanalytical theory and Erikson's psychosocial theory of development.
- Describe the common defense mechanisms used to reduce anxiety.
- Describe Piaget's theory of cognitive development.
- Describe Kohlberg's theory of moral development.
- Describe Maslow's theory of human needs.

Key Words (continued)

schema	superego
stagnation	suppression
subconscious	unconscious
sublimation	undoing

CHARACTERISTICS OF GROWTH AND DEVELOPMENT

Growth and development are natural topics of interest for most people. Curious about their beginnings and about what their futures hold, families question why one child looks more like one parent or acts more like the other. To support and guide parents, the health care worker needs to understand the normal patterns of growth and development and learn to recognize any variations from the norm. Several characteristics, patterns, and theories of growth and development are explored in this chapter.

The terms *growth* and *development* are frequently used together but have different meanings. Growth refers to an increase in physical size. Growth is quantitative: It can be measured in inches or centimeters, pounds, or kilograms. Development, however, refers to the progressive acquisition of skills and the capacity to function. Development is qualitative and proceeds from the general to the specific. Growth and development occur simultaneously and are interdependent. See Box 5.1 for universally accepted characteristics of growth and development. Development results from learned behavior and from maturation. Maturation, similar to development, is a total process in which skills and potential that are independent of practice or training emerge. Maturation is the attainment of full development of a particular skill.

Two directional terms used to explain growth and development are *cephalocaudal* and *proximodistal*. Cephalocaudal is best described as growth and development that begins at the head of the individual and progresses downward toward the feet. Proximodistal describes growth and development that progresses from the center of the body toward the extremities (Fig. 5.1). In the infant, shoulder control precedes mastery of the hands, which is followed by finger dexterity.

BOX 5.1 Characteristics of Growth and Development

- Occur in an orderly pattern from simple to complex. One task must be accomplished before the next one is attempted. For example, infants must learn head control before they can learn to sit.
- Are continuous processes characterized by spurts of growth and periods of slow, steady growth. For example, infancy is a period of very rapid growth; after infancy, the rate of growth slows down until adolescence.
- Progress at highly individualized rates that vary from child to child. Individuals have their own growth timetables, and one child's pattern of growth should not be compared to another's.
- Affect all body systems but at different times for specific structures. Although many organs mature and develop throughout childhood, the reproductive organs mature at puberty.
- Form a total process that affects a person physically, mentally, and socially.

As discussed in Chapter 1, health is influenced by both genetic and environmental factors. Genetics and environment are also the major influences on an individual's growth and development. Genetics, or heredity, includes characteristics such as hair color, eye color, and body size and shape. Heredity is discussed in greater detail in Chapter 6.

Every person goes through certain stages of development from infancy to old age. As individuals progress through these stages, they are exposed to different environmental factors that influence their inherited makeups. The resultant behavior is unique to that person and is known as personality. Personality consists of the behavior patterns that distinguish one person from another—the individual's style of behavior (Fig. 5.2). Personality traits remain

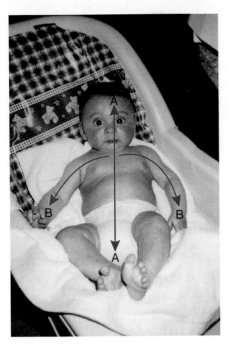

FIGURE 5.1 Principles of growth and development include cephalocaudal and proximodistal development.

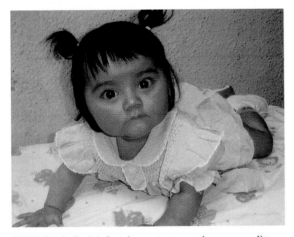

FIGURE 5.2 Each infant demonstrates a unique personality.

identifiable throughout a person's life span. A solid understanding of personality development can assist the health care worker in promoting health and delivering care.

Although no single theory explains the personality development of all individuals, several major theories provide key frameworks that help nurses understand different aspects of personality development. This chapter includes a brief overview of Sigmund Freud's psychoanalytical theory, Erik Erikson's psychosocial theory, Jean Piaget's cognitive theory, Abraham Maslow's human needs theory, and Lawrence Kohlberg's theory of moral development.

Most of these theories are covered in greater depth in the chapters that follow. Freud's theory provides the foundation from which other theories developed. We chose to present his theory in this chapter because nurses need to have a basic knowledge of personality development. This will enable them to identify the behaviors that are associated with the various stages and better understand whether the behavior is appropriate or inappropriate for a particular developmental level. Unlike later theorists, Freud believed that infancy and childhood are the critical periods for development and change. Freud's theory discusses only these stages. As authors, we believe that development is ongoing throughout the life cycle; therefore, we limited the discussion of Freud to this chapter alone but refer to other theorists in later chapters because their theories apply to each stage of growth and development.

All developmental theories are divided into stages and are considered progressive. Ideally, an individual accomplishes a task or skill at one stage before moving on to a later stage. However, conflicts and stressors can delay or prolong the completion of a task or even cause some temporary backward movement, known as regression. After the resolution of the conflict or stress, individuals usually return to their appropriate developmental levels. The specific age ranges given for these developmental stages are approximate and vary somewhat for individuals. It is even possible for stages to overlap, allowing individuals to work on several tasks at the same time.

PSYCHOANALYTICAL THEORY

Sigmund Freud made many important contributions to the understanding of personality development. Three parts of his theory include levels of awareness, components of the personality or mind, and psychosexual stages of development. According to Freud, the levels of awareness include the conscious, subconscious, and unconscious. The conscious level refers to all those experiences that are within one's immediate awareness. It is based in reality and logic. The subconscious, or preconscious, level of awareness stores memories, thoughts, and feelings. These can be recalled with a little effort and brought into the conscious level. The unconscious level refers to that part of the mind that is closed to one's awareness. These stored memories are usually painful and are kept in the unconscious to prevent anxiety and stress. Freud believed that behavior could be understood by delving into the forces of the unconscious mind. The levels of awareness became the basis for Freud's theory of psychoanalysis.

Freud further believed in the three functional components of the mind known as the id, the ego, and the superego. The id refers to the body's basic primitive urges. Primarily concerned with satisfaction and pleasure, the pleasure principle, or libido, is the driving force behind most human behavior. The id operates according to the pleasure principle. The id demands immediate satisfaction of its drives. The ego, also known as the "executive of the mind," is the part that is most closely related to reality. This part develops as a result of the demands of the id and the forces in the environment. Through interactions with the environment, the child learns to delay immediate satisfaction of his or her needs. This learned behavior is the development of the ego. The superego is a further development of the ego. It judges, controls, and punishes. It dictates right from wrong and acts in a similar way to what is thought of as a conscience. These three components—id, ego, and superego—are in constant conflict with one another.

Ideally, a balance or compromise should be reached between them. Someone once attempted to explain what each of these components is trying to communicate. The id says, "I want it now!" The superego states, "You can't have it." And the ego attempts to compromise by saying, "Well, maybe later." Unrestrained id dominance can result in a breakdown of the personality, leading to childlike behavior persisting throughout adult life. An extremely harsh superego can cause the blockage of reasonable needs and drives. Figure 5.3 illustrates Freud's components of the mind.

DEFENSE MECHANISMS

Defense mechanisms, also known as mental mechanisms, are techniques used at all stages of the life cycle to help individuals cope with the threat of anxiety. Many of these mechanisms were first recognized by Sigmund Freud as a way to protect one's ego. Most mechanisms are at the unconscious level, with the exception of suppression. Depending on the frequency of their use they can be helpful or harmful.

On a short-term basis the use of a defense mechanism may help the person by allowing her or him time to adjust to a stress while developing acceptable coping methods. Overuse or maladaptive use of defense mechanisms prevents the individual from achieving personal growth and satisfaction. The frequency and intensity of their use will determine whether defense mechanisms help or hinder by distorting reality.

Suppression is the one mechanism that operates on the conscious level. This is best described as the conscious putting out of awareness of one's distressing feelings. These feelings can be brought back into focus any time at will. All individuals use suppression as a means of concentrating on what is at hand. For example, the person who just had an argument with his or her spouse goes to work and says, "I can't think about my anger while working."

Rationalization is the defense mechanism that is most widely used by all ages. It is used to justify or excuse undesirable actions or feelings. It is a face-saving technique that may or may not deal with the truth. This mechanism can prevent the individual from confronting reality and learning to deal with it constructively. An example of rationalization is the student who blames the teacher for his failing grade when in reality he did not study or prepare adequately for his exam.

Identification is a mechanism in which one takes on the personality traits of another person, usually one held in high esteem. This mechanism is used by the child during sexual role identification. The young boy assumes the masculine characteristics admired in his father. The nursing student may copy behavior and mannerisms of a professor held in high esteem.

Sublimation is another mental mechanism in which the individual channels or redirects unacceptable impulses into socially acceptable outlets. Most of these mechanisms involve primitive drives or pleasurable feelings that are channeled and expressed in socially appropriate ways. An example of sublimation is demonstrated when the jilted lover expresses his longings in poetry or song. The youngster who becomes enraged at his teacher takes his hostile feelings and punches the punching bag as his outlet. Sublimation is considered to be a positive, effective coping mechanism.

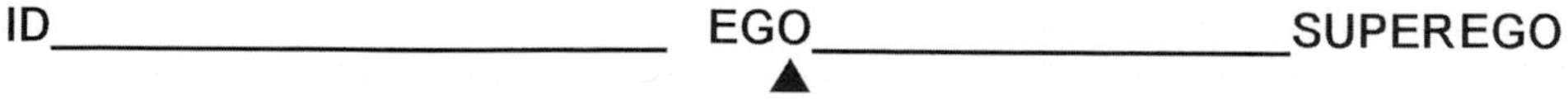

ID_____ EGO_____SUPEREGO
▲

FIGURE 5.3 Freud's three functional components of the mind.

Regression is a mental mechanism in which the individual facing a conflict returns to an earlier, more developmentally secure stage. The previously toilet-trained young child facing the stress of the birth of a new sibling starts having accidents and wetting the bed. This retreat to an earlier stage of development allows the person to feel more comfortable and less threatened.

Denial is a mental mechanism that is used totally on the unconscious level. Individuals automatically use this technique when they are unexpectedly confronted with some sort of unbearable news. With this mechanism the individual is unable to recognize the event or emotions surrounding the occurrence. An example of denial is illustrated in the story of the woman who, when faced with the news that her husband was just killed in an accident, rejects the news and goes to call him in his office.

Displacement is another mechanism that transfers emotions associated with a person or an object to another, less threatening person or object. A classic example of displacement is the man who is angry at his boss but yells at his wife instead. This may protect the man from losing his job, but it creates displaced hostility toward his wife.

Projection is often referred to as the blaming mechanism. In projection the individual rejects unacceptable thoughts or feelings and attributes them to another person. The man is projecting when he accuses his wife of flirting and being unfaithful when it is he who has an attraction to another woman.

Compensation is a mental mechanism that allows the person to make up for deficiencies in one area by excelling in another area. The school-age boy tries to excel in class to compensate for his lack of athletic abilities. This technique helps maintain his self-esteem.

Undoing is a mechanism in which the individual acts in a manner that symbolically cancels a previous unacceptable thought or action. In this way the individual attempts to make up for something that is unacceptable. An example of undoing is when the teacher compliments the student's new hairstyle after being overcritical of his homework.

Reaction formation, sometimes called *overcompensation,* is another mechanism. In reaction formation unacceptable feelings or thoughts are kept out of one's awareness and replaced with opposite feelings or thoughts. For example, the man who dislikes dogs meets his friend in the park who is walking his two dogs. The man acts openly friendly to his friend's dogs.

Conversion is a mental mechanism that converts unconscious feelings and anxiety into a physical symptom that has no underlying organic basis for the complaint. Conversion is illustrated by the soldier on the front line of the battlefield who finds himself unable to move his arm and hold his weapon. Refer to Table 5.1 for a summary of adaptive and maladaptive use of the common defense mechanisms.

TABLE

5.1   Adaptive and Maladaptive Defense Mechanisms

Adaptive	Maladaptive
Rationalization The student says, "I didn't want to be a nurse anyway."	"I'm not going to study because I know I won't pass the test."
Identification The young boy says, "I'm going to be just like Daddy when I grow up."	"Those gang members are really cool. I hope to be just like them."
Sublimation The hostile, angry teenage boy is successful as a boxer.	Usually adaptive.
Regression The hospitalized 5-year-old boy starts to suck his thumb again.	The woman has a tantrum after not getting her way.
Denial The woman just informed of her terminal illness tells her family that she will outlive all of them.	The parents have kept their deceased son's room intact for the past 10 years and speak of him as if he were going to return home.

Continued

TABLE 5.1   Adaptive and Maladaptive Defense Mechanisms—cont'd

Adaptive	Maladaptive
Displacement Immediately after getting a traffic ticket the mother scolds her two children.	The rape victim becomes afraid of intimacy and men.
Projection The young male accuses another male friend of making sexual advances toward him when he himself has unconscious feelings toward the person he accuses.	The angry young man believes that people are out to harm him.
Compensation The sibling of a very popular sister becomes well known for her superior athletic ability.	Usually adaptive.
Undoing The youngster after his time-out goes and picks flowers for his mother.	After a very strict, rigid upbringing the young man is obsessed with washing his hands whenever he has sexual urges.
Reaction formation The child molester actively works toward passing legislation to protect children.	The physically abusive mother acts overprotective after injuring her child.
Conversion The nursing student is unable to take her final exam because of a headache.	The witness to a horrific crime suddenly becomes blind and unable to identify the suspect in the police lineup.
Suppression While driving the car, the woman says, "I'll think about paying the bills later."	Usually adaptive.

FREUD'S STAGES OF PSYCHOSEXUAL DEVELOPMENT

Freud described five stages of psychosexual development: oral, anal, phallic, latency, and genital. Each stage is associated with particular conflicts that must be resolved before the child can move on to the next stage. He also believed that the experiences a child has during the early stages of growth determine later adjustment patterns and personality traits in adult life (Fig. 5.4).

Oral Stage

The oral stage lasts from birth to the end of the first year of life. The infant's mouth is the erogenous (sexually arousing) area and the source of all comfort and pleasure (Fig. 5.5). If the infant's oral needs are met, the infant gains satisfaction. The infant receives pleasure by sucking and biting, using the mouth as the center of gratification. By the end of the first year of life, the infant begins to see that he or she is separate from the mother and other objects in the environment.

Anal Stage

The anal stage lasts from the end of the first year of life to the third year. At the beginning of this stage, the mouth continues to be an important source of satisfaction for the child. By the beginning of the second year, the center of pleasure is shared between the mouth and the anus. Instead of being repulsive to the child, the process of defecation gives the child pleasure and satisfaction. Toilet training is initially experienced as a conflict between the demands of the parent and the child's biological needs. Resolution of this conflict gives the child a sense of self-control and independence. Recommendations for toilet training will be discussed in a later chapter.

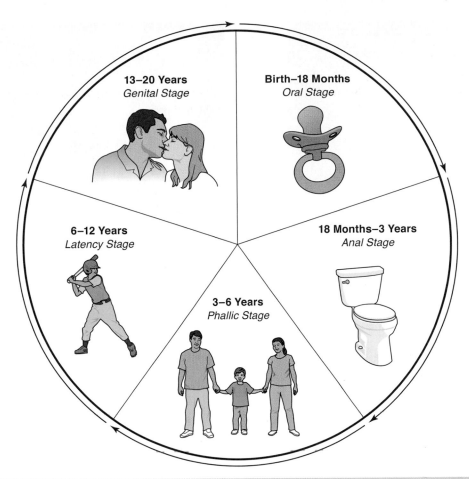

Major Developmental Tasks

Oral—Relief from anxiety through oral gratification of needs
Anal—Learning independence and control, with focus on the excretory functions
Phallic—Identification with parent of same sex; development of sexual identity; focus on genital organs
Latency—Sexuality repressed; focus on relationships with same sex peers
Genital—Libido reawakened as genital organs mature; focus on relationships with members of the opposite sex

FIGURE 5.4 Freud's stages of psychosexual development.

Phallic Stage

The phallic stage lasts from ages 3 to 6. At this stage, the child associates both pleasurable and conflicting feelings with the genital organs. During this period the child devotes a lot of time to examining his or her genitalia. Masturbation and interest in sexual organs are normal. Exhibitionism is also typical at this age. The child appears comfortable with his or her body and likes to undress and parade around naked. Parental disapproval of the child's preoccupation with the genitals can result in feelings of confusion and shame. The Oedipus and Electra complexes develop at this stage. The Oedipus complex refers to a boy's unconscious sexual attraction to his mother. He wishes to have his mother to himself and sees his father as a rival for his mother's affection. To win his mother's affection, he resolves the conflict by eventually taking on the father's characteristics. This process begins sex-role identification. The Electra complex occurs when a young girl is attracted to her father and wishes to get rid of her mother. Through imitation, the child copies the mothering role and eventually gains the father's affection and approval. Resolution of the Electra complex produces sex-role identification for the female child.

Latency Stage

Latency lasts from ages 6 to about 12. During this time the child's sexual urges are dormant. The sexual energies are being channeled into more socially

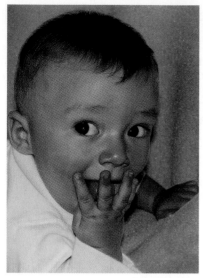

FIGURE 5.5 The infant's mouth is the source of comfort and pleasure.

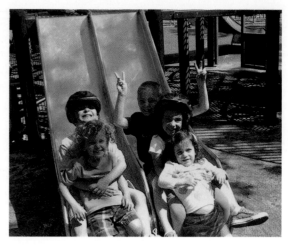

FIGURE 5.6 Outdoor activities are attractive to young children.

acceptable means of expressions. School-age children focus mainly on intellectual pursuits. Peer relationships intensify between children of the same sex. Sports and other such activities help in the development of these peer relationships (Fig. 5.6).

Genital Stage

The genital stage begins with the onset of puberty. During **puberty** many physical changes occur that prepare the body for reproduction. Hormonal activity and maturing of the sex organs result in the awakening of sexual attraction and interest in heterosexual relationships. The child continues to struggle with a desire for independence but still has a need for parental supervision.

PSYCHOSOCIAL THEORY

Erik Erikson, a psychologist and close follower of Freud, broadened Freud's theory of personality development. Erikson identified eight stages that span the full life cycle from infancy to old age. He studied the child within a larger social setting beyond the immediate family. He believed that at each stage certain critical tasks have to be accomplished. The successful completion of each task enables individuals to increase independence and feel good about themselves and others. Erikson's eight stages of psychosocial development are discussed in the following section and are listed in Table 5.2.

TABLE
5.2 Stages of Development in Erikson's Psychosocial Theory

Age	Stage	Major Developmental Tasks
Infancy (Birth–18 months)	Trust vs. mistrust	To develop a basic trust in the mothering figure and be able to generalize it to others
Early childhood (18 months–3 years)	Autonomy vs. shame and doubt	To gain some self-control and independence within the environment
Late childhood (3–6 years)	Initiative vs. guilt	To develop a sense of purpose and the ability to initiate and direct own activities
School age (6–12 years)	Industry vs. inferiority	To achieve a sense of self-confidence by learning, competing, performing successfully, and receiving recognition from significant others, peers, and acquaintances

TABLE
5.2 **Stages of Development in Erikson's Psychosocial Theory—cont'd**

Age	Stage	Major Developmental Tasks
Adolescence (12–20 years)	Identity vs. role confusion	To integrate the tasks mastered in the previous stages into a secure sense of self
Young adulthood (20–30 years)	Intimacy vs. isolation	To form an intense, lasting relationship or a commitment to another person, cause, institution, or creative effort
Adulthood (30–65 years)	Generativity vs. stagnation	To achieve the life goals established for oneself while also considering the welfare of future generations
Old age (65 years–death)	Ego integrity vs. despair	To review one's life and derive meaning from both positive and negative events while achieving a positive sense of self-worth

Source: Townsend, MC: Psychiatric Mental Health Nursing: Concepts of Care, ed. 4. FA Davis, Philadelphia, 2003, p 38, with permission.

Trust Versus Mistrust (Birth to 18 Months)

At birth the child is helpless and totally dependent on others to meet his or her needs. When these needs are met in a timely fashion, the child develops trust in people and in his or her environment. Trust is built by having consistency and sameness from care-givers. This helps infants cope with their needs and urges and learn trust in self. Trust is the foundation of a healthy personality.

Autonomy Versus Shame and Doubt (18 Months to 3 Years)

The child begins to gain control over his or her body and develop a sense of independence or autonomy (Fig. 5.7). **Autonomy** is characterized by the acquisition of skills involving feeding, mobility, dressing, and control of elimination. Developing independence strengthens the child's self-concept. Without loving support from the environment, the child develops feelings of shame and doubt.

Initiative Versus Guilt (3 to 6 Years)

During this stage the child begins to explore his or her environment and try different roles. Imagination and curiosity allow the child to further expand and develop his or her potential. Parents and caregivers need to permit the child to explore within safe

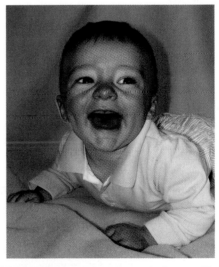

FIGURE 5.7 Infants master good upper-body control before crawling.

boundaries. Without this freedom the child may develop guilt and feelings of inadequacy.

Industry Versus Inferiority (6 to 11 Years)

During this stage the child acquires many new social and physical skills. School-age children have the maturity to concentrate on learning and working with others. They strive for praise and recognition. Family life should support and prepare the child for school endeavors, and school must continue with these efforts. Without these positive responses, children may develop a sense of inferiority.

Identity Versus Role Confusion (12 to 20 Years)

This stage is transitional between childhood and adulthood. It is characterized by both physiological and emotional changes that create turmoil for both the child and the family. One of the chief concerns of this period is the individual's emerging sexuality and the need to find his or her place in society. Many demands are placed on the adolescent in terms of career, vocation, education, and peer relationships. Role confusion results if the individual does not have love and support.

Intimacy Versus Isolation (20 to 30 Years)

A goal of this stage is to establish a close meaningful relationship with another person. The individual must be able to give of himself or herself and be committed to another. This is learned from within the family unit during the growing years. Close ties with family members and intimate relationships are essential to the well-being of the young adult. Failure to accomplish a meaningful close relationship results in loneliness and isolation. Some individuals have many superficial relationships that leave them unfulfilled. Commitment and drive are also needed for career choice and success.

Generativity Versus Stagnation (30 to 65 Years)

Erikson defines **generativity** as the process by which the middle-aged person focuses on leadership, productivity, and concern for future generations. Individuals reflect on their accomplishments and become involved with their new family roles. Generativity takes on different forms. Some adults engage in nurturing their children or grandchildren; others become involved in community projects. Still others begin new careers at this stage. Inability to establish generativity results in stagnation. Stagnation occurs when a person is unconcerned with the welfare of others and is preoccupied with himself or herself.

Ego Integrity Versus Despair (65 Years and Over)

During this period, life experiences are reviewed. Ego integrity is achieved if the person reaches a level where he or she is able to accept past choices as the best that could be accomplished at the time. The individual has a sense of dignity from his or her life accomplishments. Ego integrity implies that the individual has resolved the tasks of earlier stages and has little desire to relive his or her life. Dissatisfaction with life review leads to feelings of despair. The person may wish to start over and have another chance. Despair produces feelings of worthlessness and hopelessness.

COGNITIVE THEORY

Jean Piaget's contribution to the field of psychology is cognitive development. He was concerned with how the individual acquires intellect and develops thought processes. Piaget believed that intelligence was an innate ability that further developed as the child adapted to the environment. Piaget believed there are three major concepts: schemas, assimilation, and accommodation. The term schema refers to patterns consisting of a number of organized ideas that grow with a child's experiences. Initially infants have several schemas such as sucking and grasping. These schemas act as a guide that interacts with their environment. Eventually, as the infant's experiences expand, new patterns emerge. This can be demonstrated by the infant's ability to suck. Assimilation is Piaget's second concept, which can be described as the ability to absorb new information into the existing schemas. The infant broadens the schema of sucking to include sucking on anything within his or her reach, such as a blanket, pacifier, toy, or fingers. Piaget's third concept is accommodation, which occurs with new experiences that no longer fit or can be assimilated into existing schemas. As a result, schemas are changed to merge with the new information. This can be seen by the infant no longer just sucking food off a spoon but opening his or her mouth when the spoon approaches. Piaget believed that the child's cognitive abilities progress through four stages: sensorimotor, preoperational, concrete operational, and formal operational (Table 5.3).

Sensorimotor Stage (Birth to 2 Years)

At birth the infant begins by responding to the environment primarily through reflexes. Schemas have object permanence or are limited to what the child can see, hear, or touch—what is out of sight will be

TABLE
5.3 Piaget's Stages of Cognitive Development

Age	Stage	Major Developmental Tasks
Birth–2 years	Sensorimotor	With increased mobility and awareness and development of a sense of self as separate from the external environment, the concept of *object permanence* emerges as the ability to form mental images evolves.
2–6 years	Preoperational	Learning to express self with language; developing understanding of symbolic gestures; achieving object permanence.
6–12 years	Concrete operations	Learning to apply logic to thinking; developing an understanding of reversibility and spatiality; learning to differentiate and classify; socializing and applying rules.
12–15 years and up	Formal operations	Learning to think and reason in abstract terms; making and testing hypotheses; expanding and refining logical thinking and reasoning; achieving cognitive maturity.

Source: Townsend, MC: Psychiatric Mental Health Nursing: Concepts of Care, ed. 4. FA Davis, Philadelphia, 2003, p 42, with permission.

out of mind (Fig. 5.8). Gradually the infant acquires knowledge by exploring the environment and attaches meaning and recognition of things. Through trial-and-error behavior, the child perfects sensory and motor reflex skills. By the completion of this stage, the child is able to see himself or herself as separate from other objects in the environment.

Preoperational Stage (2 to 6 Years)

The child is concerned with the development and mastery of language. This stage is characterized by egocentrism. The child sees himself or herself as the center of the universe and is unable to accept other viewpoints. He or she uses language skills and gestures to meet his or her needs. At this time objects are singular and one-dimensional to the child. This means that the child can create a mental picture of an object or person. The child lacks the ability to do reversible mental processes. An example is seen by asking a young girl, "Do you have a sister?" The girl answers, "Yes, I do." You respond, "Does your sister have a sister?" and the child answers, "No, she doesn't." Thinking is described as animistic, which causes a child to believe that objects, tables, the sun, and trees have feelings and motives. For example, when the child trips near the table he cries, "Bad table."

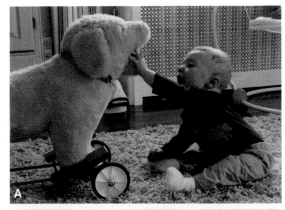

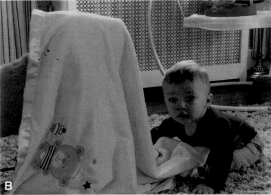

FIGURE 5.8 The child in photo B thinks the object no longer exists. Can you explain why, according to Piaget?

Concrete Operational Stage (6 to 12 Years)

The increased acquisition of cognition allows the child to think and converse on many topics. The child is beginning to think logically and solve problems to some degree but is unable to deal with hypothetical or complex abstract situations. The child is less egocentric and more social. Concepts of reversibility and spatiality are developed. Children at this age can understand that water can be in liquid or solid form and can change back and forth. Children at this stage can classify objects using several characteristics. For example, they see a car not simply as a car but as a 2010 Ford Taurus.

Formal Operational Stage (12 to 15 Years)

The individual has the ability to think logically in hypothetical and abstract terms. He or she demonstrates both form and structure in organizing thoughts and is capable of scientific reasoning and problem solving.

HUMAN NEEDS THEORY

Abraham Maslow described human behavior as being motivated by needs that are ordered in a hierarchy (Fig. 5.9). At the bottom are basic survival needs (physiological needs, safety, belonging), and

at the top are more complex needs (self-esteem, self-actualization). Maslow believed that people must meet their most basic needs before they can move up the hierarchy to the highest level.

Physiological Needs

The most basic needs are physiological and include the need for oxygen, food, water, rest, and elimination. Maslow also included sexual needs, which are important for survival of the species, among the basic needs. When these basic needs are met, an individual is free to move to the next stage. However, if these needs are not met, an individual will continue to be preoccupied with them. For example, a hungry child may lack interest in school (or anything other than food) until he or she is no longer hungry.

Safety Needs

The need to feel secure, safe, and free from danger is the next need to be met, but one cannot think of safety until physiological needs have been met. The young child must have feelings of security in the home and family before he or she can venture out into the larger community and school environment.

Belonging

Belonging is feeling loved and accepted by another person. To enter into any relationship, a person must first feel secure. Love and affection begin with bonding at the time of birth and continue throughout human development. All individuals need affection and meaningful relationships.

Self-Esteem

People need to feel good about themselves and their accomplishments. To arrive at this place, each person must receive approval and recognition of his or her own worth. Self-esteem is first built by parental approval and acceptance. During the school years teachers and other social contacts can further strengthen a person's self-esteem.

Self-Actualization

Self-actualization means self-fulfillment, the achievement of one's full potential. Maslow did not believe that everyone can be completely self-actualized. He thought that as people continue to achieve and develop healthy relationships, they progress toward this goal. As people move toward self-actualization, they become more comfortable with themselves and who

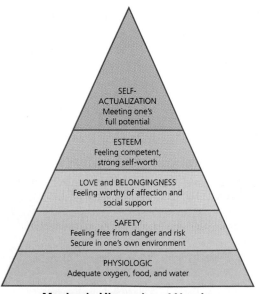

Maslow's Hierarchy of Needs

FIGURE 5.9 Maslow hierarchy diagram.

they are. At this level people are self-directed in ideas and actions. Self-actualizers must be oriented to reality, flexible, and able to change as needed. Although part of a group, a self-actualized person maintains his or her own individuality. Creativity, a sense of humor, and respect for the welfare of others are fundamental to this level of achievement.

THEORY OF MORAL DEVELOPMENT

Lawrence Kohlberg introduced his theory of moral development by expanding Piaget's stages of cognitive development. Kohlberg believed that the child progressively develops moral reasoning as he or she gains the ability to think logically. Kohlberg identified three levels of moral development, which are further subdivided into six stages of acquired moral reasoning, beginning at age 4 and extending to adulthood (Table 5.4).

Level I: Preconventional Thinking (4 to 10 Years)

The child learns reasoning through the parents' demand for obedience. To avoid punishment the child begins to recognize right from wrong. A 4-year-old child might think, "If I'm mean to my brother, I will be punished."

Level II: Conventional Thinking (10 to 13 Years)

The school-age child begins to seek approval from society. Kohlberg believed that the child at this stage is influenced by external forces in interactions with his or her peers and environment. A 12-year-old child knows that it is wrong to cheat in school and wishes to win the approval of both family and teachers.

Level III: Postconventional Thinking (Postadolescence)

Adolescents develop their own moral codes. Moral reasoning is based on the individual's own principles rather than on external forces. Kohlberg further believed that some individuals never attain this higher level of moral reasoning. Those who operate at the level of postconventional thinking usually act according to their internal codes of beliefs. Most people stop at a traffic signal even when traffic is clear and they know that no one is watching them.

Carol Gilligan, one of Kohlberg's students, is one of the most outspoken critics of Kohlberg's theory of moral development. Gilligan expresses concern that the research from which Kohlberg developed his theory failed to explore unique female experiences as they pertained to morality. She further argues that his research was biased against women because all of the subjects in his study were males.

TABLE
5.4   Kohlberg's Stages of Moral Development

Level/Age*	Stage	Developmental Focus
Preconventional (common from 4–10 years)	1. Punishment and obedience orientation 2. Instrumental relativist orientation	Behavior motivated by fear of punishment Behavior motivated by egocentrism and concern for self
Conventional (common from 10–13 years and into adulthood)	3. Interpersonal concordance orientation 4. Law and order orientation	Behavior motivated by expectations of others; strong desire for approval and acceptance Behavior motivated by respect for authority
Postconventional (can occur from adolescence on)	5. Social contract legalistic orientation 6. Universal ethical principle orientation	Behavior motivated by respect for universal laws and moral principles; guided by internal set of values Behavior motivated by internalized principles of honor, justice, and respect for human dignity; guided by the conscience

*Ages in Kohlberg's theory are not well defined. The stage of development is determined by the motivation behind the individual's behavior.
Source: Townsend, MC: Psychiatric Mental Health Nursing: Concepts of Care, ed. 5. FA Davis, Philadelphia, 2006, p 43, with permission.

According to Kohlberg, males function at a higher moral reasoning level than females. Gilligan purports that female moral development is different from, not inferior to, that of males in that females develop a morality of caring and responsibility. She believes this is true because she feels that females are more concerned than males with relationships, caregiving, and intimacy. According to Gilligan, male moral development is more concerned with morality and justice. Furthermore, Gilligan states that men make more decisions based on abstract reasoning and principles, whereas women are more concerned with how their decisions affect others.

Gilligan presents her own theory of moral development in the same way as Kohlberg's, with three stages of moral development: preconventional, conventional, and postconventional. At the preconventional stage the child is mainly selfish, dominated by survival goals. As the child grows she or he moves from this selfishness to more responsibility. During the conventional stage the child sees sacrifices as goodness. Children now begin to place more interest in relationships, and as a result they start to put others first. At the postconventional level individuals learn to think and consider others in addition to themselves.

Gilligan's theory has also come under criticism by other scholars. It has been said that Gilligan's research is limited in that it cannot be duplicated and validated. Recently theorists have indicated their belief that both men and women exhibit some degree of justice and caring that affects their moral reasoning. Refer to Table 5.5 for an illustration of Gilligan's theory.

Understanding moral development is important for nurses to better understand moral issues that affect patients at different stages in development. An understanding of moral reasoning may also assist nurses in making ethical decisions in clinical practice. Box 5.2 is a guide to moral decision making.

TABLE 5.5 Gilligan's Theory of Moral Development

Stage	Characteristics
Preconventional	Self-centered
Conventional	Interest and concern for others
Postconventional	Socially responsible for oneself and others

BOX 5.2 Guide to Moral Decision Making

The following questions will assist you in moral decision making:

1. What characteristics make an act right or wrong?
2. How do rules affect moral acts?
3. What action should be taken in this specific situation?

SUMMARY

1. Growth and development, terms often used together, have different meanings. Growth refers to an increase in size; development refers to acquisition of skills.

2. Growth and development occur simultaneously and are interdependent.

3. Maturation is the total process in which a child's potential unfolds, regardless of practice.

4. The two major influences on growth and development are heredity and environment. Hereditary characteristics are all those transmitted by the genes. All other factors that affect the unborn and born child are environmental.

5. The five universally recognized basic assumptions about growth and development are that they:
   • Progress in an orderly manner from simple to complex
   • Are continuous processes
   • Occur at highly individualized rates
   • Affect all body systems and stages
   • Together form a total process

6. Each individual has a unique behavior known as personality. Understanding the different theories of personality development helps the nurse promote health and provide health care to individuals.

7. These personality theories describe stages of development. The stages are generally progressive—that is, it is necessary to complete an earlier stage before moving on to the next. However, at times an individual may temporarily regress to an earlier stage.

8. Defense mechanisms are techniques used at all stages of life to assist persons in coping with anxiety.

9. Freud described five stages of psychosexual development: oral, anal, phallic, latency, and genital.

10. Erikson developed a theory of psychosocial development that covers the entire life span. Certain tasks need to be accomplished in each of the eight stages: trust versus mistrust, autonomy versus shame and doubt, initiative versus guilt, industry versus inferiority, identity versus role confusion, intimacy versus isolation, generativity versus stagnation, and ego integrity versus despair.

11. Piaget's theory focuses on cognitive development using three concepts (schemas, assimilation, and accommodation), which proceeds through four stages (sensorimotor, preoperational, concrete operational, and formal operational).

12. Maslow believed that human behavior was motivated by human needs arranged hierarchically from the most basic to the most complex. Beginning with physiological, these needs progress to those for safety, belonging, self-esteem, and self-actualization.

13. Kohlberg's theory of moral reasoning identified three levels of moral development: preconventional, conventional, and postconventional. Moral development progresses within these stages in an orderly sequence. However, one does not attain the highest level of moral reasoning.

14. Gilligan proposes her theory of moral reasoning from a feminine perspective.

CRITICAL THINKING

Exercise #1

Jane and Bill bring their 4-month-old baby girl, Tayna, to the hospital. She is admitted for vomiting and dehydration and is not permitted anything by mouth. Both parents work and must leave the baby in the nurse's care during the day. Using the information given and the material in this chapter, respond to the following questions or problems:

1. Identify Tayna's psychosexual level of development according to Freud's stages.
2. What psychosocial task, according to Erikson, would Tayna be struggling with at this stage?
3. Based on Maslow's human needs theory, what need would be of primary concern to Tayna?
4. List one nursing action that would help Tayna in meeting the need identified above.

Exercise #2

Jeremy, age 2 years, is playing at the park with his mother. When his mother tells him it is time to go home, Jeremy responds by crying "No!" and refusing to leave.

1. At what stage of development is Jeremy?
2. How can Jeremy's mother best handle this situation?

MULTIPLE-CHOICE QUESTIONS

1. Growth can be defined as:
   a. The progressive acquisition of skills
   b. An increase in cognitive ability
   c. An increase in physical size
   d. The rapid development of language

2. According to Freud, what part of the mind acts as one's conscience?
   a. Id
   b. Ego
   c. Superego
   d. Libido

3. According to Erikson's stages of development, which of the following tasks would Roger, age 9, be completing?
   a. Trust
   b. Industry
   c. Initiative
   d. Autonomy

4. At the completion of Piaget's sensorimotor stage of cognitive development, the child:
   a. Can problem-solve
   b. Can reason hypothetically
   c. Has abstract thinking ability
   d. Recognizes himself or herself as separate

5. Theories of personality help the nurse to:
   a. Place judgment on the patient
   b. Direct patient goals
   c. Provide individual health care
   d. Limit ego development

6. Maslow's humanistic approach to development emphasizes the importance of:
   a. Basic goodness in humans
   b. The pleasure principle
   c. Developmental tasks
   d. Conditioning

7. The term most associated with Maslow is:
   a. Pleasure principle
   b. Psychosocial task
   c. Self-actualization
   d. Concrete operations

8. According to Freud's theory, the rational portion of the mind that tries to balance id impulses with the demands of the superego is:
   a. Conscience
   b. Ego
   c. Libido
   d. Oedipal period

9. The purpose of defense mechanisms is to:
   a. Perceive boundaries between self and others
   b. Explain life situations
   c. Reduce anxiety
   d. Provide pleasure and gratification

10. Which of the following defense mechanisms is considered to be a positive method of coping?
   a. Projection
   b. Displacement
   c. Reaction formation
   d. Sublimation

11. Moral development:
   a. Is the first stage of personality development
   b. Occurs in an orderly sequence
   c. Is a disorderly process
   d. Is the same for all individuals

DavisPlus | Visit www.DavisPlus.com for Student Resources.

CHAPTER 6

Prenatal Period to 1 Year

Key Words

acrocyanosis

Apgar score

apnea

attachment

blastocyst

bottle-mouth syndrome

cervix

chromosomes

circumcision

cleft palate

colostrum

conception

conscience

deciduous teeth

dental caries

dilation

dominant genes

effacement

embryo

engrossment

fertilization

fetus

fine motor skills

fontanels

genes

gross motor skills

involution

karyotype

lanugo

meconium

milia

molding

mongolian spot

morula

key terms continue on page 74

Chapter Outline

Heredity
  Genetic Counseling
Environment
The Prenatal Period
Physical Characteristics
  Head and Skull
  Length and Weight
  Skin
  Genitals
  Face
  Abdomen
  Extremities
Neurological Characteristics
Vital Signs
Developmental Milestones
  Motor Development
    Gross Motor Skills
    Fine Motor Skills
  Psychosocial Development
    Attachment
    Temperament
    Parental Guidance

Cognitive Development
Moral Development
Communication
Nutrition
  Breastfeeding
  Bottle Feeding
  Weaning and Introduction of Solid
  Foods
Sleep and Rest
Play
Safety
Health Promotion
Summary
Critical Thinking
Multiple-Choice Questions

Learning Objectives

At the end of this chapter, you should be able to:

- List three factors that promote a healthy pregnancy.
- Name four factors that may have an adverse effect on pregnancy.
- Describe the steps in prenatal development from fertilization to implantation.
- Describe physical development for infants from 1 to 2 months.
- Describe skin manifestations such as vernix caseosa, lanugo, mongolian spots, milia, and acrocyanosis.
- List five reflexes present at birth.
- Name the normal range for vital signs for the newborn.
- Compare the pattern of fine and gross motor skill acquisition.
- Give an example of cognitive development for this stage.
- State the process of language acquisition during infancy.
- Describe the nutritional needs of developing infants.

objective continue on page 74

Learning Objectives (continued)

- Describe the advantages and disadvantages of breastfeeding and bottle feeding.
- Distinguish between the stools of breastfed and formula-fed infants.
- State the normal sleep patterns for the neonate.
- List three interventions used to promote infant safety.
- Name the immunization schedule for the newborn.
- List two concerns for health promotion during the infancy period.

HEREDITY

Two factors that have a large influence on the health of the developing baby are heredity and environment. Each sperm and ovum contributes 23 **chromosomes** to the new entity, which is a single-celled **zygote**. The sex of the zygote is determined by the combination of X and Y chromosomes. The ovum always contains an X chromosome, whereas the sperm may contain either an X or a Y chromosome. If the ovum is fertilized by an X chromosome sperm, the zygote will be female; if a Y chromosome sperm fertilizes the ovum, a male zygote will result (Fig. 6.1).

Chromosomes carry the **genes,** which transmit all the genetic information or hereditary characteristics from the parents to the child (Fig. 6.2). The genes are found on strands of deoxyribonucleic acid (DNA) within the nucleus of the cell. Some genes are dominant. **Dominant genes** are capable of expressing their traits over other genes. **Recessive genes,** however, can transmit their traits only if they exist in like pairs. If one gene of a pair is dominant and one is recessive, the dominant gene will exert its influence over the recessive gene. Eye color is an example of a trait that is affected by the dominant–recessive pattern of inheritance. In other words, if a brown eye color gene

is paired with a blue eye color gene, the dominant brown gene will govern. More than 700 different diseases are the result of defects carried on recessive genes. Sickle-cell disease, Tay-Sachs disease, and hemophilia are some examples of recessive disorders. To inherit a recessive trait or disorder, the child must

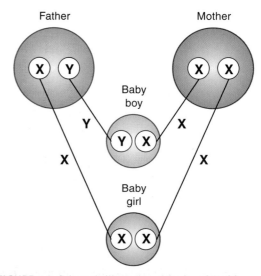

FIGURE 6.1 Schematic illustration of the sex of the fetus, which is determined at the time of conception.

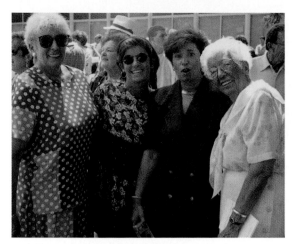

FIGURE 6.2 Heredity characteristics can be easily seen in a family unit.

inherit the recessive gene from both parents. The chromosomal structure of an entity is known as its **karyotype.** Karyotyping—mapping the chromosomal structure—can help predict the transmission of certain genetic disorders and is useful in counseling prospective parents.

Genetic Counseling

Genetic counseling may be suggested for individuals and couples so that they understand hereditary disorders, their risk, and measures to prevent and treat these disorders. Genetic screening for certain diseases should be considered for individuals of specific cultural descents, such as sickle-cell disease in African Americans and Tay-Sachs disease in European Jewish descendants. Genetic counseling includes the entire family and is a long process that may take weeks for results. A common blood sample test may be done for genetic testing. Prenatal testing includes chorionic villus sampling, umbilical cord sampling, amniocentesis, carrier detection, and ultrasonography. Amniocentesis is done only if further testing is needed. Postnatal diagnosis may be determined using physical examination, chromosomal and DNA analysis, and other testing. Health care workers can be most helpful in supporting families during this process by guiding them to select healthy lifestyle choices. Advising patients to follow a proper diet and avoid smoking and alcohol use may help lead to positive outcomes.

ENVIRONMENT

From the moment life begins, the environment begins to exercise its influence on the newly formed entity. Good health practices contribute to the development of a healthy baby. The quality of the mother's diet affects her health and that of her baby. A balance of rest and exercise is crucial for a healthy pregnancy. As a rule, a woman can continue any exercise that she has regularly participated in before her pregnancy. Walking is the best exercise during pregnancy, and women should be encouraged to walk daily. Before beginning any new form of sport or exercise, the pregnant woman should check with her physician.

Both harmful and life-sustaining substances are transmitted from the mother to the developing baby through the placenta. Chemical or physical substances that can adversely affect the unborn are known as **teratogens.** Tobacco, alcohol, and many drugs are teratogens. As soon as a woman starts to try to become pregnant, she should eliminate all known teratogens to reduce the risks associated with these substances. Bacterial, protozoan, and viral infections may also damage the fetus. The rubella virus presents great risk to the fetus if the woman contracts it during her pregnancy. This virus has been shown to cause serious fetal abnormalities. HIV may also be transmitted to the unborn child. Toxoplasmosis, a common parasite found in many animals, may cause harm to the developing fetus if contracted by the pregnant woman. Pregnant women may avoid this condition by eating well-cooked meats and by avoiding contact with cat litter.

Pregnant women should avoid any intake of any alcohol during the course of their pregnancy. Alcohol by-products can cross the placental membrane and fetal blood–brain barrier. Ingestion of alcohol during the first trimester appears to present the greatest risk for developing fetal alcohol syndrome (FAS). Miscarriages, stillbirths, prenatal and postnatal growth restriction, and central nervous system abnormalities are some of the problems associated with FAS. Prevention and education are key to eliminating these abnormalities. Early detection of FAS and proper intervention may assist the child in reaching his or her full potential.

Cigarette smoking has also been shown to have teratogenic effects on the unborn. Both low birth weight and growth restriction have been linked to smoking during pregnancy.

The mother should avoid pesticides, chemicals, radiation, and other environmental hazards because of their teratogenic effects. The pregnant woman must follow good health practices and have close medical supervision to ensure her own and her child's health and well-being.

THE PRENATAL PERIOD

The period from fertilization to birth is called the *prenatal period*. From the time of menarche in puberty until menopause in middle age, the female ovaries produce **ova,** or female sex cells. Roughly every 28 days an ovum matures and is released in a process known as **ovulation.** From puberty on, the male testes produce **sperm,** or male sex cells, which are released at the moment of ejaculation. Pregnancy begins with the union of the female ovum and the male sperm cell. This is known as **conception** or **fertilization;** all inherited characteristics are determined at this moment.

After fertilization, which normally takes place in the woman's fallopian tube, the zygote undergoes a series of cell divisions and forms a cell mass known as a **morula.** The morula continues to divide and change as it travels down the fallopian tube to the uterus, where it implants itself in the uterine wall. At the point of implantation the entity is called a **blastocyst.** The total process, from fertilization to implantation, takes about 7 days (Fig. 6.3). After implantation, the multicelled structure, now referred to as an **embryo,** continues to develop. By the end of the eighth week of development, all essential structures are formed and the embryo is now termed a **fetus.** The estimated length of pregnancy is approximately 40 weeks (9 calendar months or 10 lunar months). Prenatal development may be divided into three stages: pre-embryonic, embryonic, and fetal. The pre-embryonic stage begins with fertilization

and lasts for about 2 weeks. The embryonic stage begins 2 weeks after fertilization and ends after the eighth week. The fetal stage begins with the ninth week and ends with the birth of the baby. A summary of the process of fetal development is shown in Figure 6.4.

Approximately 280 days after conception, labor begins (Fig. 6.5). Several different hormones are believed to be involved in the process of labor, including progesterone, oxytocin, and prostaglandins. *Progesterone* is produced by the ovaries (female sex glands). It is the hormone that maintains pregnancy and helps stimulate uterine contractions at the end of the pregnancy. *Oxytocin* is produced by the hypophysis, the posterior lobe of the pituitary gland. Oxytocin has two functions: It stimulates uterine contractions and prepares the breasts for breastfeeding. *Prostaglandins* are hormones that are produced in various tissues throughout the body. Like oxytocin, uterine prostaglandins help stimulate contractions.

The labor and delivery period has three distinct stages. Stage 1, the stage of dilation, is usually the longest, lasting an average of 12 to 24 hours. This stage begins with the onset of regular rhythmic uterine contractions and ends with the complete **dilation** (widening) of the **cervix** (the lower portion of the uterus). During this stage, **effacement,** or a shortening and thinning of the cervix, occurs. Stage 2, the expulsion stage, lasts about 1½ hours, but it is the most difficult stage. It begins with the complete dilation of the cervix and ends with the birth of the baby. Stage 3 is the shortest stage, lasting from 5 to

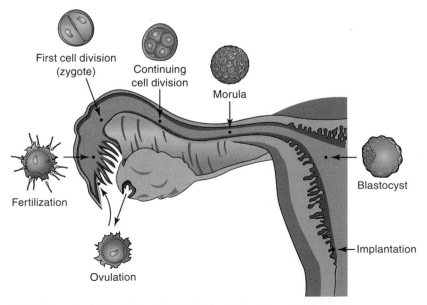

First cell division (zygote)

Continuing cell division

Morula

Fertilization

Blastocyst

Ovulation

Implantation

FIGURE 6.3 Ovulation, fertilization, and implantation.

Week 4
End of first lunar month

Length: ¼ in. (0.6 cm)
Weight:
Appearance: Curled upon itself with head touching tail.
Signs of formation of arm and leg buds.
Liver formed.
Heart present. Begins to pulsate about the 14th to 24th day.
Primitive blood cells present.
Beginnings of brain present.

Weeks 6–8
Second lunar month

Length: 1 in. (2.5 cm)
Weight: 1/30 oz (1 g)
Chambers of heart develop.
Rapid brain development occurring.
Primitive limbs present. Fingers and toes begin to form.
Face develops. Eyes, ears, nose appear. Palate and upper lip forming.
Gastrointestinal tract developing. Part of intestine still in umbilical cord.
Urogenital systems forming.
Head disproportionately large due to rapid brain development.
Organogenesis completed.

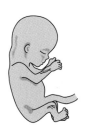

Weeks 9–12
Third lunar month

Length: 3 in. (7.5 cm)
Weight: 1 oz (28 g)
Growth and maturation of structures continues.
Head disproportionately large.
Brain shows structural features.
Eyelids fused.
Nail beds form on fingers and toes.
Bile present in intestines.
Spontaneous movements present.
Ossification centers in bones begin to appear.
Enamel-forming cells and dentin forming.
Kidney secretion by 10th week.
Bone marrow begins to form blood cells.
Distinguishing sexual traits evident.
Respiratory-like movements (reflex activity) present.
Intestines retracted from umbilical cord into abdomen.
Palate completed fused.
Neck well defined.

Weeks 13–16
Fourth lunar month

Length: 6 to 7 in. (15.2 to 17.7 cm)
Weight: 4 oz (112 g)
Fetus active. Mother may experience quickening.
Skeleton calcified and visible on x-ray film.
Downy lanugo on head.
Placenta distinct.
Blood vessels visible beneath transparent skin.
Heart actually circulating blood through fetal body.
Increasing amount of respiratory movements can be detected by sonogram.
Enzymes ptyalin and pepsin being secreted.
Fetal thyroid gland begins functioning by the 14th week.
Total body blood volume: Less than 100 mL.
Amount of amniotic fluid present: 150 to 280 mL.

FIGURE 6.4 Fetal development.

Continued

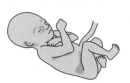

Weeks 17–20
Fifth lunar month

Length: 10 in. (.5 cm)
Weight: 8 to 10 oz (224 to 280 g)
Fetal heart sounds evident with stethoscope.
Scalp hair visible.
Lanugo present, especially on shoulders.
Skin less transparent.
Eyebrows present.
Vernix caseosa present.
Fingernails and toenails apparent.
Some fat deposits present.

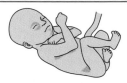

Weeks 21–24
Sixth lunar month

Length: 12 in. (30.5 cm)
Weight: 1-1/2 lb (672 g)
Skin wrinkled, pink, translucent.
Increasing amounts of vernix caseosa present.
Eyebrows and eyelashes well defined.
External ear soft, flat, shapeless.
Lanugo covering entire body.
Some breathing effort evident.

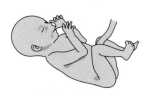

Weeks 25–28
Seventh lunar month

Length: 15 in. (37.5 cm)
Weight: 2-1/2 lb (1120 g)
Skin red, wrinkled, covered with vernix caseosa.
Looks like a "little old man."
Membranes disappear from eyes. Eyelids open.
Scalp hair well developed.
Fingernails and toenails present.
Subcutaneous fat present.
Testes at internal inguinal ring or below.

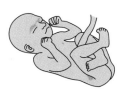

Weeks 29–32
Eighth lunar month

Length: 15 to 17 in. (37.5 to 42.5 cm)
Weight: 3-1/2 to 4 lb (1568 to 1792 g)
Skin pink and smooth.
Areola of breast visible but flat.
Testicles begin descent down inguinal canal (may be in scrotal sac), or
Labia majora small and separated, clitoris prominent.
Hair fine and wooly.
One or two creases evident on anterior portion of soles.
Deposits of subcutaneous fat present.
Can be conditioned to respond to sounds outside of mother's body.

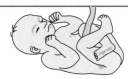

Weeks 33–36
Ninth lunar month

Length: 19 in. (47.5 cm)
Weight: 5 to 6 lb (2240 to 2688 g)
Increased fat deposits give body and limbs a more rounded appearance.
Skin thicker, whiter.
Lanugo disappearing.
Sole creases involve anterior two thirds of foot.
Breast tissue develops beneath nipples.

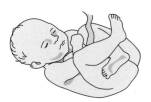

Weeks 37–40
Tenth lunar month

Length: 20 in. (50 cm)
Weight: 7 to 7-1/2 lb (3136 to 3360 g)
After 38 weeks, considered full term.
Body plump.
Lanugo gone from face.
Vernix caseosa disappearing, present in varying amounts.
Testes in scrotum, or
Labia majora meet in midline and cover labia minora and clitoris.
Ear well defined. Erect from head.
Uniform color to eyes (a slate hue).
Acquires antibodies from mother.

FIGURE 6.4—cont'd

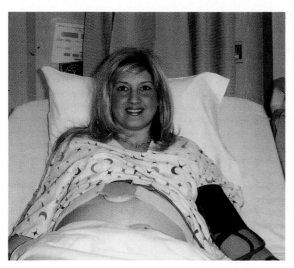

FIGURE 6.5 Length of labor and birth vary with each individual.

30 minutes. It begins with the birth of the baby and ends with the delivery of the placenta. The exact length of time for these three stages varies with the individual. Factors such as the number of previous pregnancies and deliveries affect the duration of each stage.

The culture and society to which individuals belong help influence childbirth practices and beliefs. Childbirth practices in Western civilization have changed over time. Before the mid-19th century, childbirth was a family event that took place at home. After the Industrial Revolution, childbirth shifted from the home to hospital-centered care. Physicians were the primary caregivers. Gradually, the natural childbirth movement evolved and became popular. This resulted in a decreased use of medications and instruments and a shift to family-centered care. Today many hospitals have birthing centers, which attempt to povide comfort in an "at home" atmosphere. In addition, some individuals have selected to give birth at home, often under the care of a midwife, with their family playing an active part in their birth experience. Education, preparation, and support are necessary to make the childbirth experience a safe and positive one for all involved.

During pregnancy, a protective sac of fetal membranes surrounds the developing fetus. Amniotic fluid fills the sac. Amniotic fluid acts as a protective cushion, maintains even body temperature, allows for movement of the fetus, and provides a fluid source for the fetus. Mother and fetus are linked through an organ called the **placenta.** During pregnancy this structure serves many functions, including producing hormones, transporting nutrients and wastes, and protecting the baby from harmful substances. The **umbilical cord** is the link between the fetus and the placenta. At birth it appears to be whitish blue and is covered by a glistening membrane. In the delivery room the cord must be assessed for the presence of three vessels—two arteries and one vein. Any deviation from this usually indicates some serious cardiac abnormality. In fetal circulation, oxygen and nutrients reach the fetus by way of the umbilical vein, and waste and deoxygenated blood return to the placenta for oxygenation by way of the umbilical arteries.

Fetal circulation ends at birth, when the umbilical cord is tied off and the newborn infant, or **neonate,** takes its first breath. At 1 minute after birth, and again 5 minutes later, the neonate is assessed and given an **Apgar score** (Table 6.1). Five essential categories of functioning are assessed, including color, reflex irritability, heart rate, respiratory rate, and muscle tone. The Apgar score gives an immediate clinical picture of the newborn's overall status.

PHYSICAL CHARACTERISTICS

Head and Skull

At birth the newborn's head is large in proportion to the rest of its body, typically one-fourth of the total body length. A newborn's average head circumference is 13 to 14 inches (33 to 35.5 cm)—about 1 inch larger than the chest. The head circumference increases by about 3 inches during the first 8 months of life. The skull consists of six soft bones: one occipital, one frontal, two parietal, and two temporal bones (Fig. 6.6). The skull bones are separated by bands of cartilage, called **sutures.** Located at the anterior and posterior of the infant's skull are two spaces or soft spots, called **fontanels.** These fontanels are very visible and even appear to pulsate when the infant cries. The skull should be palpated for the presence of sutures and fontanels. The small triangular-shaped posterior fontanel closes by the infant's fourth month. The larger, diamond-shaped anterior fontanel closes when the child is 12 to 18 months old. These spaces allow the skull to accommodate the rapid brain growth that takes place in this period. The newborn's skull may appear misshapen or elongated as a result of **molding,** which occurs as the head passes through the narrow birth canal. This is a temporary condition that disappears naturally in a few days.

TABLE
6.1   Apgar Scoring Chart

Sign	0	1	2	1 minute	5 minutes
Heart rate (beats per minute)	Absent	<100	>100	—	—
Respiratory rate (breaths per minute)	Absent	Slow, irregular	Good, crying	—	—
Muscle tone	Limp	Some flexion of extremities	Active motion	—	—
Reflex irritability: Catheter in nostril	No response	Grimace	Cough or sneeze	—	—
Slap to sole of foot	No response	Grimace	Cry and withdrawal of foot	—	—
Color	Blue, pale	Body pink; extremities blue	Completely pink	—	—

Frontal suture
Frontal bone
Anterior fontanel
Parietal bone
Sagittal suture
Posterior fontanel
Occipital bone

FIGURE 6.6 Infant's skull showing sutures and fontanels.

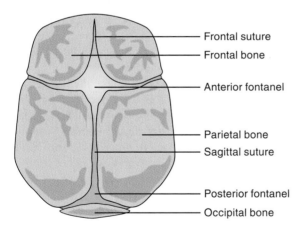

FIGURE 6.7 Physical characteristics of the newborn include a short neck and tightly flexed limbs.

Length and Weight

The average length of the newborn measured from head to heel is 20 inches (50 cm). Normal length for newborns ranges from 19 to 21 inches (48 to 53 cm). Usually, infants grow 1 inch per month for the first year. At 12 months the child's brain is approximately 2.5 times as big as it was at birth, the head and chest are equal in circumference, and the child is 1.5 times longer than at birth.

The newborn's head appears to rest on its chest because its neck is short and has deep creases (Fig. 6.7). The arms and legs are proportionately short and kept in a tightly flexed position. At birth, the newborn weighs an average of 7.5 pounds (3,400 g); the

normal range is from 5.5 to 10 pounds. Boys are generally slightly larger than girls at birth. The newborn loses 5% to 10% of its birth weight in the first few days of life. This occurs because the infant is given nothing by mouth for the first few hours and, therefore, the infant's output exceeds its intake. This is known as **normal physiological weight loss.** When the mother's breast milk comes in or formula feeding begins, the neonate regains its initial weight loss in approximately 10 days. Thereafter the newborn will gain 5 to 6 ounces per week for the first month; infants will double their birth weight by 5 to 6 months of age and triple their birth weight by their first birthday. Approximately 75% of an infant's body weight consists of water. For this reason infants with vomiting and diarrhea may suffer a rapid loss of total body fluid and possible dehydration.

Skin

The newborn's skin at birth is thin and appears pale. Some temporary acrocyanosis (blueness of the hands and feet) may be present as a result of poor peripheral circulation; this is usually transient and disappears a few hours after birth. Pigmentation may be more pronounced in certain areas of the body, such as the earlobes, scrotum, and back of the neck; full pigmentation develops several days later. The neonate's color varies according to the amount of melanin present in the skin. In general, infants of northern European descent vary from pink to red; infants of African descent vary from pink to dark red; infants of Asian descent vary from rosy red to yellowish tan; those of Hispanic and Mediterranean descent may be yellowish brown; and Native American infants vary from light pink to reddish brown. Infants with relatively more melanin in their skin may be born with a mongolian spot, a flat, irregular, pigmented area in the lumbar-sacral region. The mongolian spot usually fades and becomes less noticeable at about age 4.

Many newborns have a covering of fine hair over the body. This covering, known as lanugo, vanishes in the first few days after birth. The newborn's skin creases have a white, cheeselike, oily covering called vernix caseosa, which protects the fetus's skin during pregnancy.

Milia, small clusters of pearly white spots mostly on the infant's nose, chin, and forehead, may also be present at birth. These spots are caused by the retention of sebaceous material within the sebaceous glands and disappear spontaneously without treatment.

Some infants develop a yellow tinge to their skin known as icterus neonatorum, or physiological jaundice. Physiological jaundice frequently occurs in newborns within 48 to 72 hours after birth. At birth the neonate's red blood cell (RBC) count is higher than that of the normal adult—usually 6 million per mm^3 of blood. A few days after birth the RBC count begins to decrease as the body destroys these unnecessary excess cells. This releases a high amount of bilirubin (a component of RBC), producing the jaundiced appearance in the infant. Physiological jaundice should not be confused with jaundice related to blood incompatibilities, which is usually present immediately at birth and requires prompt medical intervention and treatment.

Genitals

Maternal hormones of pregnancy present in the neonate's bloodstream may cause certain physiological anomalies. The breasts of neonates of both sexes may be swollen. This condition will disappear without intervention. The scrotum of male neonates may appear large and edematous. The scrotum should be palpated for the presence of testicles, which usually descend from the abdominal cavity into the scrotal sac during the seventh month of fetal life. If the testicles have not descended, the infant will be observed to see if descent occurs over the next few months. Undescended testicles can be treated with a short course of drug therapy or surgery. The newborn's penis is inspected for the location of the urethral opening. Normally this opening is just at the tip of the head of the penis under the foreskin. Circumcision, the surgical removal of the foreskin, may be performed after birth for hygienic or religious reasons. Any deviation should be noted and reported to the physician for follow-up treatment.

The labia in the newborn female may appear swollen. A blood-tinged mucous vaginal discharge known as pseudomenstruation may be noted. These conditions are related to maternal hormones and disappear without treatment.

Urine is normally present in the bladder at the time of birth. The newborn should void within 24 hours after birth and 8 to 10 times a day thereafter. The initial voiding may appear rust-colored because of the presence of uric acid crystals. This condition generally disappears without treatment.

Face

The newborn's face is small, and the eyes may appear swollen. The eyes are treated after birth with antibiotic application of erythromycin or silver nitrate as a preventive against blindness caused by gonorrhea. Eye color varies from slate gray to dark blue. Permanent eye color is not determined until 3 to 6 months of age. No tears are produced until 4 weeks of age, when the lacrimal ducts (tear ducts) are developed.

The neonate usually has a flat nose and a receding chin. The neonate's mouth is usually examined closely for any defects or abnormalities, particularly cleft palate, the incomplete formation and nonunion of the hard palate. This condition can be corrected through surgical repair. The gums should be pink and moist. The first teeth, called deciduous teeth or primary teeth, begin to erupt when the infant is

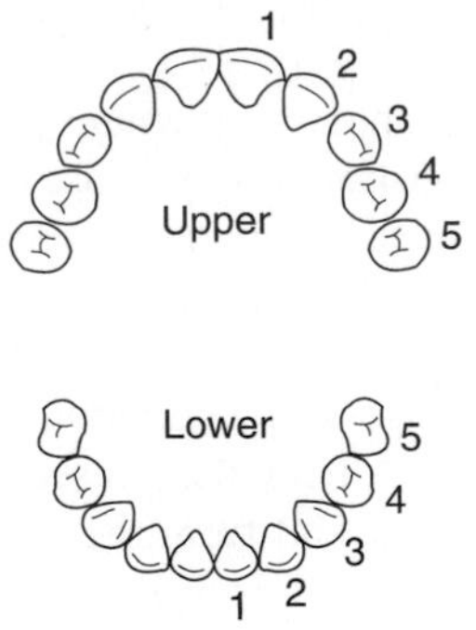

	(Upper)	(Lower)
1 Central incisor	8–12 mos.	5–9 mos.
2 Lateral incisor	8–12 mos.	12–18 mos.
3 Cuspid	18–24 mos.	
4 First molar	12–18 mos.	
5 Second molar	24–30 mos.	

FIGURE 6.8 Approximate ages for the eruption of deciduous teeth.

about 6 or 7 months old (Fig. 6.8). Usually the first teeth to appear are the two lower central incisors; they are followed by the two upper central incisors. By age 12 months the baby will have about six or eight teeth.

Abdomen

The neonate's abdomen appears large and flabby. Immediately after birth the umbilical cord is tied and cut. After a few days the blood vessels of the cord become dry or thrombosed. This is accompanied by a change in color from dull yellowish brown to black. By the tenth day the dried cord falls off and the navel is completely healed. Tub bathing is avoided until the navel is fully healed.

At the time of birth the newborn can swallow, digest, metabolize, and absorb nutrients. The newborn can metabolize only simple carbohydrates. For this reason, whole milk, which contains complex sugars, is not given to the newborn. The newborn's stomach can hold 1 to 3 ounces of fluid; by 10 months, it can hold about 10 ounces. The neonate's cardiac sphincter is underdeveloped; therefore, it is important to allow the infant short periods of feeding, followed by "bubbling" or burping for the release of swallowed air.

Bowel movements of healthy infants vary in number, color, consistency, and general appearance. The

HELPFUL HINTS

Do not use liquor or apply aspirin to the teething infant's irritated and swollen gums.

HELPFUL HINTS

To hasten cord healing, fold diapers away from the cord stump, apply alcohol to the area around the cord, and report any signs of redness or drainage to the pediatrician.

mother's diet or the type of formula given will also influence the infant's stools (Table 6.2). Within 10 hours after birth the newborn should pass his or her first stool, known as **meconium.** Meconium is thick, green–black, tarry, and odorless. Breastfed infants have stools that resemble light, seeded mustard. Stools of formula-fed infants are commonly semisolid and tan or yellowish in color. Some infants have four to six bowel movements a day. An infant is constipated if stools are very hard and can be passed only with much effort. Adding some additional water or strained fruits to the diet may prevent constipation.

Extremities

The newborn's extremities are short in proportion to the rest of the body and are kept in a tightly flexed position. They should be examined for range of motion, symmetry, and reflexes. The lower extremities are examined closely to determine if there is an extra gluteal fold, which usually indicates a congenital hip dysplasia (Fig. 6.9). Any abnormality should be reported immediately to the physician for further evaluation. The toes and fingers are counted and inspected for abnormalities. In full-term infants the soles of the feet and palms of the hands are deeply creased. Preterm infants have only very fine lines on their palms and soles.

NEUROLOGICAL CHARACTERISTICS

A neurological assessment in the newborn focuses on reflexes, posture, movement, and muscle tone. At birth the nervous system is immature, and the newborn responds to his or her environment through a series of reflexes. The presence of certain reflexes indicates a normal neurological system and also helps estimate gestational age. Several reflexes are protective; these include blinking, sneezing, swallowing, and the gag reflex. Other reflexes present include Moro, or startle, reflex; rooting; grasp; Babinski; and tonic neck reflex. Rooting and sucking help the infant secure food. Table 6.3 describes these reflexes in detail.

TABLE 6.2   Stool Patterns for Newborns

Stool	Age	Description
Meconium	First 2 days	Greenish-black, tarry, odorless
Transitional	2–3 days	Brown to yellow to green
Formula-fed	From day 2 or 3	Pasty yellow or tan, distinct odor
Breastfed	From day 2 or 3	Light, seeded mustard, sweet odor

The newborn's spinal column is inspected to make certain that there are no masses, cysts, or openings. The presence of any spinal defect necessitates immediate medical intervention.

The five senses (sight, hearing, taste, touch, and smell) are present at birth and function at a primitive level. Neonates can track objects at birth; they appear to prefer bright lights and yellow, green, and pink objects and large geometric shapes. The neonate's pupils react to light by dilating and contracting. The newborn's vision is 10 to 30 times less acute than normal adult vision of 20/20. By the time the infant is 6 months old, vision should be 20/100 or better. Movement of the eyes is usually unequal owing to immature cilliary muscles; it is not uncommon for a neonate's eyes to cross or for one eye to drift when focusing on an object. This is known as **nystagmus.** These deviations are temporary and should disappear without treatment. By 4 months of age infants have binocular vision: They can focus both eyes simultaneously to produce one image. Depth perception at first is limited to grasping for items out of reach and becomes more precise at about age 7 to 9 months. At this point the infant is able to reach for items more accurately and purposefully.

The ears are positioned on the sides of the head, with the top of the ear about the level of the eyes. At birth the newborn's ears are generally filled with either vernix or birth fluid, which dissolves within a few days. The infant hears and responds to loud, low-frequency sounds. A sudden loud sound will produce a startle response. By the age of 6 to 8 weeks, infants recognize their mother's voice and turn their heads in response to it. A 1-year-old child can discriminate between different sounds and often recognize the source.

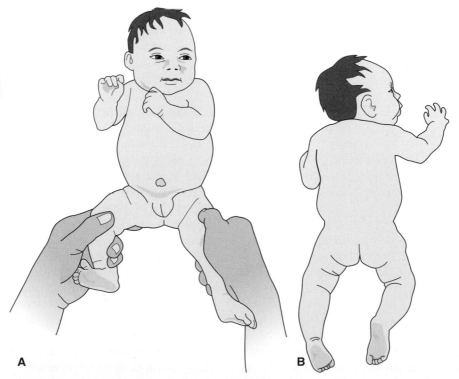

A   **B**

FIGURE 6.9 Assessment of the gluteal and popliteal folds of the hips. The folds should be symmetrical. **A:** Limited abduction. **B:** Asymmetry of the shin folds.

TABLE

6.3   Reflexes Present in the Normal Neonate

Reflex	Action	Disappearance/Extinction
Moro	Sudden movement or jarring of position causes extension and adduction of extremities.	By age 3 or 4 months
Tonic neck	If head of back-lying newborn is turned to one side, infant will extend arm and leg on that side.	By age 5 months
Rooting	When newborn's cheek is gently stroked, infant turns toward that side and opens mouth.	By age 4 to 6 months
Sucking	Newborn makes sucking movements when anything touches lips or tongue.	Diminishes by age 6 months
Babinski	When newborn's sole is stroked, toes hyperextend and fan outward; big toe turns upward.	By age 3 months
Palmar grasp	Newborn briefly grasps any object placed in hands.	By age 3 months (present from age 6 weeks)

Newborn infants can discriminate among different tastes. If they are given a sweet solution, they will begin to make sucking movements. When given something sour, they will respond with a grimace or pout. The 1-year-old child has developed a capacity to taste and has preferences for certain flavors. The sweet taste appears to be universally pleasing. The young child should be introduced to a wide variety of tastes and textures. This exposure helps to mature the child's sense of taste.

The sense of touch is keenly present at birth. The face is most sensitive, especially around the mouth. The hands and soles of the feet are also sensitive. Infants like to be touched and rocked because of the calming effect. Pain perception is present in the newborn and is witnessed when an injection is given. The typical reaction to pain is loud crying and thrusting the whole body and extremities. The 1-year-old child demonstrates withdrawal from pain but may not be able to recognize the source of the pain. For example, the child may touch a hot pot and quickly respond by withdrawing the hand and crying. However, the child might repeat the action another time, not understanding the cause and effect.

Studies indicate that newborns have a sense of smell. Newborns have been tested and found to react to strong odors by turning away. It has also been documented that newborns can recognize the smell of breast milk. One study showed that infants can even distinguish their own mother's breast milk from that of others.

VITAL SIGNS

The newborn's temperature immediately after birth may be slightly below normal. This is a result of an immature temperature-regulating mechanism and heat loss caused by the cooler environment in the delivery room. The newborn should be dried off and placed under a radiant warmer to help raise his or her body temperature. In addition, the neonate's head should be covered to prevent further heat loss from evaporation. Once stabilized, the neonate's normal axillary temperature ranges from 97.7°F to 99.5°F (36.5°C to 37.5°C). The newborn's temperature should be measured using the axillary route to prevent possible rectal perforation.

Pulse should be taken by listening to the chest for an apical pulse for 1 full minute (Fig. 6.10). The apical heart rate ranges from 120 to 160 beats per minute. Slight variations in the heart rate are common. During periods of rest the rate may slow down to 100 beats per minute; during crying periods the rate may increase to 180 beats per minute.

Blood pressure (BP) readings provide a baseline and can be used to assess the infant for cardiac abnormalities. Average BP using oscillometry (Dinamap) is 65/40 mm Hg. Blood pressure will increase and heart and respiratory rate will decrease as the child gets older.

Respirations should be counted for 1 full minute. The respirations of the newborn are normally irregular, shallow, and diaphragmatic, with brief periods of **apnea** (absence of breathing). Infant respirations

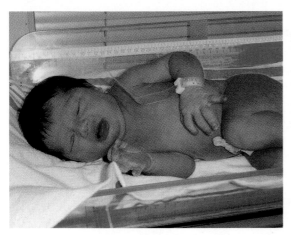

FIGURE 6.10 The newborn is measured and identified before leaving the delivery room.

can be counted by watching the abdomen rise and fall. The normal respiratory rate is 30 to 60 breaths per minute. Marked deviations in these normal ranges may indicate congenital abnormalities and warrant further investigation.

DEVELOPMENTAL MILESTONES

Motor Development

The neonate's movements and behavior appear purposeless and uncoordinated, but all newborns have distinct behavioral characteristics and physical traits that make them different from other neonates. Every infant has his or her own growth timetable. Growth and development should be assessed based on the infant's own individual progress.

Gross Motor Skills

Gross motor skills are movements of the large muscles of the arms and legs. Following a cephalocaudal pattern, head control develops by 2 months; by 3 months the infant can briefly hold its head up. At 4 months the infant can raise the head to a 90-degree angle from the prone position. Rolling over from the abdomen to the back occurs at 4 months. By 6 months old, the baby can roll both ways, sit with support, and hold the head erect. Sitting alone occurs at the seventh month. The 10-month-old infant can change position from the prone (facedown) to the sitting position. Crawling, a primitive movement in which the infant's abdomen is on the floor, is usually achieved by infants at about 9 months. Creeping is a more advanced form of movement that requires the infant to rise up on all four limbs. Some infants progress to this style of locomotion by 10 to 11 months. At about 8 months babies can pull themselves up to a standing position. Standing is followed by cruising, which is a form of stepping while holding on to some object or surface for support. Walking unassisted is achieved between the ages of 12 to 15 months (Fig. 6.11).

Fine Motor Skills

Fine motor skills include the movements of the hands and fingers. Initially, grasp is actually a reflex action involving the whole arm in a swiping movement. The neonate exhibits the palmar grasp reflex, grabbing any object that is placed in the hands. Finger and hand control develop after shoulder and arm control, demonstrating the principle of proximodistal development. Purposeful reaching and grasping using the whole hand occur by the fifth month of life. It is common to see infants take hold of objects and immediately bring them to their mouths. For this reason, it is important that safety measures be taken to prevent accidental aspiration of small objects.

The 6-month-old infant is able to hold a bottle, a cracker, or dry toast and bring it to the mouth. At this stage of development, many babies enjoy biting on a hard food object; this can be soothing to their swollen gums. Hand preference usually does not appear until the seventh or eighth month, when the baby can transfer an object from one hand to the other. The 7-month-old infant continues to make progress with self-feeding. He or she can hold the bottle and now has the use of the pincer grasp, which permits the opposition of thumb and forefinger. At this time it is typical for babies to grasp and then release small objects. This action usually delights the child because it causes the caregiver to retrieve the object so the action can be repeated. By 9 months, babies are able to drink from a cup and attempt to use a spoon. In early attempts, the spoon may be inverted and the contents spilled. The 1-year-old child can hold a writing object, make scribbling marks on paper or other surfaces, and build a tower of two blocks.

Psychosocial Development

Erik Erikson believed that each child needs to accomplish a particular task at each stage of development. The resolution of each task permits the child to move on to a new stage. For an overview of Erikson's stages of growth and development, refer to Chapter 5. According to Erikson, the infant is working on completing the task of trust. The infant

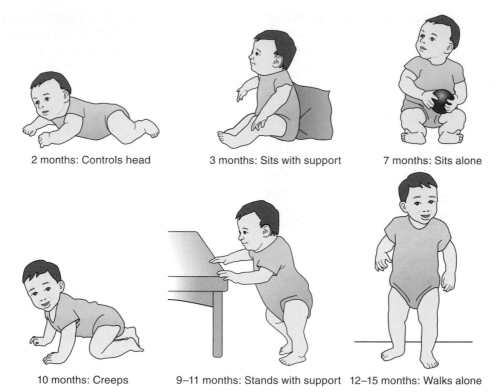

2 months: Controls head   3 months: Sits with support   7 months: Sits alone

10 months: Creeps   9–11 months: Stands with support   12–15 months: Walks alone

FIGURE 6.11 Developmental milestones.

will feel secure and develop a sense of trust when the environment consistently satisfies his or her basic needs for food, comfort, and love. This first stage lays the foundation on which future stages will be built. Depriving the infant of basic needs can result in the development of mistrust and hinder the further development of the infant's full potential.

Attachment

The parent–child relationship begins with fetal development and continues after birth. Emotional bonds between the mother and child are known as **attachment** (Fig. 6.12). This can be evidenced by the way the mother holds, talks to, and looks at the baby. This attachment, or bonding, process serves to strengthen the infant's sense of security and self. This process is reciprocal between infant and parent. Bonding is felt by the parent during the first period of touching and gazing at the infant. Touch, skin to skin contact, and seeing the infant's features as resembling other family members helps solidify this feeling of attachment. The process of bonding is referred to as **engrossment**. Bonding is as important to the father as to the mother. Encouraging fathers to participate in the pregnancy and birthing process can initiate the foundation for engrossment. After birth, bonding can be strengthened by involving the father in child care.

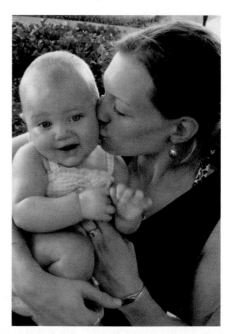

FIGURE 6.12 Parent–child bonding.

Temperament

Babies are born with their own unique temperaments, which determine their moods and their responses to stimulation. Temperament is inborn, whereas personality is shaped and affected by the environment. An infant's willingness to interact with others is a part of his or her temperament. Some babies are very social, and others are shy. Babies with difficult temperaments are more fretful and cry a lot. These infants are not easily soothed. Other infants have an even temperament, which allows them to adapt to their surroundings with little fussing.

Parental Guidance

As infants begin to develop their means of locomotion, the need for discipline increases. For the first 6 months parents may use the art of distraction. The baby who continues to look and reach for the knobs on the stove can be given an age-appropriate toy as a substitute. In the second 6 months, as the infant's memory and cognition increase, discipline must be more direct. The 10-month-old infant can be told "No" firmly when he or she reaches for something unsafe. The child at this stage is able to understand the tone of repeated admonitions. Verbal cues alone without supervision cannot prevent accidents. Parents and caregivers must be advised that discipline should not be harsh and should focus on praising the positive, desirable behavior while deemphasizing the negative, undesirable behavior. An important goal of discipline is to teach the child impulse control and to set limits. The need for discipline will expand and continue throughout childhood and into adolescence.

Cognitive Development

Piaget proposed that the infant begins life with no understanding of the world. The child then must learn about the environment through observation and sensory perception. For example, the baby begins to understand objects by touching, tasting, seeing, hearing, and smelling. See Figure 6.13. Piaget described infancy as the stage of sensorimotor development. Initially, infants respond to stimuli in the environment by reflex action. At about 8 months, infants begin to plan and coordinate their actions. For example, the infant knows that if he or she shakes a toy, it will produce a sound. By the end of the first year, infants are able to form bonds with certain people and recognize and attach meaning to objects. They begin to be able to understand some repeated actions. For example, the 10-month-old infant has learned that when mother goes to the pantry or refrigerator, she might be getting something to eat. This learning is stored, and when it is repeated, it helps to develop the child's ability to think.

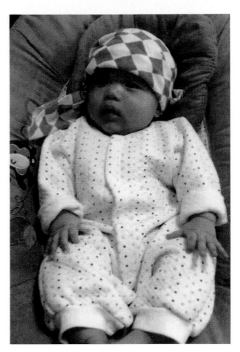

FIGURE 6.13 Infants learn about the environment through observation.

Moral Development

Moral development is not present at birth; the infant has no conscience, or system of values. The motivational forces guiding behavior are based on satisfaction of needs rather than moral beliefs. Infants do what pleases them and are not aware that their acts can affect others. They react to pain and love, and they judge behavior on the basis of how it affects them.

Communication

The infant at birth communicates primarily by crying to make needs known. Studies indicate that crying has different sounds and meanings. Differences can be noted in the type and amount of crying in newborn infants. Caregiver responses can decrease or increase the amount of an infant's crying. Picking

---

HELPFUL HINTS

- Infants who cry fretfully with their fingers in their mouth are indicating hunger.
- Infants who cry fretfully, draw their legs up in a flexed position, and pass flatus usually have colic.
- Infants with a high-pitched, shrill cry usually have injury to the central nervous system.

up an infant and holding, rocking, or using soothing sounds may decrease the amount of crying. Some cries may signal discomfort or pain. Determining and eliminating the source of the discomfort will lessen the crying.

Before they acquire speech, infants communicate in other ways. At 2 months, the infant responds to familiar voices with pleasure and a smile. See Figure 6.14. Cooing or soft throaty sounds occur at 2 months. Later, the repetition of certain sounds becomes associated with objects or persons. This is known as babbling and is the use of consonants and vowels loosely connected. Babbling occurs between 3 and 6 months. The sequence of sounds made in babbling is universal.

Disease affecting the infant's mouth, tongue, and throat can delay babbling and language development. The 8-month-old child is able to imitate simple sounds such as "dada," much to the parents' delight. Other consonant sounds are more difficult; therefore, words like "mama" will be learned later. One-year-old children have an expressive vocabulary of about four to six words. They are able to understand the meaning of many more words by association with the objects or by tone of voice. Talking and reading to infants helps increase their language comprehension and verbal ability.

All infants develop according to their own growth timetables. We have provided a rough timetable for each developmental skill for the first year of life. If marked delays in the acquisition of these skills are noted, parents should consult the physician for further evaluation. See Box 6.1 for a list of signs that should be discussed with the physician.

NUTRITION

Infants' sucking, swallowing, and rooting reflexes enable them to search for and secure their food. The infant's nutritional needs can be met during the entire first year by breastfeeding or by using iron-enriched formula. Many factors influence the mother's decision to breastfeed or bottle feed. Some of these factors include knowledge, support, financial considerations, cultural beliefs, and employment. In some cultures modesty or the belief that there is little value in colostrum influences some mothers to choose not to breastfeed. Teaching parents about breastfeeding advantages may help result in informed choices, but health care workers should ultimately support a woman's decision about how to feed her baby. While breast milk is considered the best nutritional value for infants and is recommended, breastfed and bottle-fed infants thrive equally well. Table 6.4 lists the advantages and disadvantages of both feeding methods.

Breastfeeding

The American Academy of Pediatrics (AAP) and the U.S. Surgeon General recommend breastfeeding for at least the first 6 months of life.

One immediate nutritional benefit of breastfeeding is the ingestion of colostrum. **Colostrum** is the precursor of breast milk and is present in the mother's

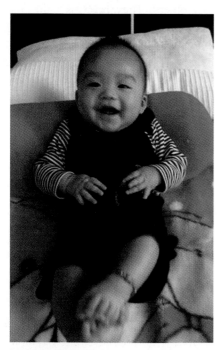

FIGURE 6.14 Infants may respond with smiles and laughter.

> **BOX 6.1 Signs of Infant Developmental Delay**
>
> Discuss the following with the physician:
>
> - Moro reflex persists after 4 months.
> - Infant does not smile in response to mother's voice after 3 months.
> - Infant does not respond to loud sounds.
> - Infant does not reach or grasp by 4 months.
> - Infant still has tonic reflex after 5 months.
> - Infant cannot sit without help by 6 months.
> - Infant does not roll over in either direction by 5 months.
> - Infant does not stand by 11 months.
> - Infant cannot learn simple gestures such as waving bye-bye or shaking the head yes and no by 1 year.
> - Infant cannot point to objects or pictures by 1 year.

TABLE

6.4 Breastfeeding Versus Bottle-Feeding	
Breast	**Bottle**
No preparation required	Requires preparation
Inexpensive or free	More costly
Mother must be present, or milk must be expressed from breast in advance	Frees up mother's time
Milk more easily digested; causes less gastrointestinal upset; less possibility of allergic reaction	Formula not as easily digested as breast milk
Low in saturated fat	High in saturated fat
Promotes bonding with mother, but does not allow other people to feed baby (except if pumped or formula is supplemented)	Allows father to feed and bond with baby
Baby gets immune factors from mother	Mother's diet does not affect baby
Mother's uterus contracts; involution hastened; menstruation delayed	
Amount baby ingests is not known	Amount taken at each feeding can be readily determined

breast as early as the seventh month of fetal life. It contains more protein, salt, and carbohydrate but less fat than regular breast milk. In addition to these nutrients, it contains immunoglobulins to help protect the newborn until its own immune system is more developed.

Some infants are placed at the breast immediately in the delivery room (Fig. 6.15). This practice has a number of positive effects for both mother and infant.

1. It promotes bonding or attachment between mother and child. Early signs of bonding are evidenced by the face-to-face interaction between infant and caregiver. Other early signs of bonding include talking, smiling, and playing with the infant.
2. It hastens **involution** (return of the uterus to its nonpregnant state) by stimulating uterine contractions and helping to restore muscle tone in the uterus.
3. It promotes the production of colostrum.

Actual breast milk appears on the third day after delivery; at this time the new mother will notice that her breasts are very firm or engorged. A visit with a lactation consultant can help new mothers learn

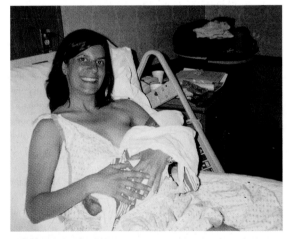

FIGURE 6.15 The infant can be put to the breast immediately after delivery.

how to successfully breastfeed their infants. Many hospitals provide consultations before the mother is discharged from the hospital.

Bottle Feeding

Mothers who cannot or do not wish to breastfeed can bottle feed with formula. Bottle-fed infants are usually given nothing by mouth for the first few hours of life. The first feeding begins with glucose and water; if this is tolerated, the infant progresses to the formula of choice. Bottle-fed newborns require a feeding every 3 to 4 hours at first and then according to their individual hunger patterns. The caregiver should never prop the bottle and leave the infant unattended. The baby should never be allowed to sleep with a bottle that contains anything other than water. Putting juice or milk in a nighttime bottle can lead to **bottle-mouth syndrome,** which is **dental caries** caused by sugar in the milk or juice that weakens the tooth surfaces. By 8 or 9 months, infants are ready to be weaned—that is, they can accept the cup in place of the bottle or breast.

Weaning and Introduction of Solid Foods

Weaning should be done gradually, one feeding at a time. The noon bottle is usually a good feeding to eliminate first; the baby isn't too tired or hungry to attempt learning to use the cup.

In addition to breast milk or formula, many pediatricians recommend the introduction of solid foods after the fifth month. Adding food to the baby's diet earlier is believed to add to digestive problems and possible food intolerances. One dietary concern after 5 months is that the infant's stored iron reserve is reduced. For this reason, iron-rich foods such as cereals, vegetables, and meats should be added to the diet. A daily supply of vitamin C helps to enhance the body's absorption of iron. The first solid food introduced into the infant's diet is usually rice cereal mixed with formula. It is recommended that only single-grain cereals be used at first and that egg whites, wheat, and citrus fruits not be used in the first year. These foods have been known to cause allergic reactions in many infants. It is best to introduce only one new food at a time for several days to detect any adverse reactions.

A general rule is to add 1 to 2 teaspoons of each new food, gradually increasing the amount to 1 tablespoon of each food item for each year. The 1-year-old baby eats three meals per day. Table 6.5 shows a schedule of foods for the first year of life. Box 6.2 shows a sample menu for the 10- to 12-month-old child.

SLEEP AND REST

The neonate sleeps a great deal, as much as 20 out of 24 hours. The faster the rate of growth, the more sleep is required. By 1 year of age, the baby will

need only about 12 hours of sleep a day. The newborn's sleep pattern is not continuous but is characterized by periods of light sleep marked by stirring movements and noises (Fig. 6.16). Sleep patterns may be interrupted by discomfort and hunger. A bedtime routine will help to establish a nighttime sleeping pattern. This consistent approach to bedtime helps to reduce anxiety and make the infant feel more secure. Early on, help infants learn to distinguish day from night by interacting during the day hours and by keeping talking, cuddling, and interactions to a minimum at night. Infants should be placed awake in their cribs so that they learn to soothe themselves and fall asleep on their own. During the first year most infants require both a morning and an afternoon nap to replenish their stamina. Table 6.6 summarizes the newborn's sleep patterns.

Sudden infant death syndrome (SIDS) is responsible for the death of about 1 out of every 500 babies, most commonly between the ages of 1 and 4 months. Although the exact cause of SIDS (also known as "crib death") is still unknown, recent research indicates an association between SIDS and sleep patterns. Death usually occurs between midnight and 6 a.m. The American Academy of Pediatrics recommends as a preventative measure that healthy infants sleep on their backs and sides and not on their stomachs. It also has been suggested that parents should offer a pacifier to infants to reduce the risk of SIDS. Studies have suggested that infants who sucked a pacifier during sleep were at less risk of developing SIDS. In addition, infants should be put to sleep in cribs that meet current safety standards. Parents should not use soft materials such as quilts, comforters, or pillows in the sleeping area. Co-sleeping arrangements in the parents' bed may pose the danger of suffocation or entrapment for the infant. In these cases special care must be taken to avoid placing the bed against a wall

TABLE
6.5   **Schedule of Foods, Birth to 12 Months**

Age	Food Selections	Rationale
Birth–6 months	Give only breast milk or iron-fortified formula.	Sucking and rooting reflexes allow infants to take in milk and formula; infants cannot accept semisolids because their tongues protrude when a spoon is put into their mouths.
	Add water.	Small amounts may be offered in hot weather or if the infant has diarrhea.
5–6 months	Add iron-fortified instant cereal; begin with rice cereal; avoid wheat cereal for first year.	Infants are now able to swallow semisolid food; cereal adds iron and vitamins A, B, and E.
	Add plain, unsweetened fruit juices, fortified with vitamin C; dilute with equal parts water.	Fruit juices provide vitamin C.
7–8 months	Add plain, strained fruits and vegetables; plain yogurt; strained meats; avoid combinations.	Fruits and vegetables introduce new flavors and textures; meats provide iron, protein, and B vitamins.
	Add zwieback, toast, crackers.	They provide iron, protein, and B vitamins.
	Continue with iron-fortified formula, infant cereal, and fruit juices.	Infants still need iron because they are not yet consuming large amounts of meat; this prepares the infant for weaning from bottle or breast.
9–10 months	Add finger foods: cooked, bite-sized pieces of meat; vegetables, soft fresh or canned; unsweetened fruits; yogurt; cottage cheese; continue with iron-fortified formula, infant cereal, and fruit juices.	These encourage self-feeding for motor skill development, and they introduce new textures and flavors; as formula or breast milk consumption decreases, other sources of calcium, riboflavin, and protein are needed.
11–12 months	Add soft table foods: dry, unsweetened cereals, cheese slices, and noodles.	Motor skills are improving; the infant is now ready for whole foods that require more chewing. The infant is also now relying more on whole foods and less on breast milk or formula for nutrients.

or using a railing or headboard, which may cause the infant's head to become trapped between these surfaces.

PLAY

Play is important to a child's growth, development, and socialization. The goal of play in the first year of life is nonsymbolic in that it helps the infant gain information about objects, their quality and function, and the immediate effects they produce.

Different play activities help infants explore their environments. Important in the first year is choosing toys that stimulate the child's senses. In addition, it is important to select play activities that challenge and encourage musculoskeletal development. The neonate begins interacting with the environment first by following bright lights and objects.

Play during the infancy stage is solitary—that is, infants do not require another person to play with them (Figs. 6.17 and 6.18). Infants frequently have play interactions with parents, who provide attention and stimulation. Brightly colored objects, objects

BOX 6.2 Sample Menus for Child, 10–12 Months

Breakfast
Scrambled egg yolk
Or
½ cup cereal
¼ cup cut-up fruit
4–6 ounces of formula
Snack
½ cup fruit juice or fresh fruit
Lunch
¼ cup cooked diced poultry
¼ cup yogurt
¼ cup cooked diced vegetables
Or
Fresh vegetables
4–6 ounces of formula
Snack
½ cup fruit juice or fresh fruit
1 teething biscuit or cracker
Dinner
¼ cup noodles, pasta, rice, or potato
¼ cup green or yellow vegetables
¼ cup poultry or other meat, tofu, or cheese
4–6 ounces of formula
Snack
4–6 ounces of formula
(Follow with water or brush teeth before bedtime)

that produce noise, and objects with different textures are appealing to this age group. Safety concerns must be considered when selecting playthings for the infant.

All toys must be carefully inspected for sharp edges and small removable parts that may potentially be ingested or aspirated. Table 6.7 lists appropriate toys for different stages of development.

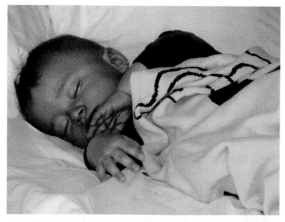

FIGURE 6.16 Infants have variable sleep patterns.

SAFETY

Because the newborn is totally helpless, the caregiver must meet all of its needs for safety and protection. At this age, most injuries and many deaths are the result of preventable accidents. Safety measures include the use of approved cribs, car seats, and car beds and the prevention of drowning, suffocation, and aspiration. An infant should never be left unattended. As babies develop and begin to have a means of locomotion, they are at risk for different types of accidents. They must be watched constantly to prevent falls; this is especially important when they are old enough to roll from side to side and later when they are placed in high chairs. Advise parents that if they must turn their back even for a moment, they should secure the infant or place him or her on the floor if nothing safer is available. If falls occur, parents should notify the child's physician if the injury results in nausea, vomiting, or lethargy. Babies learn and explore by putting everything in their mouths; therefore, to reduce the risk of aspiration, inspect all toys and small items and keep harmful items out of the baby's reach. It is the ultimate responsibility of the caregiver to set limits on behavior and supervise all activities to ensure safety in and around the home.

Parents should be instructed to support the infant's head and neck and never to shake or jiggle the newborn. Shaking causes the infant's brain to move back and forth within the skull. The brain is fragile with delicate blood vessels that may rupture. This causes the brain to swell, increasing the intracranial pressure. Shaken baby syndrome results, causing seizures, cerebral palsy, paralysis, and/or death. Shaken baby syndrome most often occurs as a result of caregiver frustration and inability to calm a crying baby. Prevention and caregiver support are key to eliminating shaken baby syndrome. Refer to Table 6.8 for information on infant safety.

Lead poisoning is a possible environmental hazard for infants and young children. Exposure may occur in older homes that often have lead plumbing or paint. If the paint is allowed to chip and peel, teething infants may pick up paint chips and chew on them. High levels of lead in the bloodstream have been associated with hyperactivity, irritability, aggression, and attention disorders. Eventually, lead can be toxic to the brain.

HEALTH PROMOTION

Health promotion is aimed at assisting the infant in movement toward optimal growth and development.

TABLE 6.6   Newborn Wake–Sleep Patterns

Type of Sleep	Activity	Duration	Intervention
Normal sleep	Eyes closed; respirations normal; occasional intermittent jerking of the body	4–5 hours per day in 20-minute cycles	Allow infant quiet rest periods; will wake if there is a sudden loud noise
Irregular sleep	Eyes closed; respiration irregular; jerky body movements; occasional groaning	12–15 hours per day in 45-minute cycles	Normal noise levels may wake child
Drowsiness	Eyes open or partly open; respiration irregular; active movement of limbs	Pattern is inconsistent	Can be easily awakened; can be removed from crib
Awake	Active movement of body and limbs; follows objects with eyes	2–3 hours per day	Position infant to interact with family members continuously; position toys so infant can play; provide other basic needs
Awake and crying	Begins with small whimpering sounds and progresses to loud crying with thrashing of limbs	1–4 hours per day	Soothe infant by holding and rocking; remove excess stimuli

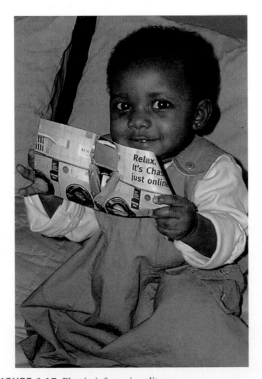

FIGURE 6.17 Play in infancy is solitary.

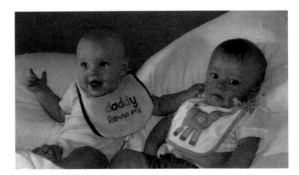

FIGURE 6.18 Infants develop at their own rate.

The nurse best accomplishes these goals by encouraging education, good health practices, and proper use of health services during prenatal development and after birth. Early assessment of the neonate can lead to early diagnosis and treatment of any abnormality. It is recommended that infants visit their health provider once a month for the first year of life (Fig. 6.19). The following is a list that can be used as a guide to seeking medical attention:

• Fever greater than 100.4°F
• Difficult, labored breathing

Newborn–1 month	Infant gazes at audible objects.
	Dangle bells 8–10 inches above infant's crib.
	Introduce rattle.
	Play music from radio or music box.
2–3 months	Infant puts hands in mouth.
	Seat infant with an upright view of the environment.
	Provide reach-for objects and an unbreakable hand mirror.
4–5 months	Infant grasps objects and brings them to the mouth.
	Offer soft toys or a blanket to squeeze.
	Talk to infant and mimic sounds.
	Offer brightly colored toys.
	Jump or bounce infant on lap.
6–9 months	Baby drops food or object and waits for it to be retrieved.
	Offer squeaky toys, stuffed toys, or toys with movable parts.
	Play pat-a-cake and peek-a-boo.
	Name body parts.
	Take for rides in stroller.
10–12 months	Baby stacks one block on top of another.
	Baby scribbles with crayon on paper.
	Baby enjoys pull toys.
	Introduce book with animal pictures; read nursery rhymes.
	Play simple games with large ball.
	Blow bubbles in a cup.

- Unexplained rash
- Absence of stools or urine
- Persistent vomiting, diarrhea, or both
- Extreme lethargy or hyperirritability

Regular visits to the health center promote good health practices and health screening and allow the administration of necessary immunizations. Immunity is the body's ability to defend itself against foreign invaders such as bacteria and viruses. For the first 6 months of life, most infants have temporary natural immunity to measles (rubella), mumps, poliomyelitis, diphtheria, and scarlet fever. At present there is no immunization against certain infections, such as the common cold. For this reason, infants must be kept away from individuals with active infectious processes. See Appendix B for the complete recommended schedule of immunizations for this age group. Infants should receive the immunizations according to the prescribed schedule unless they have fever, a history of immunosuppression, or a history of allergy to the vaccine or its contents.

H E L P F U L   H I N T S

The following are some possible side effects to routine immunization:

Minor Signs
- Localized tenderness
- Irritability
- Erythema (redness)
- Swelling at site

Major Signs
- High fever (greater than 102°F)
- Loss of consciousness
- Paralysis
- Persistent, inconsolable crying

H E L P F U L   H I N T S

Caution

Acetaminophen should be used in place of aspirin for fever or discomfort because the use of aspirin for fever caused by viral infection may lead to Reye's syndrome.

TABLE
6.8 Infant Safety

Type of Accident	Prevention
Suffocation	Use firm mattress without plastic cover. Place infant on back; do not use pillows. Keep oven and refrigerator door closed.
Falls	Provide continuous direct supervision unless infant is in crib with guardrails raised.
Choking	Keep small sharp objects out of infant's reach. Avoid giving child such foods as nuts, hard candy, or seeds.
Poisoning	Keep medicines and household cleaning products out of reach.
Drowning	Do not leave unattended in tub or baby bathtub.
Burns	Provide direct continuous supervision around stove, fire, or faucet. Use flame-resistant clothing and bedding. Place guards over electrical outlets and around heating sources. Keep matches and lighters out of reach. Do not carry hot liquids while carrying or near baby.
Car accidents	Use car seat restraints that are federally approved for baby's or child's age; do not hold on lap in moving car. When using stroller, do not go behind a parked car; cross intersections with care.
Pet injury	Do not leave infants and young children unattended with pets.
Brain injury	Never shake an infant; shaking may cause brain injury.

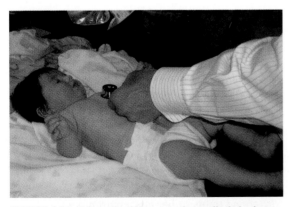

FIGURE 6.19 Infants should have regular medical checkups.

Another area of health promotion concerns the family and its support system. The birth of a baby adds stress to the other family members and changes the dynamics and roles the individuals play. Chapter 2 presents a complete description of the family during the childbearing stage. All health care workers should be alert to signs of family stress or possible child neglect or abuse. Child abuse—physical, emotional, and sexual mistreatment—can be manifested in many different ways. It is not isolated to any one family type or social class. All signs of possible abuse should be reported at once to the proper authorities. See Table 7.2 in Chapter 7 for a list of signs of abuse.

SUMMARY

1. Inherited characteristics are determined at the time of conception.

2. Any substance that can adversely affect the developing child is called a teratogen.

3. The period from fertilization to birth is called the prenatal period.

4. Immediately following fertilization, the new structure is called a zygote. It becomes a blastocyst at the time of implantation.

5. The developing structure is referred to as an embryo for the first few weeks and as a fetus thereafter.

6. Labor begins about 280 days after conception.

7. There are three distinct stages of labor: dilation; expulsion, or birth of the baby; and delivery of the placenta. The length of each of these stages varies with the individual.

8. Immediately after the delivery of the infant, the umbilical cord is clamped. This action ends fetal circulation and marks the infant's first breath.

9. The Apgar score is the first assessment of the newborn and is done at 1 and 5 minutes after birth. The Apgar scale assesses infant color, reflex irritability, heart rate, respiratory rate, and muscle tone, indicating the general neurological status of the newborn.

10. The infant's head is large in proportion to the rest of the body. The skull bones are soft to permit passage through the birth canal.

11. The infant's anterior fontanel should close by 12 to 18 months; the posterior fontanel closes by the fourth month.

12. An infant's average birth weight is 7.5 pounds. Average newborn length is 20 inches. Boys tend to be slightly larger than girls.

13. The newborn's skin is thin and delicate and varies in pigmentation. Common characteristics and skin conditions include vernix caseosa, milia, lanugo, mongolian spots, and physiological jaundice.

14. The newborn has the ability to swallow, digest, metabolize, and absorb nutrients. The first stool is passed within 10 hours after birth and is called meconium.

15. Primitive reflexes that are evident in a normal newborn include protective reflexes such as swallowing, gagging, sneezing, blinking, rooting, Moro, grasp, Babinski, and tonic neck.

16. The normal range for neonate vital signs is as follows: axillary temperature, 97.7°F to 99.5°F (36.5°C to 37.5°C); pulse, 120 to 140 beats per minute; blood pressure, 65/40 mm Hg (Dinamap); and respirations, 30 to 60 breaths per minute.

17. Gross motor skills involve the large muscles of the extremities. Growth and development follow an orderly cephalocaudal pattern, progressing downward from the head to the feet.

18. Fine motor control of the hands and fingers follows the proximodistal directional pattern; shoulder movements are mastered before hand and finger movements.

19. According to Eriksonian theory, the infant must master the critical task of trust to achieve healthy psychosocial development.

20. Cognitive development is evidenced by the cause-and-effect method the infant uses to respond to his or her new environment.

21. Infants begin to communicate with their caregivers soon after birth by smiling and babbling. By mimicking words, infants begin to build a vocabulary. By the time babies are 12 months old, they have a vocabulary of approximately 4 to 6 words.

22. The newborn's nutritional needs can be met by either breast milk or formula. Generally, solids are not offered before the fifth month to prevent food allergies or intolerances. When adding new foods to an infant's diet, it is best to add one new food at a time over the course of several days.

23. The typical newborn sleep pattern includes periods of light sleep marked by stirring movements and noises. Newborns typically sleep 20 out of 24 hours.

24. SIDS, or crib death, has been associated with abnormal infant sleep patterns. This condition occurs most frequently in the first 5 months of life. To decrease the risk of SIDS, it is recommended that healthy infants be placed on their back and sides, not their stomach, to sleep.

25. Play activities help infants explore and learn about their environments. Play during infancy is solitary. Infants need bright-colored toys free of small parts that could be accidentally ingested or aspirated.

26. Most injuries and deaths at this stage of development occur from preventable accidents. Supervision can help to decrease accidents and ensure safety. Health promotion is aimed at helping infants achieve optimal growth and development, which can be accomplished through good health practices, regular medical checkups, and immunization.

CRITICAL THINKING

Exercise #1

Joyce Whitaker, age 25, has been married for 2 years and wants to have children. Joyce is attending parenting classes at the local community hospital.

1. List two critical pieces of information you would share with Joyce to help her prepare a healthy internal environment for the fetus before she becomes pregnant.
2. Once Joyce becomes pregnant, what other measures would promote the delivery of a healthy baby?

Exercise #2

Sarah Greenoff, age 28, has been married for 8 years. Two months ago she gave birth to a baby girl named Tara. After Tara's birth, Sarah and her husband expressed concern about being effective parents. The couple was referred to the wellness clinic by the pediatric nurse practitioner.

1. Outline an assessment plan for the Greenoff family's first visit to the wellness clinic.
2. List the immunizations that are recommended for a 2-month-old infant.
3. Sarah Greenoff tells the nurse that her neighbor's baby died while asleep without any apparent warning. She is worried that the same thing might happen to Tara. Describe what information the nurse might share with Sarah to help relieve her anxiety.

Exercise #3

A woman delivers a full-term baby boy weighing 7 pounds, 4 ounces. Two days after discharge this breastfeeding mom is concerned because her infant now weighs 6 pounds, 10 ounces. The nurse's best explanation and advice is: _____

MULTIPLE-CHOICE QUESTIONS

1. Among European Jewish descendants you are more likely to see an increased incidence of:
   a. Cancer
   b. Diabetes mellitus
   c. Tay-Sachs disease
   d. Alcohol abuse

2. The period of development that begins 2 weeks after fertilization and lasts 8 weeks is known as the:
   a. Embryonic stage
   b. Fetal stage
   c. Pre-embryonic stage
   d. Blastocyst stage

3. Apgar scoring measures:
   a. The development of the fetus
   b. The newborn's neurological state
   c. The newborn's coping ability
   d. The gestational age of the neonate

4. The average length of a fully developed newborn baby is:
   a. 30 cm
   b. 40 cm
   c. 50 cm
   d. 60 cm

5. Which stool type is considered normal in breastfed babies?
   a. Solid, tan-colored stools
   b. Light, seeded-mustard stools
   c. Reddish-black stools
   d. Creamy-white stools

6. At birth most infants are:
   a. Able to hear sounds
   b. Nonreactive to smell
   c. Unresponsive to touch
   d. Unable to show taste preference

7. A 26-year-old woman gave birth to her first child, an 8-pound baby boy, 36 hours ago in a normal delivery. The health care worker reports that attachment is normal because of which of the following responses by the mother?
   a. Refuses to care for her child
   b. Frequently weeping and withdrawn
   c. States the baby looks like her sister
   d. When awake turns her back to the baby

8. The nurse can best help the mother of a newborn who decides to breastfeed her baby by (select all that apply):
   a. Telling her that all mothers should breastfeed
   b. Supporting her actions
   c. Providing education on breastfeeding
   d. Reminding her not to breastfeed the baby in public places
   e. Sharing with her that breastfeeding will prevent her from ever having postpartum depression

9. Which of the following activities demonstrates that Jeremy, age 6 months, has mastered the pincer grasp?
   a. He picks up a small morsel of food.
   b. He reaches out to grasp bright-colored objects.
   c. He brings his fingers to his mouth.
   d. He rolls over from his abdomen to his back.

10. Most infants with normal motor development can sit alone at age:
    a. 4 months
    b. 5 months
    c. 6 months
    d. 7 months

11. The typical 12-month-old child will:
   a. Coo
   b. Babble
   c. Say a few words
   d. Have fluent speech

12. The purpose of play during infancy is to:
   a. Promote toilet training
   b. Decrease hyperactivity
   c. Generate self-defense
   d. Aid exploration of the environment

13. The parents of a newborn infant should be
taught when handling their infant to support
the infant's head and avoid shaking to prevent:
   a. Seizure and death
   b. Difficulty feeding
   c. Intestinal bleeding
   d. Blood dyscrasia

14. Genes that can transmit their trait only if they
exist as a pair are known as:
   a. Dominant
   b. Recessive
   c. Karotype
   d. Heterozygous

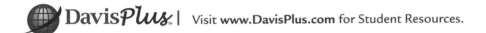

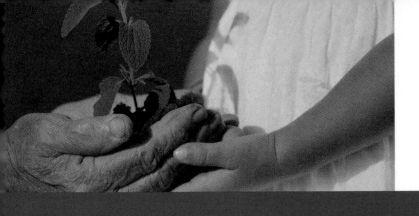

CHAPTER 7

Toddlerhood

Key Words

acuity

ambivalence

amblyopia

autonomy

child abuse

egocentric

eustachian tube

lordosis

negativistic behavior

object permanence

ossification

parallel play

regression

ritualistic behavior

separation anxiety

sibling rivalry

socialization

Chapter Outline

Learning Objectives

At the end of this chapter, you should be able to:

- Describe the main physical characteristics common to toddlers.
- Name three developmental skills that the toddler can master independently.
- Describe the psychosocial task of the toddler as outlined by Erikson.
- List one method of discipline useful in resolving conflicts during this stage.
- Describe the stage of cognitive development for the toddler as presented by Piaget.
- List two factors that help toddlers develop language skills.
- List three feeding recommendations for parents of toddlers.
- Describe the type of play typical of toddlers.
- Name five common safety hazards for this period of development.

The toddler period usually refers to the period from 1 to 3 years of age. After the fast growth spurts of infancy, the growth rate of the toddler is slow and steady. Many new skills are being developed, including both fine and gross motor skills related to dressing, feeding, toileting, and walking. Another accomplishment during this period is related to language development. These newly acquired skills serve to strengthen the toddler's newfound autonomy.

PHYSICAL CHARACTERISTICS

Height and Weight

The toddler usually grows an average of 3 inches (7.5 cm) per year. The average height of the child at 2 years is 34 inches (86.6 cm); at 3 years it is 37.25 inches (95 cm). The toddler gains an average of 4 to 6 pounds (1.8 to 2.7 kg) per year during this period. By age 2, the toddler's weight averages 27 pounds (12 kg). At 3 years, the child usually weighs 32 pounds (14.6 kg).

Body Proportions

The child's extremities grow much faster than the trunk, resulting in a more proportionate appearance for the body as a whole. The typical 2-year-old child has a potbellied appearance—a large belly and an exaggerated lumbar curve, known as lordosis. By the end of the third year, the child is taller and more slender, with stronger abdominal muscles and a more erect posture. Head growth slows down in comparison to the rate of growth in the body and extremities.

Face and Teeth

The face and jaw increase in size to permit room for more teeth. At 2½ years the child can be expected to have 20 teeth, which is a complete set of deciduous or primary teeth. Children at this age should visit the dentist for a preliminary dental examination and dental supervision (Fig. 7.1). Parents should discuss with their dentist the child's possible need for fluoride treatments, depending on their local water supplies. Parents should also help the child learn proper oral hygiene. Toddlers should brush their teeth at least twice a day under parental supervision. Some toddlers may continue a habit of thumb-sucking that may have started early in infancy. Experts vary in their opinions of the harmful effects of this habit.

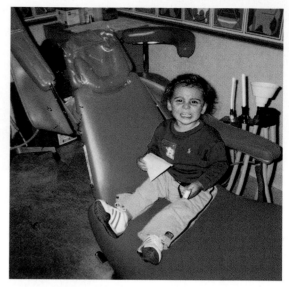

FIGURE 7.1 Toddlers should visit the dentist regularly.

Thumb-sucking may lead to malposition of the teeth. There is no easy, sure way of interrupting this habit; it is usually self-limiting. If it persists into the preschool years, parents should seek advice from a specialist.

Bone Development

Like the child's general growth, bone growth and development are greatest in the first year and then gradually slow down. As the child grows, the bones increase in density and hardness. Cartilage is gradually replaced with bone tissue. This process, known as ossification, will not be completed until puberty. The hardening of the soft, spongy tissues is gradual and occurs at different rates for different parts of the body. For example, by 18 months the toddler's anterior fontanel is closed, although other bones remain soft and pliable. This explains why infants and young children appear more flexible and can bend and put their toes into their mouths. In fact, this also explains why some young children develop a type of bone fracture known as a "greenstick fracture." In this fracture the bone is angulated beyond the limits of normal bending, similar to the bend in a green, unripe stick.

Sensory Development

The toddler's visual acuity changes gradually. The eye muscles strengthen, a process that further develops binocular vision. The toddler's vision may be 20/40—and better—when large objects are placed at a distance of 6 feet (2 m). Visual acuity will improve to 20/20 by the end of this stage. Depth perception improves as the child enters toddlerhood but is not fully developed until later during the preschool period.

Some children have a condition called "lazy eye," or amblyopia. Children with amblyopia have double vision but have no way of knowing it because they have nothing to compare it to. It is imperative that toddlers undergo vision screening to help detect this condition (Fig. 7.2). The current treatment for amblyopia involves patching the stronger eye to force the child to use the weak eye. Corrective lenses and exercises also help correct this condition. Untreated amblyopia can lead to blindness in the affected eye. *Strabismus,* or crossing of the eyes, may be seen from time to time; if it persists, professional attention is indicated.

Hearing in the toddler is fully developed. Routine physical examinations should include periodic hearing tests to detect any changes from the norm. Frequent monitoring should be done in a child with delayed speech or who has repeated ear, nose, and throat infections. One structure of the ear, called the eustachian tube, connects the middle ear to the oral pharynx. This structure is shorter and wider in toddlers than in older children, allowing easy passage of microorganisms from the upper respiratory tract to the middle ear. This accounts for a higher incidence of ear infections in the young child compared to the older child. Children with a history of ear infections can be at risk for hearing loss. A common sign of an ear infection in young children is unrelenting crying and rubbing or pulling of the affected earlobe.

VITAL SIGNS

The toddler's temperature-regulating mechanism is more stable and more fully developed than that of the infant. For this reason, the toddler is not so sensitive to environmental changes. The toddler's body temperature is maintained at the normal range of 98°F to 99°F (36.6°C to 37.2°C). The heart rate slows down because the heart is larger and more efficient. The average toddler's pulse rate is between 90 and 120 beats per minute. Respirations slow down to 20 to 30 breaths per minute as a result of increased lung efficiency and capacity. At this stage the average blood pressure measurement is 99/64 mm Hg.

DEVELOPMENTAL MILESTONES

Motor Development

The acquisition of skills in the toddler is based on the further development and refining of the crude gross and fine motor abilities achieved during infancy. The motivational force behind the development of these skills is rooted in the child's search for independence. By the end of toddlerhood, the child will have developed skills related to independent

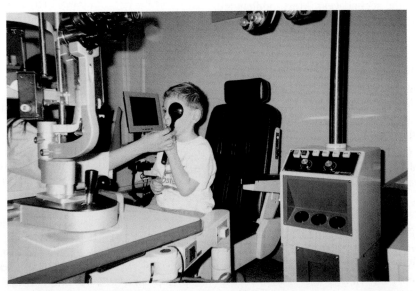

FIGURE 7.2 Eye examinations may detect vision problems.

functioning, including walking, eating, toileting, dressing, and using language.

Gross Motor Skills

Gross motor skills depend on growth and maturation of the muscles, bones, and nerves. Until a state of readiness is reached, teaching the child developmental skills such as walking, skipping, or hopping is of little value. Once readiness occurs, the child needs to be given ample time to practice and master each new skill attempted.

Walking, first with an unsteady gait, may begin for some children by their first birthday and for others several months later. Typical skills of the average 15-month-old toddler include walking alone without assistance, limited balancing, and creeping up stairs. The 18-month-old child typically can walk up stairs with both feet and sit down on a chair. The 18-month-old toddler runs clumsily, which results in frequent falling. The 2-year-old child can climb the stairs alone using two feet on each step, run with a wide stance, and kick a large ball without losing balance and falling. At this age, the typical child can walk down stairs with assistance, jump in place with both feet, and sit on a chair independently. The 3-year-old can hop, stand on one foot, and walk a few steps on tiptoe.

Fine Motor Skills

Fine motor skills include self-feeding, dressing, and playing. By 15 months, a toddler can more deftly grasp a spoon and insert it into a dish, but he or she will likely continue to invert and spill its contents until the end of the second year. Most toddlers are fascinated with dining utensils, but the majority use their fingers and prefer finger foods.

The 1-year-old child can usually remove his or her socks, shoes, hat, and mittens. By the end of the second year, the typical child can remove all of his or her clothing and will attempt to put some items back on, but only if he or she chooses to. Toddlers usually have enough fine motor dexterity to allow them to wash themselves. This is often seen as a pleasurable activity, but they frequently wash only the face and stomach while ignoring the rest of the body.

The 3-year-old child's fine motor coordination improves to permit him or her to now hold a crayon with the fingers instead of the fist. Three-year-old children can control drawing to include both vertical and circular strokes. There is slight evidence of hand preference during the first year of life. Usually infants reach for objects with both hands or with the hand closest to the object. Right- or left-hand dominance is evident by 15 months. Table 7.1 lists developmental milestones for a typical 3-year-old child.

Toilet Training

Using Freud's theory of *psychosexual* development, the toddler is at the anal stage, with the pleasurable area being the anus (see Chapter 5). Toilet training is often more important to the parents than to the young child. Successful toilet training depends on a certain degree of maturity in the toddler's muscles, including sphincter control, and maturation of the sensory centers of the brain. Furthermore, toddlers must develop a system of communication that allows them to alert parents of their needs (Fig. 7.3). The child uses either gestures or words to convey his or her need for toileting. Toddlers will learn bowel control before mastering bladder control. Usually children do not have this control until the second year—after walking for several months.

TABLE 7.1	Developmental Milestones for the 3-Year-Old Child
Gross motor	Balances on one foot Jumps on both feet Walks up steps using both feet Runs Rides a tricycle
Fine motor	Puts simple puzzles together Builds a tower of blocks Copies a circle or vertical line Turns knobs and opens lids
Psychosocial	Tolerates short separations from mother Dresses and undresses self Is possessive of own property Is nearly fully toilet trained
Cognitive	Searches and finds toys Locates body parts Knows relationship between things and persons Gives full name
Language	Uses words and gestures to indicate needs Uses two-word sentences Imitates sounds and words Sings simple songs Has increased vocabulary

Most children achieve daytime dryness long before nighttime dryness. Children of this age need help undressing and with the whole toileting process. By the time the child is 3½ years old, he or she is usually bladder trained. Changes in schedules, emotional stress, fatigue, or illness can often cause setbacks in toilet training. It is best to expect accidents at times when children are engrossed in play or simply miss the signals. These accidents should be handled in a matter-of-fact manner, without punishment, to help build the child's self-esteem.

Psychosocial Development

Autonomy

According to Erik Erikson, autonomy, or independence, is a major psychosocial task of the toddler (see Chapter 5). In particular, toddlers are trying to master independence in their daily activities, such as toileting, dressing, feeding, and taking care of their belongings (Fig. 7.4). Encouraging children to make simple decisions fosters a sense of independence. Freedom of choice, however, often sets the stage for conflicts between parent and child—that is, fostering autonomy does not preclude parental guidance. Many activities, particularly those concerning the child's safety, such as playing in the street, are nonnegotiable. How these conflicts, and mishaps

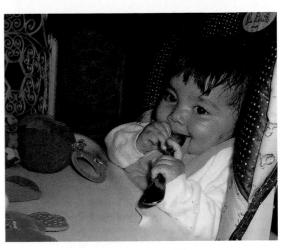

FIGURE 7.4 Self-feeding is an early skill to master.

and successes, are handled is critical to the toddler's developing self-esteem. If the toddler is punished for accidents and made to feel worthless, he or she develops a sense of shame and doubt. For example, if toddlers have accidents and soil their clothing, parents should not get angry and scold them. They should try to have a change of clothing handy and treat the accident as a minor event, saying, "You'll do better next time." Even with nurturing guidance, toddlers often develop conflicting emotions or feelings of ambivalence as they learn independent behaviors. For instance, toddlers may experience feelings of both love and hate for their caregivers when being reprimanded or disciplined. Toddlers may get angry with parents and say, "I hate you," but still want to be held and comforted.

Parents should be careful not to take over dressing the child who is attempting to carry out this skill. Although it is quicker for the parents to dress the toddler, it is better to support development of the child's independence by allowing him or her to practice these skills. Box 7.1 lists principles for understanding behavior.

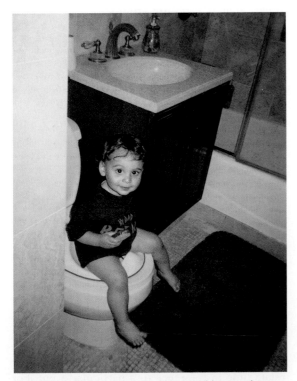

FIGURE 7.3 Toilet training should be a positive experience.

BOX 7.1 Principles for Understanding Behavior

- Behavior must be understood in the context in which it occurs by looking at all related factors.
- All behaviors have objectives and serve a purpose.
- The child's self-concept influences his or her behavior.
- Behavior helps the child maintain psychological equilibrium.
- The child's perception and interpretation of behavior influence his or her actions.

Discipline

Toddlers need discipline because they do not have enough information to understand what is acceptable or unacceptable behavior. A simple, direct "No" followed by some diversion will help lay the foundation for learning impulse control. It is crucial that caregivers be consistent and repeatedly reinforce limitations. Discipline should not deny the child freedom but rather give the child a greater opportunity to explore and learn within safe limits. Discipline should guide, correct, strengthen, and improve the child's choices. Nonnegotiable issues include items such as not hurting themselves or others, not destroying property, and not placing themselves in unsafe conditions such as a street. With these nonnegotiable issues the parents should give clear, simple instructions, such as, "Bobby is a friend to play with, not to hit!"

Sometimes discipline triggers temper tantrums or rebellious behavior. This **negativistic behavior** occurs as a result of frustration that the child encounters when his or her needs or wants are not met immediately (Fig. 7.5). The toddler is eager to take control and be independent beyond what skill or judgment allows. Toddlers have a limited vocabulary; this makes it difficult for them to express their feelings and may result in outbursts of kicking, screaming, and breath holding when they cannot

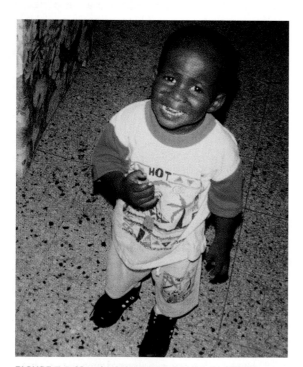

FIGURE 7.5 Negative behavior is related to the child's frustration.

have their way. Temper tantrums are commonly seen between ages 2 and 3 and diminish in intensity and frequency by ages 4 and 5 years. To avoid conflicts, parents can place less emphasis on minor issues and allow the child to make some choices. For example, the parents may find it better not to rush or hurry the dawdling child, or they may allow the child to postpone dressing until after breakfast. Giving choices when possible may help to reduce the number of conflicts and temper tantrums. If a tantrum occurs, the parents should ensure the child's safety and, if possible, leave the child in his or her room or limit the number of onlookers.

Another intervention that may be used to resolve a conflict of wills is the concept of "time-out." The child is usually removed from the center of activity to a quiet place where he or she can regain some control. Time-out should be immediate and used only for a few minutes. Following the time-out, the parent and child should talk about the events leading up to the conflict and possible solutions. This teaches the child to talk about what he or she is feeling and helps the child learn alternative solutions to problems.

The natural curiosity of toddlers makes it necessary for parents to identify and eliminate temptations. It is very common for 2-year-old children to demand that things go their way. It is usually best not to share plans in advance of an expected event. If the parent or caregiver promises to take the child to the park on the following day, the child may demand fulfillment of these plans regardless of bad weather or other happenings. Sometimes parents need to ignore attention-seeking behavior when it does not put the child at risk or in danger. Caregivers should remember to offer praise and positive reinforcement for desired behaviors. See Box 7.2 for tips on discipline.

Special Psychosocial Concerns

Toddlers are affected by what is called **separation anxiety**. As they become more independent, they can tolerate only brief periods of separation from their parents. Children in this age group are naturally warm and affectionate (Fig. 7.6), but they are still somewhat fearful of strangers unless they are accompanied by a family member. Parents should be honest about leaving or going out without the child and telling them when they will return. This helps reinforce to the child that his or her parents will come back as they said they would. Toddlers do not have a clear concept of time; rather, they relate time in reference to a particular event. For

Positive Parenting

Avoid saying:

- "Stop acting like a baby." This uses a negative label that hurts the child's feelings. It is better to focus on the behavior by saying, "You're crying because you're upset and mad at . . ."
- "There's no reason to be afraid." This makes the child feel that his or her worry is not important. It is better to acknowledge the fear and reassure with a simple explanation such as, "The noise you heard isn't a monster. It's the wind blowing against the window."
- "Why did you do that?" Very often young children don't understand *why* they acted in a certain way. Asking them why may be something that they are unable to explain. It is better to offer them an explanation for their behavior: "You grabbed the child's toy because you were angry with him." Or, "Can you tell me a better way to act?"

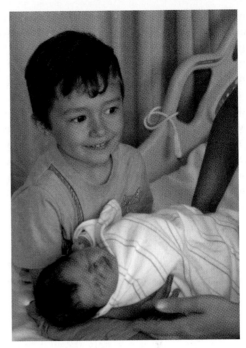

FIGURE 7.6 Toddlers are warm and affectionate.

7.2   Tips on Discipline

- Try to understand the reason for the misbehavior.
- Respect the child as a person.
- Be firm but kind.
- Be patient.
- Reward and praise often.
- Encourage open expression of feelings.
- Ignore negative behavior when safety allows.
- Provide a healthy environment.
- Listen and be attentive.
- Encourage independence.
- Avoid pity.
- Maintain control of emotions.
- Allow for trial and error.
- Reinforce consequences.
- Use familiar routines when possible.
- Model desired behaviors.
- Offer choices.

Giving Up Comfort Items

- Recognize the transitional object as a part of the child's journey toward independence.
- Try to offer a substitute item rather than insisting on removing the object.
- Allow enough time for the child to reach a state of readiness.

example, toddlers do not understand when noon is, but they can relate to lunch time. For this reason, when parents must leave they can best reassure their toddler that they will return after lunch or after their nap.

Toddlers sometimes use certain "comfort items" to decrease their anxieties. These items are often blankets, soft toys, or other common household items. These transitional objects, as they are sometimes called, are important to the child but often a concern to the parents. Children should not be expected to give up their transitional objects all at once. Significant changes in the child's life, such as arrival of a new sibling, a move, or the onset of preschool or day care, may cause stress and result in the need for the comfort item.

The birth of another child often creates **sibling rivalry**, or feelings of jealousy and insecurity in the toddler. It is difficult for a 2- or 3-year-old child to share time, attention, and parental affection with a brother or sister. Angry outbursts or regressive behavior may be seen in the toddler trying to deal with changes in the family brought about by the birth of a new baby.

Regression, a return to an earlier form of behavior with which the child felt comfortable and secure, can occur at any stressful time. It is not uncommon for the toilet-trained child to regress and have accidents, particularly following an illness or separation from parents. When this form of regression occurs, parents should minimize the significance and be confident that once the stressful period is over the child will return to normal behavior patterns. Sometimes after the birth of a new baby, the toddler may regress and want to use a bottle or be carried around like the newborn child. Parents should expect some regression and plan for special time alone with the older child to make him or her feel as important as the new baby.

Cognitive Development

Cognition continues to develop by trial and error. At 2 years of age the child begins what Piaget described as preoperational thought (see Chapter 5). The toddler's problem-solving abilities are limited. For example, the child may correctly identify a garbage receptacle but indiscriminately throw everything into the receptacle. The child also responds to the total situation rather than to a part. In other words, when objects and things have common elements, the child responds to them as if they were all the same. As memory begins to develop, many behaviors are imitated. The toddler's interpretation of new experiences is based on memory of previous happenings. For example, the toddler recognizes familiar objects and people and responds to them with pleasure but may demonstrate a fear of unfamiliar things and strangers.

Toddlers begin to experiment by trying out new ideas or actions. As the child's understanding of object permanence develops, his or her thinking follows a simple and direct pattern. Object permanence refers to the understanding that things will not disappear even if they cannot be seen. The child uses the further development of memory to create mental images. These mental images have a magical quality and are usually incorporated into the toddler's play. Events are seen as having a simplistic causal relationship. For example, toddlers believe that their own feelings can directly affect events. Some children are concerned that their angry thoughts may cause bad things to happen. Toddlers have an egocentric view of the world—that is, they cannot sense the world from any point of view other than their own. For example, a child grabs a toy from another child but cannot understand that this may hurt the other child's feelings. It is best for caregivers to simply explain that this behavior is not acceptable.

Time is still incompletely understood or can be interpreted by events within the child's own frame of reference. It is best to avoid using words like *tomorrow*, *yesterday*, or *next week*. It is clearer to the child if the speaker uses a familiar event to relate to a particular happening—for example, "We will go out to the park after your lunch." This is more meaningful than saying, "We will be going to the park in the afternoon."

Moral Development

As they grow, children learn their moral values based on their parents' moral codes and by imitating parental behavior and teachings. Parents begin to teach toddlers what is right and wrong. For example, toddlers are taught that it is wrong to stand in the car and that instead they must always be buckled and seated in their safety seats. Parents must use their own seat belts when driving or riding in a car. This sets a good example for children and helps to teach them right from wrong. Repeated instructions and consistency reinforce moral decisions. All caregivers should work together as a team to help instill the same principles. Respect between the parent and child teaches the toddler that justice is reciprocal. Reasonable discipline that draws on the respect for others is an integral part of the child's own moral development. Learning socially acceptable behaviors is a long, slow process that begins in this stage and extends through adolescence. Refer to Box 7.3 for tips on promoting self-esteem.

Communication

Language acquisition is automatic and spontaneous. Language skills are enhanced with practice. Encouraging children's speech and reading to them help build language skills. The language of toddlers is based on symbolic function and memory. This means that their words not only name things, but

---

B O X
7.3   Promoting Self-Esteem

- Attend to the child's needs immediately.
- Spend special time with the child.
- Ignore minor mishaps.
- Listen attentively.
- Convey positive regard.
- Label behavior, not the child.
- Give positive feedback.
- Be congruent with communication.
- If indicated, offer an apology.

also show understanding of the meaning. In other words, when the child uses the word "potty," he or she means the process of toileting. Cognitive development and imitation play important roles in early language acquisition. Children understand what is said to them before they are able to put their thoughts into words.

Early on, sentence structure may not be correct and pronunciation may be unclear, but toddlers are still able to complete their intended messages. Sometimes only the immediate caregivers can understand the child's language. The first sentences consist of a noun or a verb. Toddlers quickly develop the ability to use nouns or verbs in a two-word sentence. "Me go" is an example of an early sentence. To make the two-word sentence clearer, most toddlers use hand gestures to support the meaning of their words.

Most 2-year-old children are able to use words to represent their actions and make their needs known. For example, if a toddler is thirsty, he or she may repeatedly say, "juice" until the need is met. When the toddler learns the use of the word "why," he or she often uses it to challenge adults and keep them talking. This dialogue ultimately helps the child to learn more about the world. By 2½ to 3 years of age, the toddler begins to use short, three-word sentences. Toddlers often confuse the pronouns "I" and "me." "Mine" becomes a part of the child's vocabulary rapidly thereafter because at this time the child begins to show awareness of ownership. Everything becomes "mine." From a vocabulary of 50 words at age 2, the child moves rapidly to a vocabulary of 1,000 words by age 3. The 3-year-old child can put a noun and verb together to create a short sentence such as, "I go" or "Give it to me."

Young children living in a bilingual family can learn more than one language at the same time. Bilingualism is possible for the toddler if both languages are used in the home. When one language is used at home and another at playgroup or nursery school, it is much more difficult for the child to learn the second language.

NUTRITION

The toddler needs to establish good eating patterns because the eating habits taught at this stage will be lifelong. Because toddlers' eating habits are easily influenced by the eating preferences of older siblings and parents, other family members need to model good eating practices. It is especially important that caregivers provide toddlers with the appropriate amounts of foods from the various categories in the food pyramid or MyPlate chart. See Chapter 1 for the MyPlate chart and further discussion.

Toddlers particularly need foods that allow muscle development and mineralization of the bones—foods containing adequate protein, calcium, iron, phosphorus, and vitamins. Three servings of vegetables and three to four servings of fruits per day will provide the needed vitamin C. Offer foods with adequate fiber, and provide iron-rich foods such as cereals, meats, and fruits. Because most children continue to like milk, its intake must be monitored and limited to 1 quart per day. The need for milk will decrease as the amount of solid foods increases. By age 2 to 3 years, the child should be eating the same foods as the rest of the family.

Most toddlers need about 1,300 calories a day, although the amount of food needed varies greatly, depending on the child and his or her activity level. The child who is very active needs more calories than the child who is sedentary.

Allowing a toddler to select junk food, including food high in sugar, is detrimental to the child's nutritional state (Fig. 7.7). Snacks, like meals, need to be nutritious. Avoid or only sparingly give candy and other sugar-concentrated foods. The calories, protein, and other vital nutrients of snacks must be considered part of the child's daily nutritional intake.

Caregivers can comply with many of the toddler's food preferences and still offer nutritious foods. Most toddlers prefer plain foods to mixtures. They will learn about textures from a variety of foods offered. Foods that are easy to manipulate and chew are among toddlers' favorites. For example,

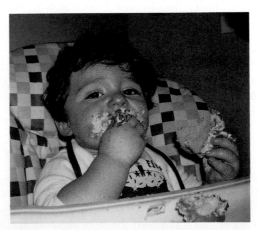

FIGURE 7.7 Sweets should be limited in the toddler's diet.

hand-held sandwiches, bite-size pieces of meats, pizza, pasta, and fruits are some of their favorite foods. Initially young toddlers bite and chew with their front teeth; however, as the back teeth (molars) appear, they will begin to chew in the back of the mouth. Because toddlers have their full set of deciduous teeth by 2½ years of age, they are able to chew and swallow all sorts of table foods.

It is not uncommon for children of this age to develop ritualistic behavior in relation to eating. For example, toddlers sometimes prefer using the same plate or cup at each meal. Their ritualistic preferences may be upsetting to caregivers, but it is best to remember that such behavior is typical for many toddlers. In addition, toddlers may develop food fads or habits. For instance, they may go for a time not eating or eating only small amounts every day. Common reasons for toddlers not eating include excitement or distraction, exhaustion, illness, lack of hunger, and attention seeking. Sometimes, a toddler will want to eat only peanut butter sandwiches day after day. Eating the same foods—although seemingly boring from an adult perspective—will not be detrimental to a child's nutrition if the foods selected contain the appropriate nutrients. Also, a food fad is likely to disappear just as suddenly as it began.

Toddlers also like consistency and familiar routines at mealtimes. These qualities foster good eating habits; thus meals should be at the same time each day. Because toddlers' stomach capacity is small, caregivers should plan for three small meals along with three nutritious snacks. See Box 7.4 for tips for nutritious snacks.

Mealtimes should be used to promote family time together and socialization of the toddler, including promotion of the child's autonomy in self-feeding. It is best at this stage to offer simple choices such as, "Would you like cereal or toast for breakfast?" This is better than offering vague choices such as, "What do you want for lunch?" Children sometimes test their autonomy by refusing to eat. Toddlers may also refuse to eat because their appetites fluctuate and they may not be hungry at mealtime. Caregivers should be careful not to offer snacks too close to mealtimes. Toddlers may also be too tired, excited, or distracted to eat. Sometimes refusal to eat is an attention-seeking behavior. It is best to ignore most refusals because they are usually short-lived: The child will eat when he or she is hungry. At times, toddlers will play with their food or dawdle. They need to be given adequate time to finish eating but not so much time that one meal runs into the next.

Caregivers should give as little attention to a toddler's negative behaviors at mealtimes as possible. To promote good eating habits and socialization of the child, mealtime should not be stressful. Parents should expect that accidents and spills will happen and react matter-of-factly to unintentional happenings. The toddler can be taught simple table manners—for example, how to use the correct eating utensils. Using the proper utensil also enhances fine motor coordination. Eating utensils can be of normal size or sized for a child, if desired. Caregivers should provide positive reinforcement for desired mealtime behaviors. Sometimes setting the table with a special cloth or with the "fancy" dinnerware helps to show toddlers that they are growing up and able to use the "grown-up stuff." See Box 7.5 for tips for fostering good eating habits.

SLEEP AND REST

Toddlers sleep less than infants and often resist sleep because they want to play and be involved in adult activities. Short nap periods during the day help prevent toddlers from becoming overtired. Bedtime should include a ritual such as reading to the child

---

B O X
7.4 Tips for Nutritious Snacks

- Snacks can be an excellent means of providing additional calories, proteins, and other vital nutrients.
- Avoid offering snacks immediately before mealtimes.
- Avoid the use of foods high in sugar with little nutritional value (for example, candy or processed baked goods).
- Choose healthy snacks such as cheese cubes, fresh fruits, raw vegetables, milk, crackers, dried cereals, dried fruits, peanut butter on bread or crackers, or plain low-fat yogurt.

B O X
7.5 Fostering Proper Eating Habits

- Encourage the toddler to taste new foods.
- Introduce new foods in small amounts along with regular foods.
- Use child-sized portions.
- Present colorful foods of different textures.
- Eat with the child.
- Never force a child to eat.
- Provide a comfortable atmosphere.
- Minimize confusion at mealtimes (for example, turn off the television).
- Recognize that accidents or spills will occur.

and allowing him or her to have a comfort toy such as a teddy bear or blanket. Ritualistic behavior or habitual acts surrounding bedtime practices can establish a familiar routine for the child to follow. Such rituals help reduce anxiety and give the child a sense of security.

Sleep disturbances caused by nightmares that awaken and frighten the child are not unusual. The child usually resists sleep after a bad dream because of fear. The events surrounding the nightmares usually appear real and lifelike, and the child needs to be comforted. The period of comfort should be brief, and it is usually recommended that parents comfort the child in the child's room rather than taking the child to their own bed. Toddlers should understand that each person in the family has his or her own space for sleeping. Taking the toddler into the parents' bed may set up a habit that later can be hard to undo. Other factors that can produce sleep disturbance in the toddler include fear of separation from the parent, illness, and physical exhaustion.

PLAY

Play is a very important activity in the toddler years and is the major means by which children continue to explore and understand the world around them. At first, play mimics the activities performed by others around the toddler, such as talking on the telephone. This type of mimicking is not only pleasurable, but also helps the toddler try out adult roles. By 2 years of age, the play appears to be symbolic rather than nonsymbolic, as is the play of infants. Nonsymbolic play is demonstrated when the young child squeezes a soft ball. Piaget described symbolic play as the emergence of make-believe and pretense. Objects become the symbol, or represent something else slightly similar. Children between the ages of 2 and 4 years most often engage in symbolic play. It is thought that symbolic play helps children to explore different possibilities, control aggression through fantasy, and pretend. An example of symbolic play is building a castle or city with blocks. Other examples of symbolic play are when a child first pretends to drink from a cup and later pretends to feed a doll. Parents have the fundamental responsibility for guiding their children's play by modeling desired activities.

Play is good in that it helps ego and development, cognition, and socialization. Many 2- and 3-year-old children are enrolled in some type of structured playgroup. Even though they cannot always interact with other children at play, they benefit from being in the presence of children of the same age group who are learning socializing skills. Playgroups may also be beneficial for the mother or caregiver, allowing them time to be with other siblings or by themselves. Children with working parents may develop similar social skills in a day-care setting. Although children are encouraged to play with other children, many confrontations occur over playthings. Toddlers usually prefer **parallel play,** in which they play alongside other children without interactions.

As toddlers develop language proficiency and the capacity to think, they are capable of incorporating their elaborate imaginations into their play activities (Fig. 7.8). Many 3-year-old children, for instance, develop imaginary playmates. Girls tend to have imaginary playmates more often than boys do. These imaginary friends are often blamed by the child when accidents or other mistakes occur. This type of play is a very normal part of development and should be treated with sensitivity by caregivers.

The selection of playthings is one of the many critical decisions parents have to make (Box 7.6). Toys foster fine and gross motor development and entertain the toddler. Push toys, riding toys, swings, and pots and pans assist with gross motor development. Finger

---

HELPFUL   HINTS

Resolving Sleep Problems

- Set a consistent routine, and remember that you cannot force a child to sleep.
- Encourage quiet rituals before bedtime.
- Use a nightlight if the darkened room frightens the child.
- Remember that not all children require the same amount of sleep.

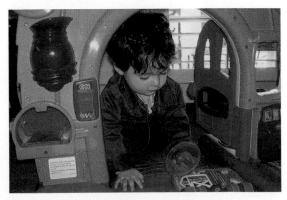

FIGURE 7.8 Toddlers use their imagination in play.

painting, drawing, puzzles, and building blocks strengthen fine motor development. Some 2-year-old children like to unscrew tops from bottles, open boxes and containers, turn pages in a book, and cut with scissors. Toddlers should use safety scissors with supervision from a grown-up. Musical instruments help provide rhythm and exploration (Fig. 7.9). Many of the objects used in these favorite activities are readily found in the home.

Electronic Devices, Television, and Toddlers

Many parents allow their infants and toddlers to use tablets and smartphones to keep the child occupied and decrease crying. The concern with infants and toddlers using these devices is that they provide no or very little sensory stimulation. They do not have a texture, smell, or taste and do not stimulate fine motor skills.

At this age children are great imitators and look to use these devices as they see others doing. Parents should limit the amount of time they spend using tablets or smartphones around their children.

BOX 7.6 Play and Playthings for Young Toddlers

Parallel play: Plays alongside other children but does not interact or share

Playthings: Uses tricycles, swings, climbers, rocking horse, color cubes, paint and brushes, and simple musical instruments such as drums or bells

---

If toddlers are allowed to play with these devices, parents should choose applications that allow the child to draw, color, or arrange puzzles. Parents should play along with the child and teach colors and vocabulary, remembering that the more parents talk to the child, the more he or she will learn.

About 90% of parents report that their child under the age of 2 years watches some form of electronic media or television. Some programs may be beneficial to children under 2 years, but there is no scientific proof. What research *has* shown is that overuse of media can cause language delay. As a result of these findings the American Academy of Pediatrics has suggested limiting the use of media to less than 2 hours per day, parental review of program content, and never placing a television in the child's bedroom.

SAFETY

Because of their natural curiosity and explorative behavior, toddlers are prone to accidents (Fig. 7.10 and Fig. 7.11). Accidents are the leading cause of death in children of this age and the most frequent reason why medical services are sought. Most accidents are preventable, and prevention requires parental education. The toddler requires constant supervision because there are many hazards both inside and outside the home. Toddlers are incapable of recognizing danger or threats to their safety; this, along with their curiosity, places them at great risk for injury.

Recent statistics indicate that, in this age group, more than half of all accidents that result in death or

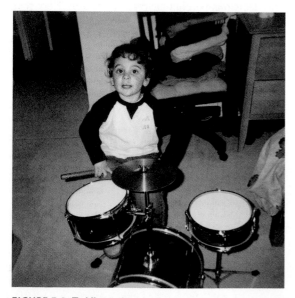

FIGURE 7.9 Toddlers enjoy musical instruments.

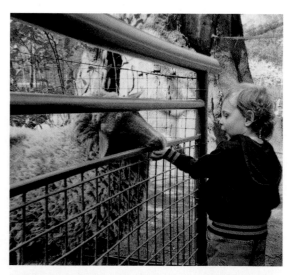

FIGURE 7.10 Toddlers show an interest in animals at the zoo.

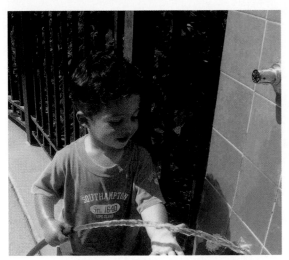

FIGURE 7.11 Toddlers are fascinated by water and a hose.

serious injury are motor vehicle accidents. Car safety seats and restraints are regulated and strictly mandated by state laws to reduce the numbers of injuries and deaths. Children must be taught what is expected of them with regard to car safety. For example, the child must know that he or she is expected to be seated in the proper seat and restrained when in any vehicle.

Car windows and door handles should be off-limits to all young children. However, many car seats are installed next to the window in the back seat, putting the door handle and window controls within the child's reach. Child safety locks for car doors and windows are standard on most cars sold in the United States. When used correctly, the window buttons and door handles are disabled and prevent curious toddlers from opening their doors or windows. These locks must be activated by the driver. A consistent approach to rules pertaining to car safety, or safety in general, will better ensure a child's compliance.

In this age group, injuries resulting from burns rank second to those from motor vehicle accidents. Safety in the kitchen includes removing stove knobs and turning pot handles toward the back of the stove to prevent spills. Cover electrical sockets with safety caps when not in use to prevent shocks. Children are at risk for burns from hot liquid spills, hot bath water, or playing with matches.

Play areas should be carefully selected to provide child safety. Children should not play near roads or in active driveways. Continuous watchful supervision is necessary to prevent accidents. No child of this age can be trusted to remember all the safety rules or be able to recognize potential dangers.

The ingestion of poisons is another safety hazard as the toddler begins to climb and open drawers and closets. Special care must be taken in storing household cleaning agents, garden products, car products, and prescription and nonprescription drugs. These agents should be stored on a high shelf out of the reach of children and securely locked. Parents should never refer to medicine as candy or say that it tastes good; otherwise, toddlers may be tempted by it. Parents should make it a point not to take their own medications in front of their children so that their behavior is not copied. All caregivers should have the national poison control number (800-222-1222) readily available in the event of accidental poisoning.

Choking or aspirating a small object is a continued concern for this age group, just as it is for infants, particularly because toddlers often eat food on the run. Certain food items have been identified as frequent offenders. They include hard candies, popcorn, fruit pits or seeds, and large pieces of meat. Other potential safety hazards are toys with small removable parts that can be placed in the child's mouth and either swallowed or aspirated. This kind of toy should not be given to young children. Suffocation can be avoided by advising parents not to use plastic coverings on beds or furniture. Balloons have been implicated in many toddler deaths: While attempting to blow up a balloon, toddlers may accidentally inhale the deflated balloon into the windpipe, obstructing the airway.

Drowning accounts for high numbers of deaths in this age group. Drowning can occur in the bathtub, swimming pool, or another body of water—even in only a few inches of water. Supervise toddlers at all times during bathing. Adult supervision and teaching children to swim can make water a safe, fun activity (Fig. 7.12).

HEALTH PROMOTION

Regular physical examinations should be scheduled for toddlers. These examinations include monitoring the child's growth patterns, health screening, identification and correction of any deviation, education, and disease prevention. Visits to the health provider should be scheduled when the child is 18, 24, and 36 months old. A history and physical examination is done at each yearly visit; it should include an assessment of the child's growth and development. At the 24-month checkup, the child will need to be screened for tuberculosis. To strengthen parenting

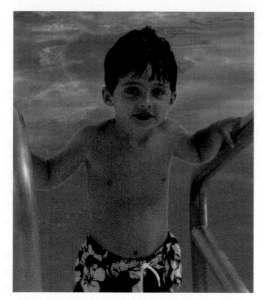

FIGURE 7.12 Water safety is important

TABLE 7.2	Signs of Child Abuse
Physical abuse	Bruises, welts (may be at different stages of healing)
	Signs of multiple fractures at different stages of healing
	Lacerations or tears
	Cigarette or immersion burns on extremities or buttocks
	Head injuries
	Swollen, blackened eyes
Sexual abuse	Difficulty walking or sitting
	Bruises or bleeding from genitalia
	Recurrent urinary tract infections
	Symptoms of sexually transmitted diseases
	Inappropriate sexual behavior in young teenagers
Psychological /affective abuse	Excessive anger, aggression
	Poor peer relationships
	Negativism, loss of pleasure
	Low self-esteem, lack of trust
	Developmental delays
	Withdrawn behavior, regression

skills, child-rearing classes may be indicated. Toddlers should receive the measles, mumps, and rubella vaccine at 12 to 15 months of age. The varicella vaccine is currently recommended for 12- to 15-month-old toddlers. The complete schedule of recommended immunizations is found in Appendix B.

Child Abuse

Health care workers, caregivers, and teachers should be alert for signs of mistreatment or abuse. Abuse of any kind can occur in any family type and at any level of social standing. Child abuse can include physical, emotional, and sexual mistreatment. See Table 7.2 for the common signs of child abuse.

Child abuse is defined as any recent act or failure to act by a parent or caregiver that results in death, serious physical or emotional harm, sexual abuse, or exploitation. In some cases, the failure of the parent or caregiver to act places the child at imminent risk for serious harm. This law targets persons under 18 years old who, in the care of a parent or caregiver, suffered a sustained injury or harm. However, the law also holds all health care workers who interact with children responsible for assessing and reporting suspected abuse or maltreatment. Primary care providers are in a unique position to identify children experiencing abuse or neglect during well-child and other visits. The law does not require the health care worker to be sure the abuse has taken place; "suspicion is all that is necessary" for the abuse to be reported and child services to investigate. There are four common forms of abuse or maltreatment: physical abuse, neglect, psychological abuse, and sexual abuse.

Physical Abuse

Physical abuse is any nonaccidental physical injury that a child sustains while being cared for by a parent or caregiver. This includes bruising; hitting with any object (for example, a belt or hands); shaking, commonly seen in infancy and toddler years; burning with cigarettes, flames, or hot liquids; kicking; choking; biting; or stabbing. This category also includes any verbal threats of harm.

Neglect

Neglect is the failure of a parent or caregiver to provide for the basic physiological needs of the child, such as food, clothing, shelter, medical care, or supervision. As a result, the parent or caregiver causes harm and injury to the child's health, safety, and well-being. The first type of neglect is educational. Educational neglect describes parents or caregivers who fail to comply with a school authority complaint of chronic absence from school, a failure to enroll a child in school, or a failure to provide special education needs for a child who has been diagnosed with a learning disorder.

The second form of neglect is when a parent or caregiver places the child in an environment where there is chronic exposure to domestic violence or spousal abuse or allows the child to use drugs or alcohol.

The third form of neglect is abandonment. In some states abandonment is a form of abuse or neglect, especially when the parent or caregiver leaves the child and does not explain where the child will be, how the child can be contacted, or if (or when) the child will return. The child is left in an environment without reasonable support and as a result can sustain serious physical, sexual, or emotional harm.

Psychological Abuse

Psychological abuse describes attitudes and behavior by the parent or caregiver that interfere with the child's mental and social well-being. This includes belittling, shaming, yelling, and failing to provide the needed love and affection that will foster growth and development and the child's physical health.

Sexual Abuse

All states include sexual abuse in their definitions of child abuse. Sexual exploitation is also considered child abuse. Sexual exploitation is when a parent or caregiver allows the child to engage in prostitution or in the production of child pornography. Sexual abuse is the act of touching or introducing anything into the vaginal or anal cavity other than when providing needed care. This includes anal or vaginal intercourse, oral sex, verbal seduction, and threats. Many individuals sexually abuse children, and parents and caregivers must be mindful that offenders can be family members, friends, neighbors, babysitters, and clergy. Findings of sexual abuse include symptoms of sexually transmitted diseases; injury to the genital area; difficulty and/or pain when sitting or walking; and sexually suggestive, inappropriate, or promiscuous behavior in teenagers.

SUMMARY

1. Toddlerhood refers to the period of development from 12 months to 3 years of age.

2. Growth rates of toddlers are slower than those of infants. Growth during this period results in the body appearing more proportionate with a taller, more slender look.

3. Bone development continues with a gradual hardening or ossification.

4. By 2½ years of age, toddlers usually have a complete set of deciduous teeth. Children at this age must visit the dentist for dental examination and treatment to help ensure healthy teeth later in life.

5. Gradually, visual acuity will improve and can be enhanced with the use of large objects held at close range. Hearing is fully developed and should be tested during periodic examinations.

6. Heart rate, respiratory rate, and blood pressure readings will decrease during the toddler period.

7. Gross and fine motor skills develop further.

8. By the end of toddlerhood, the child gains skills related to walking, eating, toileting, dressing, and communicating independently.

9. Development of gross motor skills depends on growth and maturation of muscles, bones, and nerves. Teaching new skills is of little value until a state of readiness is reached.

10. Fine motor skills achieved during this stage are related to self-feeding, dressing, and playing. By the end of toddlerhood, children should be actively participating in dressing, washing, and brushing their teeth.

11. Freud's theory of psychosexual development places the toddler at the anal stage, with the pleasurable area being the anus. Toilet training can be successful once the child has achieved a degree of maturity in sphincter muscles, nerves, and language.

12. Autonomy (independence) is a primary psychosocial task of toddlers. It encourages toddlers to make decisions, especially in their activities of daily living.

13. Two-year-old children need guidance and discipline. Caregivers should be consistent and repeatedly reinforce limitations. Limits should not deny children freedom; limits should give them greater opportunity to explore.

14. Piaget suggested that toddlers interpret new experiences based on memory of previous happenings. This is referred to as *preoperational thought*.

15. Moral development depends on children imitating their parents' moral behavior and teachings.

16. Language acquisition develops along with memory and cognition. Young toddlers use one-word sentences. Three-year-old children have a vocabulary of approximately 1,000 words and use multiple words in a sentence.

17. Toddlers need a well-balanced diet and good eating habits to support muscle and bone growth. Food amounts vary greatly depending on individual activity levels. Likes and dislikes are influenced by other family members' dietary habits. Foods that are most frequently accepted are those that the child can eat as he or she moves about.

18. Sleep needs decrease during this stage of development. However, short naps are still indicated. Bedtime rituals are common; they help reduce anxiety and give the child a sense of security. Nightmares should be handled in a consistent, comforting manner.

19. Play is the major means by which the child continues to explore and understand the world. Toddlers usually prefer parallel play. Imaginary play and imaginary playmates are common and normal at this stage.

20. Electronic media, tablets, and other devices, while commonly available to young children, offer them no or very little sensory stimulation. The American Academy of Pediatrics recommends limiting the use of electronic media by toddlers to less than 2 hours per day, parental review of program content, and never placing a television in the child's bedroom.

21. Natural curiosity and the child's inability to recognize danger make accident prevention extremely important at this stage. For this reason, toddlers require continuous supervision in all of their activities.

22. Schedule regular physical examinations for toddlers. These visits should be at 18, 24, and 36 months. Dental examinations are scheduled when children have their complete set of deciduous teeth.

23. Health care workers and others should be alert for signs of mistreatment or abuse in children. Child abuse can include child neglect and physical, psychological, and sexual mistreatment. Under the law, health care works are responsible for assessing patients for abuse and reporting suspected abuse to authorities.

CRITICAL THINKING

Exercise #1

Ms. Sterdowski brings Eric, 28 months of age, to the clinic because she believes that he is not thriving. She explains that he walks alone without assistance but only attempts to say about four words. His pronunciation is unclear to anyone outside of the immediate family. She states that she has not yet been successful with potty training him. She further explains that her older child had mastered all these skills and more by this age.

1. Describe the best approach to use to reassure Ms. Sterdowski that Eric is developing normally.
2. Based on expected growth timetables, what is the best interpretation of Eric's performance?

> **CRITICAL THINKING** (continued)
>
> **3.** List three instructions that should be given to assist Ms. Sterdowski with accomplishing toilet training.
>
> **Exercise #2**
>
> The parents of a 2½-year-old toddler are anxious that they are not able to get their child to agree to their wishes. They report that all he does is say "No." What advice could you offer these parents?

MULTIPLE-CHOICE QUESTIONS

1. Toddlers' motivation to acquire and master most psychomotor skills is related to their need for:
   a. Balance
   b. Independence
   c. Sameness
   d. Dominance

2. A child usually has a complete set of deciduous teeth by age:
   a. 12 months
   b. 18 months
   c. 24 months
   d. 30 months

3. Fine motor skills that should be mastered by 3 years of age include:
   a. Holding the spoon with the fist
   b. Using a crayon to draw a circle
   c. Drawing a complete face
   d. Recognizing dangerous situations

4. Toilet training depends on the child's ability to:
   a. Sit alone on the toilet
   b. Attain sphincter control
   c. Want to please the parents
   d. Properly digest a regular diet

5. According to Erikson, the psychosocial task for the toddler is:
   a. Trust
   b. Initiative
   c. Autonomy
   d. Industry

6. Moral development in the toddler is based on:
   a. Innate instincts
   b. Mature behavior
   c. Promptly meeting needs
   d. Copying parental values

7. The type of play seen in a 2-year-old child is:
   a. Solitary play
   b. Parallel play
   c. Cooperative play
   d. Competitive or team play

8. The overuse of electronic media in toddlers may lead to:
   a. Weight loss
   b. Language delay
   c. Slowed fine motor skills
   d. Aggressive personality

9. Toddlers resist sleep because of:
   a. Overeating
   b. Fear
   c. Apprehension
   d. Curiosity

10. Parents of a 2-year-old should look around their house for potential safety hazards. They should remember that a 2-year-old should be able to:
    a. Bathe alone
    b. Use a knife safely
    c. Take medicine independently
    d. Climb up and down stairs

11. Rash, who is 2½ years old, cried when his mother had to leave him with their babysitter. The best way to tell him when she is returning home is to say:
   a. "She'll be back at 12:30."
   b. "She'll be back a little later."
   c. Don't offer a time—just distract him.
   d. "She'll be back after naptime."

12. The thinking style associated with the toddler is best described as:
   a. Imaginative
   b. Competitive
   c. Industrious
   d. Egotistic

13. Toddlers may handle periods of stress with the following coping mechanism:
   a. Denial
   b. Repression
   c. Regression
   d. Sublimation

14. Which of the following statements about child abuse is correct?
   a. Health care workers must investigate and prove child abuse before reporting it.
   b. Only strangers tend to abuse a child.
   c. Health care workers need only to report suspicion of child abuse.
   d. The child abuse law targets children from 2 to 21 years old.

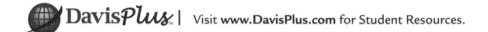

Davis*Plus* | Visit www.DavisPlus.com for Student Resources.

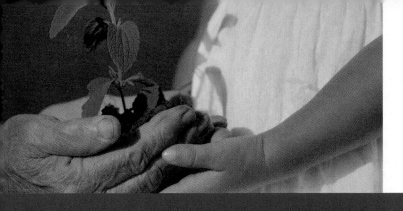

CHAPTER 8

Preschool

Key Words

adducted

centration

conscience

cooperative play

enuresis

initiative

night terrors

reversibility

Learning Objectives

At the end of this chapter, you should be able to:

- Describe the physical changes that commonly occur during the preschool years.
- List two gross motor skills characteristic of preschoolers.
- Describe the psychosocial task of the preschooler as outlined by Erikson.
- List the important guidelines useful in assessing a nursery school program.
- Describe the stage of cognitive development for the preschool child as presented by Piaget.
- List three appropriate snack foods for preschool children.
- Describe the type of play characteristic of preschoolers.
- List the safety concerns important to the preschool stage of development.
- Name two common behavioral concerns affecting preschoolers.

The preschool period generally refers to ages 3 to 6 years. The rate of growth during the preschool period is slow and steady. Preschoolers are focusing on refining their gross and fine motor skills, improving their vocabularies, and increasing their knowledge of the environment. Characteristically, children by this stage have mastered some autonomy and are moving toward a creative exploration of their potential. Preschool children are usually ready to spend more time away from their homes and caregivers and often attend preschool or nursery school.

PHYSICAL CHARACTERISTICS

Height and Weight

The trunk and body lengthen, giving the child a taller appearance. On average, preschool children gain 5 to 7 pounds (2.3 to 3.2 kg) a year. Most children grow 2½ to 3 inches (6.75 to 7.5 cm) per year.

Body Proportions

During the preschool period, children lose some subcutaneous or adipose tissue, which accounts for their more slender look. Growth patterns vary with each child. The rate of growth for the extremities is faster than for the trunk, resulting in more adultlike proportions. The protuberant abdomen and exaggerated lumbar curvature (lordosis) of toddlerhood disappear. The head and neck decrease in size in proportion to that of the rest of the body.

Muscle and Bone Development

Rapid growth in the muscles accounts for approximately 75% of the weight gain during this period. Heredity, nutrition, and actual muscle use play a role in stimulating muscle growth and increasing muscle strength.

The hips gradually rotate inward, causing a more adducted foot position. The adducted movement causes the foot to move toward the center of the body, resulting in a more erect posture and steady gait and making the child appear less awkward and clumsy.

During this stage of development, fat replaces the red marrow in the long bones. From this time on, marrow is found in the flat bones of the body such as the skull, sternum or breastbone, vertebrae, and pelvic bones. Red marrow helps the body to produce blood cells.

Teeth

Deciduous teeth are important for nutrition and because they help prepare for the child's permanent teeth. During the preschool years, many children develop dental decay and plaque buildup. Care of the teeth should include daily brushing, flossing, and visits to the dentist at least every 6 months. Proper care and dietary practices may help to avoid excessive tooth destruction. Recommendations for promoting dental health are listed in Box 8.1. Preschool children should be encouraged to eat snacks that are low in carbohydrates, such as apples, celery, carrots, and cheese. These snacks are nutritious and help prevent tooth decay.

Sensory Development

Visual acuity improves to 20/20 at about 3 years of age. The lack of depth perception contributes to some of the clumsiness that is still characteristic of the early preschool years. Depth perception and color detection are fully established by age 5. Maximum visual ability is achieved by the end of the preschool period.

Hearing matures at an earlier age. Children at this stage are better able to listen and to interpret and distinguish different sounds. Preschoolers, like toddlers, frequently develop ear infections. By the preschool years, the child may be capable of verbalizing and pinpointing ear discomfort. A simple ear examination followed by the prescribed course of antibiotics will treat an ear infection and prevent permanent hearing loss.

B O X
8.1   Promoting Dental Health

Daily dental hygiene:

- Provide a small, soft toothbrush for the child.
- Provide toothpaste with fluoride. Teach the child not to swallow fluoride toothpaste.
- Ensure the child brushes daily in the morning and before bedtime.
- Show the child how to use a back-and-forth motion while the brush is against the teeth and gum line.

Foods:

- Limit the child's intake of high-sugar foods.
- Offer fresh fruits and vegetables daily.

Health supervision:

- Schedule dental visits for the preschooler every 6 months.

VITAL SIGNS

The preschool child's cardiovascular system enlarges to meet the general demands of the body. The average pulse rate for this age ranges from 90 to 100 beats per minute. The average blood pressure is 100/60 mm Hg. Hypertension may develop during the preschool period; therefore, blood pressure should be monitored during routine annual health assessments. The normal range for the respiratory rate is 22 to 25 breaths per minute at rest. This decrease in the rate of respirations from that of a younger age is related to growth of the lungs that permits better efficiency.

DEVELOPMENTAL MILESTONES

Motor Development

Gross Motor Skills

Four-year-old children are capable of walking and running on their tiptoes. They can hop and balance on one foot for 3 to 5 seconds and use alternating feet while descending stairs. Their development improves to the point where they can pedal a tricycle and begin to quickly navigate corners and turns. A 4-year-old child likes to climb and jump from heights without demonstrating much fear, making constant supervision necessary (Fig. 8.1). A child of this age can catch a ball with extended arms and hands.

By 5 years of age muscle coordination and strength increase, permitting the child to jump rope, skip on alternating feet, walk on a balance beam, and catch a ball with both hands. Preschoolers' movements are now smoother and more efficient, and they can begin to play certain sports, including soccer, skating, and baseball. Five-year-old children are also capable of imitating and learning simple dance steps or other similar routines.

Fine Motor Skills

Four-year-old children are able to manage many of their self-care activities, including bathing, dressing, feeding, and toileting. These skills, which began in the toddler years, can now be performed with greater ease and dexterity. Although preschool children can wash and dry their hands without supervision, they still require supervision and some assistance with the task of bathing.

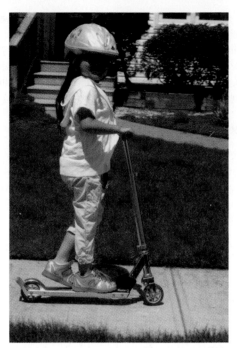

FIGURE 8.1 Gross motor skills improve during the preschool stage.

Children at this age can manipulate their clothing, including buttons, zippers, and snaps. Children of 4 and 5 years can readily recognize the front and back of their clothing. They still need help with tying shoelaces.

Preschool children can handle a spoon without inverting it, and many prefer to use a fork rather than a spoon. Many children are able to use a knife to spread butter or jelly. They still need help cutting up their food but like making their own sandwiches or pouring their own drinks. They are able to sit at the table for longer periods of time. Children of this age can learn about table manners. Preschool children usually can sit at meals for longer periods than toddlers. Whenever possible, families should eat together. Mealtime can be a time for family interaction, communication, and sharing of daily accomplishments.

At 4 years of age children are able to recognize their need to use the toilet but may require some assistance in manipulating their clothing and carrying out the necessary hygiene measures. By 5 years of age toileting has become a more independent practice. However, it is wise for parents to still supervise toileting to make certain that the child is washing his or her hands, wiping properly, and remembering to flush.

Fine motor development improves at 4 years of age to the point of allowing the child to draw a simple face and use scissors to cut along a line. Five-year-old children can control their drawing to permit copying letters and printing their names (Fig. 8.2). Their drawings are more detailed and include not only a face, but also other body parts. The 5-year-old child also has better control of scissors.

Sexual Development

During the preschool period children become aware of their genital organs and their sexual identity. As discussed in Chapter 5, children may become strongly attached to the parent of the opposite sex. They later identify with the parent of the same sex. Single-parent families should try to plan for the child to spend time with aunts, uncles, and other relatives or adult friends of the opposite sex during the preschool years. Children at this stage are also curious about the differences between the male and female bodies. Parents should respond simply and at the level of the child's understanding. For example, a preschool girl may ask why her baby brother looks different. Usually this age group is not looking for a detailed explanation, so the parents should simply explain that boys look different. The child should be told that her brother has a penis. Using the correct terms and encouraging questions about sex helps keep the lines of communication open between parents and children.

Masturbation is a common activity in both sexes, although it is usually a concern to parents. It is normal behavior, and caregivers must respond in a matter-of-fact manner to prevent instilling feelings of guilt in the child. As children mature and grow, they will develop mechanisms to channel sexual feelings, and this behavior will decrease.

Psychosocial Development

Initiative

According to Erikson, by preschool age the child has learned to trust those in the environment and has

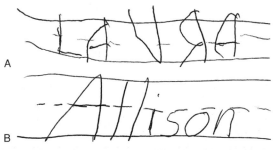

FIGURE 8.2 Progression of fine motor development from (A) 3 years to (B) 5 years.

developed a sense of independence. Preschoolers pretend, explore, and try out new roles. Erikson referred to exploration as the task of **initiative**. Children enjoy playing and pretending to be many different people in their environment. It is important that young preschool children have good role models whom they may imitate and from whom they may learn. Although parents are the primary role models, other adults in the community, such as teachers, health providers, and clergy, may also serve as role models. Caregivers must allow children freedom to explore and try out roles they desire, regardless of gender or stereotype. If not, children can develop feelings of guilt that may thwart their ability to grow and develop.

Discipline

Parents need to continue to set limits to protect children and property. Preschool children must not go into the street or hit others. As preschoolers develop a sense of initiative and guilt, they strive to follow rules and please parents. Discipline teaches children impulse control. If a child hits another child, the parents need to help the child learn to channel emotions into words. For example, a parent might say, "Stop it. You are very angry. Tell me why." This encourages the child to talk about his or her feelings.

Parents can also limit undesirable behavior by using positive reinforcement. In other words, parents can give a privilege or remove it, as the behavior warrants. Discipline should be of short duration because the child still has a limited concept of time. Time-out, as discussed in Chapter 7, can be useful in disciplining the preschooler.

Special Psychosocial Concerns
Jealousy
Jealousy, or sibling rivalry as discussed in Chapter 7, is a normal, inevitable behavior pattern seen at various stages of development. During the preschool stage, children need affection, attention, and recognition. Unlike the toddler, the child of this age is better able to share and understand that he or she is not the only person in need of the caregivers' attention. Preschoolers who are involved with nursery school and other activities outside the home seem less threatened by a new baby or younger child at home. To help minimize sibling rivalry, parents should try to understand the preschooler's feelings, set aside special time for him or her, and provide a designated space for toys and other meaningful items. Even busy parents must always try to meet the preschooler's needs. Taking time out to tell the child

a story or offer a special hug may be just enough to help the child adjust to a new baby. The child of this age can also be given little "jobs" to help assist the parent with the care of other siblings. For example, the preschool child may be able to hold the diaper bag, get the powder, or hand the parent what is needed during diaper changes. Allowing the preschooler to do these jobs helps strengthen his or her growing self-esteem.

Responses to Divorce

Divorce is one of the common stresses affecting children during the preschool period. At this age, children may interpret the failing marriage as their fault. They usually have a strong wish to reunite their parents and may fantasize about this. Parents need to try to privately resolve their conflicts and spare the child undue emotional pain. Important measures include making the child feel loved and protected by both parties. The degree of emotional fallout from divorce can be minimized by having the noncustodial parent establish consistent and orderly visiting patterns. Children should feel that they have their own space in both parents' homes. Allowing the child to leave toys and clothing at the "other home" helps to reinforce a sense of belonging. See Box 8.2 for hints for divorced parents.

Preschool Education

Preschool is rapidly becoming the norm in the United States today. The purpose of preschool education is to promote cognitive, motor, and social development. Preschool provides a place where children can form friendships and begin to learn to get along with peers. Starting school is a new experience for young children (Fig. 8.3). The first day should be brief, and the parent should stay with the child until he or she appears to be acclimated to the

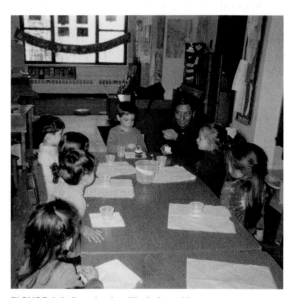

FIGURE 8.3 Preschoolers like being with peers.

surroundings. For some children acclimation is especially difficult and requires special understanding and patience from the parent. No activity should be forced on a child. If a child is not ready for preschool, socialization skills such as forming friendships and getting along with peers are unlikely to develop. Parents and school staff can work together to assess the readiness of the child. Signs of preschool readiness include mastery of toilet training, ability to tolerate brief periods of separation from parents, and increased communication skills. Children eventually gain confidence in themselves and become interested in participating with peers. To better prepare the child for preschool, parents can begin by familiarizing the child with the school location and teachers, visiting the school before the first day, and offering the child ample opportunity to discuss feelings.

Parents should consider several factors when selecting a preschool for a child. First, the parents should consider the location, cost, and schedule to make certain that the school fulfills the family's needs. Next, parents should determine what philosophy forms the basis of the preschool program.

It is recommended that the program and curriculum be driven by student needs, interests, and learning styles, not teacher desires. This type of program places the children at the center of activities. Each child should be considered unique and given diverse play experiences tailored to his or her individual needs. The philosophy must appreciate the physical, cultural, cognitive, and emotional differences among the children. To best indicate its appreciation for these differences, the school should recognize and discuss holidays, introduce foods from different cultures, and value and celebrate diversity. The National Association for the Education of Young Children (NAEYC) recommends that at least one teacher hold a degree in early childhood education. NAEYC recommends a teacher-child ratio of one adult for every four to six 2-year-old toddlers, with a maximum group size of 12, or one adult for every eight to ten 3- to 4-year-old children, with a maximum group size of 20.

The school should allow parents to visit at any time, and parents should make at least one unannounced visit. Play is very important to the development of preschool-aged children. The school should have adequate play space to allow freedom of movement. The supplies at the preschool should include blocks of various sizes and shapes and other hands-on materials such as clay, sand, wood, water, and puzzles. The entire classroom area should be clean, but it should not be an environment that is prohibitive to exploration and play. Bathroom facilities must be close by and accessible for preschoolers. Box 8.3 provides a preschool safety checklist.

Types of Preschool

Parents have many choices for preschool programs, including public, private, or homeschooling. Homeschooling education is typically run by parents or tutors rather than in formal settings. There are several reasons for selecting this form of education, including religious or moral instruction. Often it is the choice of parents who find themselves dissatisfied with public education and the school social environment.

BOX 8.3 Preschool Safety Checklist

- Playgrounds should be secured with a fence.
- Equipment must be free of sharp edges, in a good state of repair, and routinely inspected.
- Fire alarms and fire extinguishers must be present and working.
- Emergency exits and evacuation plans must be clearly posted.
- Toys must be appropriate for children's ages and in good condition.
- Staff should be trained in first aid and cardiopulmonary resuscitation.
- Bathrooms must be kept clean and easily accessible for young children.
- Water temperature in faucets must be no higher than 110°F (43°C) to prevent accidental burns.
- The sites for picking up and dropping off children should be safely secured.
- Children must be allowed to leave only with authorized caregivers.

Cognitive Development

According to Piaget, the preoperational stage of development begins in the toddler period and extends through the school-age years. It is limited in several ways. First, the preschooler is unable to focus on several aspects of a stimulus. For example, if someone is wearing a mask, preschool children do not recognize the person and instead become frightened. Piaget called this **centration** and described it as the child focusing or centering attention on only one cue. Piaget further believed that preschoolers lack **reversibility,** or the understanding of how two actions may be related to each other. For example, preschoolers may watch liquid being poured from a short, fat beaker into a tall, thin beaker but maintain that the tall beaker contains more fluid. Preschoolers are unable to understand that the physical attributes of an item remain the same despite superficial changes in its appearance. This is easily demonstrated by asking a preschooler to tell you if the amount of play clay has changed when you simply change its shape.

At this stage the child continues to develop language and memory. The preschooler is still somewhat egocentric but is now able to share, take turns, and follow rules.

Preschoolers can form general concepts but cannot reason formally. Their reasoning appears to be based on their earlier experiences. For example, preschoolers, like toddlers, become concerned when they see their mother dressing up in her "going out" clothes, knowing that this means that she is leaving. If trust and autonomy have developed sufficiently, however, the preschooler is able to tolerate separation and understand that Mommy will come back. Limited reasoning is also evident in the preschooler's concept and understanding of time.

During the preschool years children often pretend and are highly creative (Fig. 8.4). When 4- or 5-year-old children tell a story, they may use their overactive imaginations to embellish or enhance parts of the story. Their thinking style is still egotistical and also magical. They may believe that they are the center of the world and that they are all-powerful. Sometimes they develop feelings of guilt over their "bad" thoughts, which they believe may have caused an accident or other adverse happening. It is also common for preschoolers to believe that if they become ill or injured, they are being punished for their wrongdoings. Parents and health care workers need to explore preschool children's feelings to minimize their guilt and misunderstandings.

Preschoolers have longer attention spans than toddlers. This permits the preschool child to perform an activity for longer periods than a toddler can. Toddlers may have difficulty sitting still and listening to an entire story, whereas preschoolers listen attentively, often memorize the story, and do not let the reader skip even a word.

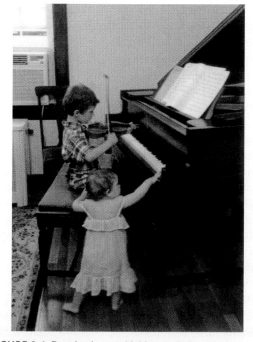

FIGURE 8.4 Preschoolers are highly creative.

Moral Development

According to Kohlberg, the preconventional stage of moral development begins at about age 4 and continues to about age 10 (see Chapter 5). Moral development is a process in which children learn by modeling and imitating adult behaviors. For this reason it is imperative that parents set good examples and have consistent patterns of interaction.

According to Freud, children at this stage begin to develop a superego, or **conscience.** The conscience gives them the capacity for self-evaluation and criticism. The superego becomes the moral dimension of the child's personality. It is at this stage that children begin to emulate beliefs, values, and ideals based on what is learned in their homes and immediate environments. Caregivers must help children understand the cause and effect that certain behaviors may have on others. Preschool children should be reminded that if they take a toy from a playmate, the action will cause an unfavorable response.

The vivid imagination of preschoolers can make it difficult for them to distinguish fantasy from reality. They often tell stories that have threads of truth woven together with untruths. Preschoolers are just beginning to recognize that deliberate lying is a bad thing to do.

Communication

A child's language and speech become more sophisticated during the preschool period. Whereas toddlers make their needs known by gestures and the use of a few words, preschoolers can use nouns, verbs, and adjectives in their sentences. At 4 years of age children can form sentences using three to four words and understand who, what, and where questions. Most 5-year-old children can form sentences containing five or more words. The 5-year-old child's vocabulary contains between 2,000 and 2,400 words.

Preschool children may exhibit some difficulty with the pronunciation of certain words. This is to be expected and should be treated by the adult by gently correcting the child's mispronunciation without criticism. Putting undue stress on the child's ability to speak clearly may lead to stuttering and hesitancy. Some hesitancy is a normal pattern of speech development.

Children who are 3, 4, or 5 years old are usually very talkative. They like monopolizing the conversation and will talk even if no one is listening or answers them. Preschoolers ask questions even when

HELPFUL HINTS

Strategies to Stimulate Language Development

Read to your child.
Encourage storytelling.
Play naming games.
Gently correct mispronunciations.

they know the answer. They can express past, present, and future with an improved understanding of time. For example, if a preschooler is riding in a car and asks for a drink, you can tell him or her that in just a few minutes you will be able to get the drink. Unlike toddlers, preschoolers can understand basic time concepts and delay their gratification. Children in this age group also enjoy talking on the telephone. At 3 years of age, children's phone skills are limited to talking without interactive conversation. In other words, the 3-year-old can tell about a happening but is not able to answer questions asked by someone on the phone. By 5 years of age, the child can converse on the telephone.

Preschool children can be taught their full name, address, and telephone number. This is the time for parents and teachers to instruct children about how to respond to emergencies. This age group can be taught how to dial 911 to initiate the emergency help system if needed.

Preschoolers learn by imitating others in their environments. Their vocabularies increase through repetition and practice. It is important that adult role models use appropriate words to instill positive

HELPFUL HINTS

Red Flags for Language and Speech Problems (Birth to Preschool)

0–3 months	Does not listen to sounds or does not coo or make throaty sounds
4–6 months	Does not notice noisy items such as vacuums
7–12 months	Does not babble or respond to name
1–2 years	Does not use one- to two-word sentences
2–3 years	Does not use two- to three-word sentences
3–4 years	Does not understand or answer who, what, and why questions

influences on a growing child. As a preschooler thinks about the right word to use, he or she may hesitate or stutter. This mannerism usually disappears within a few months. Parents should be patient and listen without hurrying or labeling the child a stutterer.

When the child repeats an unacceptable or bad word, simple correction without a fuss is needed. Drawing attention to the "bad" words serves only to reinforce the child's negative behavior.

NUTRITION

The nutritional requirements for the preschool years are similar to those for the toddler years. The child will need all of the basic nutrients outlined in the food pyramid and MyPlate. See Chapter 1 for the MyPlate chart. The average daily caloric needs for this age are approximately 1,800 calories, divided over the course of the day. Like toddlers, most preschool children do best when they have three meals and three snacks daily.

Certain issues may be a concern during this stage, including food fads carried over from the toddler years, rebellious behavior, and periods of diminished appetite. Many parents become concerned about the amount of food consumed by their child. Parents should not expect the preschooler to eat an adult-size portion of food. Some children develop strong food preferences that may limit the type of foods that they will eat. By age 5 many children begin to develop food habits similar to those of their peers. Fast foods and highly advertised foods are known favorites for this age group. Parents must exercise caution when planning meals from fast-food restaurants because many of these food choices are very high in calories and fat.

The best diet for young children includes foods containing proteins, carbohydrates, vitamins and minerals, and limited fats. Milk is still an important food because of its calcium content. Preschoolers need at least 1 pint of milk per day to meet their daily calcium requirements. It is also important that snack foods be selected for their nutritional value and appeal. Good food choices for snacks may include fresh or dried fruits, vegetables in bite-size pieces, cheese, or yogurt. It is best not to offer candy or other excessively sweet foods as snacks. These foods are not good for the health of the teeth and have a tendency to spoil the child's appetite for regular meals. See Table 8.1 for a typical preschool diet.

TABLE 8.1	Sample Daily Diet for Preschoolers	
Type of Food	**Amount per Day**	

Dairy foods

Milk	4 oz.
Cheese	½–¾ oz.
Yogurt	½ cup

Protein foods

Meat, fish, or poultry	Two servings, 1–2 oz.
Eggs	3 eggs per week
Peanut butter	1–2 tablespoons
Legumes, dried peas, beans, cooked	¼–½ cup

Vegetables and fruits

Vegetables, cooked	Four servings, 2–4 tablespoons
Vegetables, raw	Include 1 green or yellow vegetable
Fruits, raw	Several pieces
Fruits, canned	4–8 tablespoons

Grains

Bread, enriched or	1–2 slices
Whole wheat bread	1–2 slices
Multigrain crackers	3–4 crackers
Cereal, cooked or dry	¼–½ cup
Pasta, rice	½ cup

Fats

Bacon	1 slice
Butter	1 teaspoon

Mealtimes should be pleasant and allow family interaction. If the mealtime is very long, the preschooler may not be able to sit through it without getting restless and fidgety.

Obesity

Obesity is more accurately measured in infants, toddlers, and preschoolers using the weight for height chart. Any reading over the 85th percentile is considered obesity. Obesity places children at risk for cardiovascular disease, hypertension, type 2 diabetes, liver and gallbladder disease, and asthma. Researchers believe that a person can have a genetic predisposition for obesity, although other factors that can contribute to obesity include medications, consumption of fast food, and a sedentary lifestyle (such as more than 2 hours a day spent watching TV). To counteract obesity in children, the whole family must be involved in making better food choices and becoming more physically active. The adults must demonstrate healthy eating, and children should be involved in meal planning and preparation.

SLEEP AND REST

The average preschool child requires about 10 to 12 hours of sleep each night. Children in this age group are usually very active and busily engaged in some activity or game. Many are too busy and active to have time for a nap, even though they still need to rest and replenish their energy. Some children in this age group take only one nap per day, and many do not nap on a daily basis. The average nap at this age lasts 30 to 60 minutes. By evening the child is generally overtired and very much in need of an early bedtime. Many children during this stage have difficulty falling asleep at bedtime. Following a consistent bedtime routine helps minimize the conflict or debate over bedtime practices. Each child should be expected to follow the bedtime routine regardless of the day of the week or other distractions. Sometimes, however, it is necessary to limit the routine if a child tries to lengthen it as a means of putting off the inevitable.

Preschool children often wake up during the night with nightmares. Parents should gently reassure the child that he or she is safe and not alone. After sitting with the child until he or she is relaxed, the parent should then proceed with the bedtime routine and encourage the child to go back to sleep. Some children experience a more extreme form of nightmare called night terrors. When these occur, the child suddenly sits up screaming but is not fully awake. The child's appearance may be very frightening to the parents. The screaming may be accompanied by rapid breathing, a rapid heart rate, and profuse perspiration. The child may be inconsolable for a brief period. These episodes are usually followed by the child relaxing and falling back into a quiet sleep. The child is unable to recall the event in the morning. Night terrors are not thought to represent any emotional stress and disappear without intervention.

PLAY

Preschool children engage in **cooperative play,** also called associative play. Such play requires that children be able to understand limited rules. By this age children usually have developed some social skills that permit them to begin to share and take turns. Their mastery of basic communication skills enables them to express their desires. They enjoy being with peers and interacting with them during play.

When observing preschool children at play, one can clearly see different personality traits emerge. For example, some children are dominant; others are passive and follow another child's lead. Some children are more cautious and timid when trying new activities, whereas others aggressively attack any new activity without regard for danger. Still others may not interact well with peers or may even be excluded from peer activity. Unless the child is victimized or appears unhappy, he or she should be allowed to socialize at his or her own pace. Caregivers should understand that children have different personalities and different social needs. For example, some children need to be in the center of all activities, whereas some prefer to be observers or to play alone.

The preschool child uses toys such as jungle gyms, tricycles, and big wheels, and these activities help further develop gross motor skills such as jumping, running, climbing, and pedaling. See Figure 8.5. It is possible to teach a preschooler to swim, skate, and play soccer and other sporting activities. It is important, however, that parents not force their own competitive needs on their children. Just as growth patterns vary with each child, so do gross motor skills and innate abilities. Some children are more coordinated and skillful than others.

Fine motor skills are enhanced through the use of playthings such as puzzles, construction sets, and computer programs. These activities help children at this age learn to manipulate and coordinate their small motor movements. Computer programs and other interactive games also help stimulate the preschooler's thinking skills, reasoning, and memory. The preschool years are a time for building confidence. Children at this stage frequently say, "Look at my tall tower" or "Listen to me sing the ABCs." "Watch me" is a common demand. At this age they seek approval and recognition from adults.

Child-size kitchens and tool corners permit children to use their imagination, try on roles, and pretend to be grown up. Regardless of the type of plaything used, it is important that children be taught to clean up their play areas and take care of their toys. This helps to teach children responsibility and initiative, both of which can later be transferred to other situations.

Preschoolers still use symbolic play, as described in Chapter 7. A great amount of play time is spent

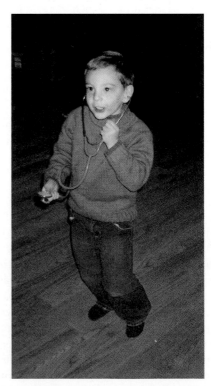

FIGURE 8.6 Preschoolers like to try on different roles.

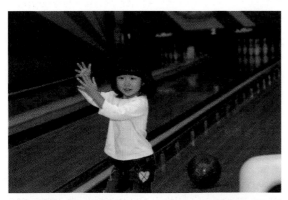

FIGURE 8.5 Play helps improve gross motor skills.

in activities that use their imaginations. Dramatic play may involve dressing up in different clothes, exploring roles, and imitating adults (Fig. 8.6). Common activities may also include playing with dolls or tools.

Television is sometimes used as a time filler and for entertainment. Parents should screen the types of programs that their children view. Many programs have educational value, whereas others may have little or none. Educational programs can foster good social relationships and help enhance the child's imagination. Television shows involving puppets have been shown to be useful in stimulating the imagination and creativity of preschool children. Preschool children may benefit from an introduction to music and instruments during this stage. This can enhance their sense of rhythm and concentration (Fig. 8.7).

SAFETY

The more coordinated preschool child is less likely to fall than the awkward toddler. This age group is also more aware of certain dangers and limitations. Most of them can recite a long list of "Nos" or things they cannot touch or do. Even so, they still need adult supervision and continual reminders about potential environmental hazards. The safety precautions outlined in Chapter 7 for the toddler also apply to the preschool child. See Box 8.4 for an overview of the recommended safety precautions for preschoolers.

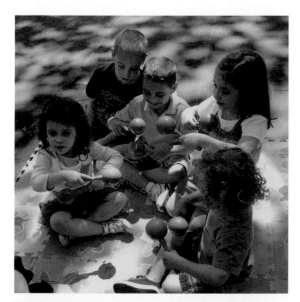

FIGURE 8.7 Children connect with both music and one another.

Clothing items must be carefully inspected to make certain that they are safe for the active child. Clothing must allow freedom of movement and be nonrestrictive. Strangulation deaths have occurred as a result of clothing strings, belts, or loops catching on playground items. It is the responsibility of both the clothing manufacturers and caregivers to help look for these potential dangers to prevent accidents. Federal regulations now require that children's nightclothes be flame-resistant as an additional means of providing for child safety in the home.

Motor vehicle accidents are the major cause of accidental death in preschool children, as they are in toddlers. Preschool children must always be restrained in proper car safety seats. Some preschool children may be big enough to use an adult safety restraint, depending on the type of car and the state in which they live. It is best to check with the car manufacturer for guidelines about use. Because preschoolers like to imitate adult behaviors, adults must always use their own car safety restraints.

As children become more active and involved in various games and activities, the number of injuries they sustain often increases. Preschool children are less likely to drown in the bathtub but more likely to get into danger outdoors near pools or other bodies of water. Preschool children should be given swimming lessons and instructions about water safety regulations.

Parents must begin to educate their children about the dangers of talking to strangers or accepting candy, rides, or money from strangers. It is also necessary to teach children about their private body parts, including the rule that no one should be allowed to touch them. The environment in the home must permit children access and freedom to discuss their concerns and worries without shame or ridicule. Many communities have enacted safety programs that fingerprint and create photographic identification of children as a preventive measure in case of abduction or for help in searching for a missing person. Parents may contact their local police department for information on or help in establishing these types of programs.

HEALTH PROMOTION

Preschool children need to receive booster shots for diphtheria, pertussis, and tetanus (DTaP) and the polio vaccine (TOPV); the measles, mumps, and

8.4 Safety Precautions for Preschoolers

Motor Vehicles:

- Car safety seats and restraints must be used at all times.
- Windows and door handles should be off-limits to all young children or locked.
- Never leave children alone or unattended in a motor vehicle.
- Children should not play near roads or in active driveways.
- Children should be actively supervised whenever near roads or motor vehicles.

Poisoning:

- Store household cleaning agents, garden products, car products, and prescription and nonprescription drugs safely away from children (for example, on a high shelf or in a locked cabinet).
- Never refer to medicine as candy, and avoid taking medication in front of children to avoid their imitation of parental behavior.
- Keep the national poison control number (800-222-1222) readily available in the event of accidental poisoning.

Burns:

- Keep the stove safe by removing stove knobs and turning pot handles toward the back of the stove to prevent spills.

Cover Electrical Sockets:

- Prevent burns from hot liquids, including bath water.
- Keep matches and lighters away from young children.

Choking or Aspiration:

- Avoid known choking hazards, including foods like hard candies, popcorn, fruit pits or seeds, and large pieces of meat.
- Avoid toys with small removable parts that can be placed in the child's mouth and either swallowed or aspirated.
- Suffocation is another safety concern. Keep all plastic coverings and bags away from children.
- Do not let children blow up balloons, as this poses an aspiration risk.

Drowning:

- Drowning can happen in just a few inches of water. Always supervise children while in the bathtub, swimming pool, or another body of water.

Safe Clothing:

- Avoid clothing that has loops, strings, or belts that could pose a strangulation risk.
- Purchase fire-resistant sleepwear.

Strangers:

- Educate children about the dangers of talking to strangers or accepting candy, rides, or money from strangers.
- Teach children about body parts that are private and that no one should be allowed to touch.

rubella vaccine (MMR); the varicella vaccine (VAR); and an annual influenza vaccine (Hib) to ensure immunity and protection against these diseases. Children at this age need yearly preventive health care visits to supervise their physical and social growth and development. See Box 8.5 for a sample of preschool health-screening assessments. Because preschoolers have increased exposure to other children, they are more likely to spread simple infections such as the common cold. They should be taught the importance of hygiene principles such as handwashing, using tissues, or sneezing or coughing into one's elbow if tissues are unavailable.

Common Preschool Concerns

Thumb-Sucking

Thumb-sucking is thought to be a primitive, instinctive behavior that may fulfill the child's sucking and comfort needs. One concern with prolonged thumb-sucking is that it may cause malalignment of the teeth. For this reason, many parents try to discourage

this habit, often unsuccessfully. Sometimes other comfort objects such as a teddy bear, soft doll, or blanket can replace the thumb and still provide the child with a sense of security. Usually by school age this behavior lessens and eventually disappears.

BOX
8.5 Preschool Yearly Health Screening

A complete examination should include the following:

- Physical examination
- Health history
- Physical, nutritional, and psychosocial assessment
- Vision and hearing testing
- Cardiac screening
- Blood screening
- Urine testing
- Immunizations
- Tuberculosis screening
- Dental supervision

Bed-Wetting

Bed-wetting, also known as enuresis, is a problem that is seen more often in boys than in girls. Enuresis is not considered to be a problem until after toilet training is well established. The cause of enuresis is not fully understood. Stress and illness in the child appear to make it worse. If this behavior persists, it is important that the child be given a complete medical examination to help rule out any underlying pathology. The best approach in dealing with the problem of bed-wetting is one that minimizes each episode and avoids making the child feel guilty or ashamed. Parents can sometimes help prevent these accidents by taking the child to the toilet in the evening hours and limiting the child's fluid intake after 5 p.m. Punishment or ridicule lowers the child's self-esteem and morale and should be avoided.

Fears

Preschool children frequently have fears of the dark, mutilation, and abandonment. All childhood fears should be approached in a similar manner. Caregivers must first acknowledge the child's fears. Reassurance and reality reinforcement are essential in helping children cope with their fears. Some preschoolers experience fear of the dark. This may cause bedtime hassles or interrupt sleep. Having a simple nightlight in the child's room or in a hallway may lessen the fear.

Fear of mutilation often becomes evident at the time of injury or during hospitalization. Bleeding from a small scrape seems particularly frightening to this age group. Bandages can help cover the site of an injury, making the child feel better.

Fear of abandonment frequently occurs at this age. Preschoolers may get hysterical if a parent is a few minutes late in picking them up at school. They respond as though the parent is never coming back. However, they show increased independence by thinking nothing of walking away from their parents in a store or on the playground. They think it is all right if they wander out of sight, but their response is different if the parent walks away. Parents may help allay the fears of abandonment by being honest with their child. For example, if parents/caregivers are going out for the evening, they should tell the child that they are leaving and when they will be back. Parents should never sneak out or lie to their child.

SUMMARY

1. The rate of growth for the preschool period is slow and steady.

2. Children grow 2½ inches per year. The average weight gain is 5 to 7 pounds a year. The trunk and body lengthen, giving the child a taller appearance and a more erect posture.

3. Care of the teeth during the preschool stage is important to promote healthy teeth in future years.

4. Visual acuity improves and hearing matures during this stage.

5. The structural makeup of the preschool child's ears continues to account for the high incidence of middle-ear infections in this age group.

6. The normal pulse rate is between 90 and 100 beats per minute, and blood pressure is about 100/60 mm Hg. The normal respiratory rate is 22 to 25 breaths per minute at rest.

7. The focus during the preschool years is on increasing motor skills, improving vocabulary, and increasing knowledge about the environment.

8. Four-year-old children are capable of walking and running on their tiptoes, hopping, and balancing on one foot. Preschoolers can pedal a tricycle and like to climb and jump. By age 5, they can skip, walk on a balance beam, and catch a ball.

9. Improved fine motor development allows 4-year-old children to accomplish self-care.

10. Preschoolers find pleasure in examining and exploring their bodies. They are now very curious about the differences between male and female bodies.

11. Masturbation is common for both sexes during this stage. Parents should respond in a matter-of-fact manner and not instill feelings of guilt in their child.

12. The psychosocial task of the preschool period is the development of initiative.

13. Preschool children need discipline to learn impulse control.

14. Preschools should be selected on the basis of philosophy, location, schedule, and cost.

15. Jealousy is a normal pattern of behavior seen at various stages of development.

16. Divorce is one of the common stresses that affect children. Preschool children often blame themselves and have a strong wish to reunite the parents.

17. Cognitive development is at the preoperational stage. The child continues to develop language and memory. The thinking style of the preschool stage is often described as magical, giving the child the feeling that he or she is all-powerful.

18. Preschool children are developing their consciences and have a beginning capacity for moral reasoning. Moral reasoning is learned mainly by imitating parents and other adults. It is therefore important that the adult role model use appropriate words and set good examples for the child.

19. Communication is more sophisticated during this period of development. Children are very talkative and can be taught their full names and addresses and how to respond to emergencies.

20. The average daily caloric need for this age is 1,800 calories, divided over the course of the day. By age 5 many children have developed food habits similar to those of their peers. The diet for this age group should include foods containing proteins, carbohydrates, vitamins, minerals, and limited fats.

21. Children at this stage are very active and require an average of 10 to 12 hours of sleep each night. All preschool children need consistency with their night rituals. Nightmares and night terrors are common during this stage of development.

22. Preschool play style is known as cooperative, or associative. Children are able to share, take turns, and follow simple rules.

23. Toys should be selected to help stimulate fine and gross motor development. Just as growth patterns vary with each child, so do motor skills and innate abilities, making some children more coordinated than others.

24. Safety continues to be a major concern for preschool children, and they still need adult supervision and constant reminders about potential environmental hazards.

25. During the preschool years, children need to be given booster shots for DTaP and TOPV to help ensure immunity and protection against these diseases. Children at this stage need yearly preventive health care visits and screening to supervise their physical, emotional, and social development.

26. Thumb-sucking is thought to be a primitive and instinctive behavior. If it becomes a prolonged habit, it may cause malalignment of the child's teeth.

27. Bed-wetting, also known as enuresis, is a problem seen more often in boys than in girls. Stress and illness in the child seem to make it worse.

CRITICAL THINKING

Exercise #1

Mrs. Hyatt attends a local community support group supervised by the pediatric nurse practitioner for new and working mothers. Mrs. Hyatt verbalizes her concern about her 4½-year-old son. He appears to be slow in mastering language. He is presently enrolled in a preschool program. Although his speech has improved since he began school, he demonstrates marked stuttering. Mrs. Hyatt also reports that her son repeatedly uses bad language. She is very upset and admits that she doesn't know how to handle this. Mrs. Hyatt assures the nurse that neither she nor her husband uses this type of language in the home.

1. What reason would you give Mrs. Hyatt for her son's:
   a. Bad language?
   b. Stuttering?
2. How would you instruct Mrs. Hyatt to respond to her son when he:
   a. Uses bad language?
   b. Stutters?

Exercise #2

You are assigned to a playroom. Explain what play activities would be appropriate for several 4- to 5-year-old children. Select activities that will stimulate their growth and development.

MULTIPLE-CHOICE QUESTIONS

1. The purpose of preschool education is to foster which of the following? (Select all that apply)
   a. Cognitive development
   b. Physical development
   c. Social development
   d. Psychological development

2. Preschool focuses on which of the following? (Select all that apply)
   a. Medical care
   b. Interests
   c. Learning style
   d. Rest

3. The erect posture and steady gait seen in preschool children may be a result of:
   a. Movement of the foot away from the center of the body
   b. Exaggerated lumbar curvature of the spine
   c. Movement of the foot toward the center of the body
   d. Increased fusion of the spinal bones

4. Ear infections are more commonly seen in children because of:
   a. Their increased exposure to infection
   b. Their earlobes, which are smaller than those of adults
   c. Their short eustachian tubes
   d. A decrease in the number of white blood cells

5. The type of play seen at the preschool age is:
   a. Parallel play
   b. Associative play
   c. Solitary play
   d. Isolated play

6. Occasional periods of masturbation in a 4-year-old child suggest:
   a. Pathology in the child's personality
   b. A normal pattern of development
   c. History of sexual abuse
   d. Impaired cognitive development

7. According to Erikson, a sense of initiative is best explained as:
   a. Finishing tasks started
   b. Establishing trust
   c. The ability to express one's needs
   d. Trying new roles without feelings of guilt

8. Preschoolers learn to handle frustration in a positive manner by:
   a. Becoming ambivalent
   b. Learning self-control
   c. Developing apathy
   d. Becoming manipulative

9. The average daily caloric intake recommended during the preschool years is:
   a. 1,000 calories
   b. 2,500 calories
   c. 1,800 calories
   d. 500 calories

10. Nightmares and night terrors differ in the following way:
   a. With nightmares, the child remains inconsolable for a long period.
   b. With night terrors, the child remembers the event in detail.
   c. Nightmares are usually accompanied by rapid respirations and rapid heart rate.
   d. With night terrors, the child has no recall of the event.

11. Sibling rivalry is best resolved by:
   a. Blaming both parties
   b. Separating both children
   c. Immediately determining the instigator
   d. Supporting the weaker child

12. According to Piaget, preschoolers lack the concept of reversibility. This can be demonstrated by:
   a. Believing that if the item is out of sight, then it doesn't exist
   b. Having the ability to solve problems abstractly
   c. Not recognizing that changing the shape of something, such as clay, does not change the amount
   d. Having the ability to learn through their senses

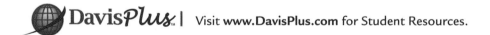

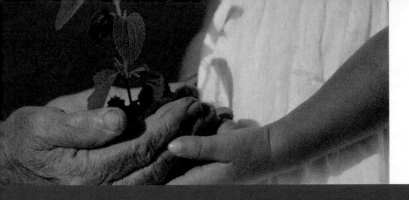

CHAPTER9

School Age

Learning Objectives

At the end of this chapter, you should be able to:

- List four physical characteristics common to school-age children.
- Describe three developmental milestones common to school-age children.
- Describe the psychosocial task identified by Erikson for the school-age period.
- Describe the cognitive levels of functioning during the school-age period.
- Describe moral development in school-age children.
- List three factors that help contribute to the health of school-age children.

The period of development known as *school age,* the *middle years,* or *late childhood* starts with the child's entry into formal education and ends with the onset of puberty, roughly from ages 6 to 11. Puberty commonly refers to the developmental period in which the body prepares for the changes necessary for reproduction. Five significant accomplishments occur during the school-age period:

1. Growth remains slow and steady.
2. Children move away from the family toward peer relationships.
3. Children become less self-centered and more goal-directed.
4. Deciduous teeth are lost, and the permanent teeth appear (Fig. 9.1).
5. Sexual tranquillity replaces sexual curiosity and preoccupation.

PHYSICAL CHARACTERISTICS

Height and Weight

The school-age period begins with slow, consistent growth and ends with a growth spurt just at the time of puberty. The average expected growth rate for the child during this period of development is 2 to 3 inches (5 to 7 cm) per year. Weight increases on an average of 4.5 to 6.5 pounds (2 to 3 kg) per year. The average 6-year-old girl measures 45 inches (116 cm) and weighs 46 pounds (21 kg); the average 10-year-old girl measures 59 inches (150 cm) and weighs 88 pounds (40 kg). Boys may appear taller and heavier in the early school-age period, but for a brief time toward the end of this stage, girls are taller and heavier than boys.

Bone and Muscle Development

Bone growth and maturation can be affected by several factors, including gender, race, nutrition, and general state of health. The bones mature 2 years earlier in girls than in boys. African American children, in general, show earlier bone development than do white children. Growth in the long bones stretches the ligaments and muscles, causing most children to experience "growing pains," mostly at night. The child's arms and legs lengthen, producing a thin, spindly appearance.

School-age children's posture changes because their center of gravity shifts downward as their muscle strength increases. The abdominal muscles also grow stronger, causing the pelvis to tip backward. The chest broadens and flattens, but the shoulders continue to appear rounded. Exercise encourages muscle development and improves strength and flexibility. Poor posture causes fatigue and may indicate minor skeletal pathology. Health screening for defects in the skeletal system is discussed in the section titled "Health Promotion."

Generally, muscle mass and muscle strength increase, but the school-age child's muscles are still relatively immature and easily injured. Fine and gross motor skills show marked improvement, allowing the child to be more independent and self-sufficient both at home and at school.

Sensory Development

Visual maturity is usually achieved by 6 to 7 years of age. Peripheral vision and depth perception improve, permitting better hand–eye coordination. School-age children no longer require large print in books and schoolwork.

Dentition

An important hallmark of this stage is the loss of the deciduous teeth and the appearance of the permanent teeth (Fig. 9.2). Children should be told in advance that they will lose their baby teeth so that

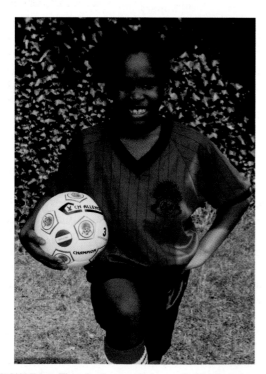

FIGURE 9.1 The school-age period is marked by the appearance of permanent teeth.

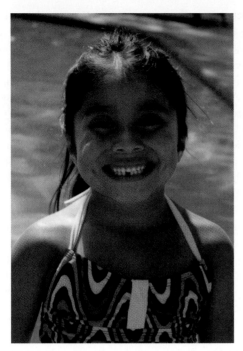

FIGURE 9.2 Loss of deciduous teeth is common at this stage.

they are not frightened when it happens. This can be done when the first tooth starts to loosen, usually at 6 to 7 years of age. Parents can emphasize that this is a sign that the child is growing up. Some parents play the "tooth fairy" game, rewarding the child with money for each lost tooth. The first tooth to fall out is the lower central incisor. Teeth should not be pulled or forced to fall out but allowed to progress naturally.

The permanent teeth grow in the same order as the deciduous teeth. They usually appear very large in relation to the rest of the facial structures. The result is what is sometimes called the "ugly duckling" stage of development. Up to 75% of children have some degree of malocclusion, or malposition, of the teeth that may affect their chewing, facial relaxation, and appearance. Children should visit the dentist regularly, at least every 6 months, to have their teeth inspected and cleaned and any dental disease corrected. Daily dental care should include regular toothbrushing after meals and before bedtime. The use of fluoride toothpaste is strongly recommended to help decrease the incidence of dental caries. Dental caries begins with the buildup of plaque around the tooth surface and margins. Regular brushing and limiting children's intake of concentrated sweets help prevent plaque formation. Certain snack foods such as apples, raw carrots, and sugarless gum can help reduce plaque formation.

Development of the Gastrointestinal and Nervous Systems

Because the gastrointestinal system matures during this stage, school-age children have fewer digestive intolerances and disturbances than do younger children. As the capacity of the stomach increases, the child needs to eat less often. Three meals a day are now sufficient.

The nervous system continues to mature, as evidenced by the child's improved motor skills and expanded cognitive processes. The senses of taste, smell, and touch fully mature, making the school-age child more discriminatory. At this stage children develop many distinct food preferences based on personal taste and peer influences.

Development of the Immune System

The school-age period is marked by the maturing of the immune system, producing a peak in the child's antibody levels. Lymphatic tissues known as the tonsils and adenoids are located in the nasopharynx. These tissues may be disproportionately large, but unless they are causing infection or obstruction, surgical removal is not recommended. When children begin school, they are exposed to a greater number of microorganisms, and as a result they often have an increased incidence of upper respiratory tract infections. Once their immune systems adjust to the increased exposure, their resistance improves. The school-age period is generally a healthy period of development.

VITAL SIGNS

Because school-age children's hearts are small in proportion to their body masses, they may feel tired after strenuous exercise. During this stage of development, the heart rate decreases to an average of 90 beats per minute. Functional (innocent) heart murmurs may be present in 50% of school-age children. These murmurs do not usually require intervention. Blood pressure readings are generally higher than at the earlier stages—usually 100/60 mm Hg—because of the development of the left ventricle. Hemoglobin and hematocrit levels also increase slightly, whereas red and white blood cell counts decrease slightly during this period of development.

The respiratory system of the school-age child continues to develop. By 8 years of age the child's alveoli (air sacs) are fully mature. The normal respiratory rate decreases; the average resting respiratory rate is 20 breaths per minute.

DEVELOPMENTAL MILESTONES

Motor Development

During the school-age period there is a marked increase in muscle mass and muscle strength and significant improvement in gross and fine motor skills. School-age children can run faster, farther, and for longer periods. At this stage they are able to jump higher and throw farther and with more accuracy than children in younger age groups. Most children are stronger and better coordinated at this stage. Gender differences exist in motor skills. On average, boys are stronger; better at running, jumping, and throwing; and have greater endurance than girls. Girls are better at balance and coordination than boys. Girls perfect their fine motor skills before boys perfect theirs. Motor accomplishments are very important to both girls and boys during this stage.

School-age children have developed enough proficiency in gross and fine motor skills to permit independence in many areas at school and home, including play and self-care. Although 6-year-old children appear grown-up and independent, they are easily frustrated and fatigued. It is not uncommon for them to cry and become irritable and infantile. Children of this age group often play on their own and select activities that they find enjoyable. Many of their newfound skills can be accomplished without parental assistance. Some of the skills that validate their independence include swimming, skating, and bicycle riding. During this stage children show competence in performing necessary self-care activities such as bathing, dressing, and feeding themselves. School-age children learn to write, draw, dance, and develop many other creative talents.

Most 6- to 7-year-old children can print letters and their names and can throw, catch, swim, and run with better control. Children of 6 and 7 years start to learn to tie their shoelaces.

The gross motor skills of 7- and 8-year-old children improve, permitting smoother movements while running, jumping, and skipping. Many at this stage are capable of using a ball and bat with greater control and accuracy.

Fine motor skills continue to improve, and by 8 years of age fine movements become steadier and more controlled. Children now prefer a pencil or pen to a crayon and can print smaller and learn script lettering. With their improved fine motor development, they can now begin to learn to play many musical instruments.

Children of 8 to 9 years are usually outgoing, talkative, and enthusiastic. They are ready to take on any project regardless of their capabilities. This fearlessness may put them at greater risk for injury. At this stage they appear more graceful and have smoother motor coordination. Their strength and endurance also increase, improving their motor performances. Eight-year-old children practice a skill longer and with more commitment. Once they master the skill, they are ready to show off their talents. Various new activities may be attempted, such as gymnastics, karate, ballet, and other dance forms. Their fine motor skills also improve to now permit mastery in the areas attempted at an earlier age. There no longer seems to be a random selection of games and activities. Instead, children select activities based on their specific interests and likes. By the end of this stage, their physical strength is almost equal to that of an adult. Endurance and skills improve through practice.

Children of 9 and 10 years show improved motor development. As their strength and endurance increase, so does their interest in sports and other activities. By this age, children can actively participate in team sports (Fig. 9.3). They are now better able to understand rules and complex plays. Fine motor coordination improves, permitting them to learn to write and print.

Sexual Development

Sexual curiosity continues during this stage. Young school-age children ask many questions. Parents need to answer the questions honestly on the level of their child's understanding, being mindful not to give more information than the child can digest or understand. Children learn much about their own sexuality and about the sexuality of others from their parents' behaviors. Critical for the child's understanding are not only the details of sexual intercourse, but also how people feel about and treat others and how they handle issues of responsibility. School-age children need to learn about respect for other people's feelings and values even if they differ from their own. They should learn never to force another child to do something simply because it is what they themselves want

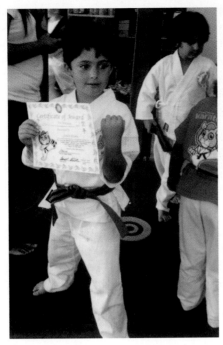

FIGURE 9.3 Skill and practice teach discipline and confidence during school age.

to do. This teaches a valuable point without even focusing on sexual content.

Parents can use issues on television or song lyrics to form the basis of conversations relating to sexuality. Children should be asked questions such as, "Does that make sense?" or "How would you feel in that situation?" Parents should provide all the information children need and keep the lines of communication open so that their children will be able to make future decisions regarding sex.

Freud describes this period as latency, a time when sexual energies are relatively dormant. During this stage children are more involved with cognitive skills and learning than with sexual concerns. Because this is sometimes thought of as a period of "homosexuality," their peer relationships are mainly with children of the same sex. The ability to establish meaningful, caring relationships at this stage helps children prepare for caring relationships in adulthood.

Psychosocial Development

Industry

Erikson believed that school-age children are able to see themselves as producers. Thus he viewed the primary task for this stage of development as industry. Children at this time are more focused on the real world and see themselves as part of a larger group, allowing them to accomplish more and get along better with others. Their motivational drive increases, and they gain satisfaction from their accomplishments. Schoolwork takes on a great deal of importance to children of this age. They often set very high standards of achievement in their academic endeavors. When they fall short of their goals, they may be very disappointed and develop a sense of failure. Some children become very upset if they do not get a grade of 100% or receive praise from their teachers for their efforts. For this reason it is important to use positive reinforcement as motivation for learning.

Children of 6 to 7 years of age are full of energy and anxious to try new skills. Many begin new projects but do not have the patience or attention span to see things to completion. For example, a mother and child may begin to bake cookies, but halfway through the task the child loses interest, leaving the mother alone to complete the task. At the beginning of this stage, children need immediate gratification for their work efforts. They are in a hurry to finish what they start and proudly show it off to others. They need praise and rewards from others to help strengthen their self-esteem and motivate them.

Nine-year-olds can initiate a task and are motivated to see the task to completion. They know what is expected of them and are more likely to conform to win the regard of adults. By age 11 most children are capable of working on more complex projects and can accept delayed rewards. Praise still helps strengthen their self-esteem. Without reinforcement and praise, children may develop a sense of inferiority.

Peer Relationships

During this period, children begin for the first time to move away from the family toward peer relationships (Fig. 9.4). These relationships are generally numerous and of short duration. Most of the time children gravitate toward peers of the same sex and openly express dislike for the opposite sex. Among 7- to 8-year-old children friendships become more intense and serious but are still mainly with children of the same gender. These friendships are made up of several children who have common needs and interests. They frequently form one strong friendship or best friend. Heroes or idols may be worshiped and fantasized about by children of both sexes. Thinking and behavior become more complex. Activity levels vary greatly, with some periods of quiet sitting and other periods of high energy and activity.

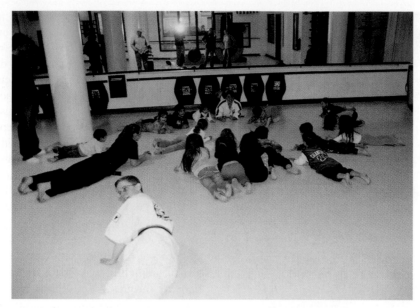

FIGURE 9.4 School-age children move toward peer relationships.

School-age children are frequently engaged in rivalry with their siblings and often wind up in tears, still wanting things to go their way. They keep track of whose cookie has more chips in it or who got to choose the radio station in the car during the last outing. Their words, anger, and level of competition seem out of proportion to the issues. For example, they might say, "I wish you were dead" to a brother or sister who is sitting in the favorite chair. Jealousy is a common emotional expression that may intensify when the child enters school and leaves younger siblings at home with undivided parental attention. Another form of this emotion occurs when the child believes that his or her peers are more accomplished. Although at all ages children need love and affection, boys of this age tend to feel that they are too old to be kissed or hugged and may resent their parents' use of endearing terms or displays of public affection.

Family relationships appear to be less important to school-age children than their new peer relationships. Inside the home they often express negative feelings and are openly hostile toward family members, whereas outside the home they firmly defend, support, and even boast about their family members. Friendships are very important and are the cornerstone of the school-age child's social world. The patterns of interpersonal relationships that are learned at this stage continue into adulthood. School-age children are able to develop reciprocal relationships with their peers. These relationships are based on genuine feelings and appreciation of the other person's unique qualities. It is common for children to establish intimacy with their friends and to share their possessions and their innermost secrets and feelings. Toward the end of this stage friendships become more intense and serious but are still mainly with children of the same gender.

Other Developments

Privacy

Privacy becomes important to children of this age group. They want their belongings and valuables to be off-limits to others. They also want privacy in self-care activities and appear modest and shy. For example, when shopping for new clothes with a parent, the child may insist on going into the dressing room alone. These feelings should be respected and not ridiculed.

Fears

It is not uncommon for children at this age to have an exaggerated fear of physical harm to themselves and to members of their families. Some of these fears may be increased by watching violence on television or in the movies. To help reduce these fears, children should be given realistic reassurance, and their exposure to violent programming should be limited. At this age they may spend time worrying about issues such as divorce, illness, and dying. As children move toward adolescence, they tend to become more nonverbal about their worries, keeping feelings to themselves.

Concept of Money

Preschool children recognize that money can buy things, but their concept of money is yet unclear. For example, they may believe that coins are worth more than paper money and that nickels are more valuable than dimes because they are larger. School-age children begin to place importance on money and possessions. Parents should establish with their children a predetermined amount of money as an allowance and use the allowance to help teach them how to handle money. School-age children are also now capable of working at small jobs; in fact, many ask, "How much will you pay me?" before doing a simple household chore. Allowances and home chores should be kept separate. Children should be taught that they are expected to help around the home simply because they are part of the family unit. This teaches them responsibility within the family setting, and these principles can later be applied to the larger environment.

Hygiene

During this period there are often conflicts regarding the child's personal hygiene and other home-care activities. School-age children frequently have to be reminded to bathe and change their clothes. They may spend a great deal of time in the bathroom but may emerge no cleaner than when they went in. By the end of this stage children frequently leave their rooms in a mess, suggesting that puberty and the teen years are rapidly approaching. Box 9.1 offers hints on preparation for puberty.

Emotions

Emotions have wide ranges of expression, depending on the child's chronological age and psychological maturity. In the early part of this stage of development, children may use simple emotions to express their feelings. Tears, for example, are still used but are quickly seen as a babyish form of expression. Some children are shyer than others. Some have many fears or worry about social acceptance or school performance. Table 9.1 lists common school-age fears. Children may express anger, a powerful emotion, in different ways. Some may

TABLE 9.1	Common School-Age Fears
Age	**Fear**
6–7 years	Strange loud noises, ghosts and witches, being alone at night, bodily injury, school
7–8 years	Dark places, catastrophes, not being liked, physical harm
8–9 years	Failure in school, being caught in a lie, divorce or separation of parents, being a crime victim
9–11 years	Becoming ill, heights, pain, evil people

be negative or sulk, others may withdraw or refuse to speak, and still others may be openly disagreeable and hostile. Anger may represent the child's frustration and need for independence.

Discipline

Discipline continues to be an important need for children of this age group. It teaches them boundaries and helps to set limits on their behavior. Children also need a certain amount of freedom to explore. The proper amount of discipline is crucial. Too much may lead to acting-out behavior, with the child attempting to prove and assert himself or herself. However, too-lenient parental control may lead to insecurity and doubt. Children need adequate praise and rewards to help reinforce desirable behavior.

Physical discipline refers to just that—using physical force such as hitting or spanking. This type of discipline leads to a decrease in the child's self-esteem. Better forms of discipline include time-outs and clear explanations of appropriate behavior. Several studies have looked at the relationship between parental physical discipline and different ethnic groups. Results have indicated that in families using physical discipline, there was a higher incidence of children having behavior problems regardless of the ethnic group. Many researchers believe that findings support parental nurturance and gentle disciplinary tactics as a means toward positive child outcomes.

School-age children are usually able to take responsibility for their rooms and possessions. They can be given small jobs around the house as part of their chores. These jobs help give children a sense of importance within the family structure and help teach them responsibility.

BOX 9.1 Preparations for Puberty

- Offer information and answer questions regarding puberty.
- Expect adult appearance to precede adult behavior.
- Promote positive self-esteem.
- Treat puberty as a positive experience.

Special Psychosocial Concerns

Television Violence

Studies have indicated that violence on television can have an adverse effect on young viewers. Even children who have no problems dealing with aggression have been shown to become more aggressive after watching violent television. The belief that television portrays real-life events further complicates the school-age child's distorted views. It is not uncommon for children of this age to imitate and idolize cartoons or other characters from television shows. Parents can help children choose shows to watch and limit their viewing of excessively violent programs. In addition, parents need to discuss values and practice nonviolent behavior.

Video Games/Internet Use

Playing video games may help develop hand–eye coordination, and some games help children strengthen their problem-solving skills. Parents can assist by helping children select age-appropriate games. Extra care must be taken not to simply rely on the rating stamped on the package. Instead, parents must view the contents before having the child use the product. Computers should be placed in an open area where the family gathers and parents can oversee the child, and time spent using games or computers should be limited. Parents must monitor the Internet sites their child visits. Children should be instructed not to go into chat rooms and give out personal information. Children should know that sometimes individuals misrepresent themselves on the Internet (Box 9.2), and that at no time should any child plan to meet in person someone that they met on the Internet.

Bullying

School-age children are often critical of others but may brag and boast about themselves. It is common to overhear them teasing, bullying, or using insulting comments when talking about others. Bullying is defined as repeated negative actions by one or more persons against chosen victims. Bullies are often children who have been bullied themselves and may pick on others to feel powerful, popular, or in control. Some children even find humor at someone else's expense. There are usually three groups involved: the bully, the victim, and the bystander. Bullies pick on individuals whose responses provide instant gratification. Male bullies are at risk for poor long-term outcomes unless counseling or other help stops their pattern of bullying. Victims of repeated bullying may begin to feel that they deserve the teasing. The bystander is the individual who just observes the bullying incident without any active involvement. This person fails to assist the victim, which may leave the bystander with feelings of powerlessness.

Bullying is more widespread than we would like to believe. If your child is a bully, it is important to emphasize that this kind of behavior is unacceptable. Some children may assume the role of the victim and fall prey to a bully. Parents can help reduce the intimidation and fear of being bullied by listening to their child and offering help. Besides bumps and bruises, signs that a child is being bullied include sleeping problems, irritability, poor concentration, problems with schoolwork, missing belongings or money, and frequent unexplained psychosomatic complaints. Box 9.3 gives parental guidelines for dealing with bullies and victims.

Cyberbullying refers to the use of the Internet, phone, or other technology to repeatedly harass or taunt persons. Parents must monitor their children's

---

BOX 9.2   Cyber Risks

- Avoid exposure to inappropriate, explicit content.
- Avoid sharing personal information.
- Limit the amount of time spent in cyberspace.
- Report "cyberbullying."
- Never share passwords.
- Avoid chat rooms and chatting with strangers.

BOX 9.3   Parental Guidelines for Bullies and Victims

For the Bully:

- Teach the child to respect the rights of others.
- Set clear, firm rules with regard to social behavior.
- Teach and use negotiation techniques.
- Set positive examples.
- Praise desirable behavior.

For the Victim:

- Offer coping strategies.
- Encourage verbalization about incidents.
- Encourage participation in activities that build self-esteem.
- Praise child for achievements.
- Avoid intervening if at all possible.

For the Bystander:

- Recognize that this is a serious problem.
- Encourage the child to shout for adult assistance.
- If that fails, leave and find adult help.
- Discuss that a lack of action may further support the bully.

Internet usage and investigate any sudden onset of school phobia, attention problems, grade slippage, or psychosomatic complaints.

"Latchkey" Children

Approximately one-quarter of all elementary school children care for themselves for a short time after school. In some inner-city areas there may be after-school programs, but in more rural areas children are more likely to be at home unsupervised. It is difficult to generalize or predict how these "latchkey" children are doing. Some of them go straight home, report to their parents, and have a schedule of duties to complete. These children are less likely to get into trouble than those who are unsupervised and just "hang out."

Cognitive Development

According to Piaget, between ages 5 and 7 most children make the transition from the preoperational stage to concrete operational thought. School-age children have grasped the concept of *conservation*. For example, by 7 years of age the child understands that someone dressed in a costume is really just another human being and not some alien being to fear. Piaget believed that the school-age child develops *causation*—that is, understands the cause and effect of relationships. For example, 8-year-old children usually know that rain does not always cause thunder. According to Piaget, school-age children can also place objects in order according to size (*seriation*). Piaget also suggested that school-age children have improved conservation and classification skills. They learn to develop their conservation skills in an orderly sequence—that is, first they understand the concept of number and then the concepts of substance, length, area, weight, and volume.

At this age they can recognize the relationships of a part to the whole and between sets and subsets. For example, 7- to 8-year-old children frequently have collections of stickers, baseball cards, books, videos, and so forth. These can be arranged and sorted according to several characteristics. Children who are 8 to 9 years old can readily recognize and name different makes and models of cars. A car is not simply a Ford; it is a Taurus sedan. They can break down items into smaller parts and then reassemble them. Children at this age can enjoy working on more complex puzzles, assembling model cars, and so forth.

School-age children can take into consideration the views of other people, thereby widening their own perspectives. Typically, they have an increased attention span and are less restless, which makes them better able to stay focused on activities for longer periods. Seven-year-old children are more serious than younger children. School-age children are very productive and adventurous. Their abilities have increased to allow a more organized style of thinking, which includes problem solving. They are better able to understand and follow rules.

School-age children can understand concepts such as time, space, and dimension with more clarity than they could at earlier developmental stages. Their increased cognitive abilities enable them to master reading, mathematics, and science. During elementary school, children begin to learn how to tackle and solve problems. School-age children have improved memory, which enhances their learning skills.

Formal Education

Starting formal education is a major accomplishment for this age group. School becomes the focus of the child's environment. In preschool the focus is on protection, play, and caring; in elementary school the emphasis is on education and learning. School offers children the opportunity to establish themselves as individuals, separate from their parents and family. Children spend more time in school than anywhere else outside the home. This is where they try on different roles within a group setting, test their negotiation skills, and experiment with learning. Adjustment to school depends on the individual child, the home setting, and the school environment. For some, leaving home is difficult and results in the onset of school phobia, which is an intense fear of going to school. The onset of various somatic (physical) complaints—stomachache, headache, or other unexplained pains—may be manifestations of school phobia and should be thoroughly investigated to rule out any underlying medical pathology or problems at school with the teacher, a bully, and so forth. Once the child has been medically evaluated, he or she should be treated if necessary, given support, and gently encouraged to return to the school routine. School places several stresses on children. They must find a classroom by themselves, speak in front of the class, or be reprimanded by a teacher. School, however, is also the place for rewards, recognition, and success.

In kindergarten, children learn to socialize and get along with their peers. Children at this age respond favorably to an authority figure, such as a teacher, and to praise and rewards.

During the early grades (1 through 4), children learn to follow routines and concentrate on specific tasks. Children 8 and 9 years old are serious about their academic performance and are more ready to take responsibility for their learning and for their actions. They are concerned about being wrong and worry about being humiliated in front of their peers. They accept the teacher with unconditional respect.

Later, during the upper grades (5 through 8), learning becomes more of an independent task. Children of this age group are more judgmental and critical. Respect for teachers and authority wanes, giving the teacher less control in the classroom. Children need clear-cut rules, with an emphasis on fairness. Box 9.4 provides guidelines for a good classroom environment.

At an earlier age, homework was considered fun, but by 8 or 9 years of age children regard homework as something to avoid, rush through, forget, or put off. Homework and studying are the basis of many arguments between parents and older school-age children. Parents of young children are very involved with the mechanics of studying, assisting with assignments, and checking completed work efforts. Children who develop a routine for doing homework are generally more successful in school than those who do not.

By ages 9 to 11, most children would rather be at home or with their friends following their interests than in school. The children who thrive and succeed in school are usually more motivated and receive positive reinforcement from both parents and teachers. Poor performance in school at this time should not be ignored by parents or teachers.

Homeschooling

Homeschooling is an alternative to formal school that some parents elect for their children. The advantage of homeschooling is the control parents gain over the environment and their child's learning. They can modify the teaching to individual learning styles and needs. Some of the disadvantages may include decreased socialization experiences for the child and time-consuming parental responsibilities that may lead to parental stress.

Moral Development

Just as school-age children are making a transition in their cognitive abilities, they are also moving from one stage of moral development to the next. According to Kohlberg, most 6-year-old children are still likely to be at the *preconventional* level of moral thought—that is, they are primarily egocentric. They react to situations mainly to be rewarded or to avoid punishment or reprimand, without concern for other moral implications. Later, children move to the *conventional* level of moral reasoning. They begin to make moral decisions based on what their families or others in society expect of them. They want to conform to what they believe will make them "good" girls or boys. By middle childhood, children can be counted on to act "the right way."

School-age children tell different types of lies than younger children do. They lie to improve their self-esteem and status and to win recognition. This lying is a type of bragging that helps them cope with new social pressures. These lies, if infrequent, should not be of concern to parents.

BOX
9.4   Desirable Classroom Environment

To create a desirable classroom environment, teachers should do the following:

- Give ample praise.
- Structure comfortable work areas.
- Encourage sharing of responsibilities.
- Stress academic achievement.
- Use positive reinforcement.
- Be positive role models.
- Promote open communication.

HELPFUL HINTS

Homework

- Try to make homework a pleasant experience.
- Set aside a specific time for homework.
- Make homework a top priority.
- Offer a lot of reassurance.
- Provide attention and contact with the child during homework sessions by offering a snack, a hug, or a reassuring touch.

Toward the end of this stage, at about age 11, children begin to balance their self-interests and needs against what they know to be right. They also begin to consider what is fair to others. Kohlberg described their concern for others as the beginning of reciprocity.

The 11-year-old child has a need to be trusted. Trust reinforces the child's concept of self-worth. At this point children demand loyalty from their friends and reciprocate this feeling. School-age children also learn self-regulation and control of their behavior.

Some studies have supported Kohlberg's views on moral development and have indicated that children's moral thinking is stimulated when they are involved in ethical discussions or in decision making. Other studies suggest that moral development is different for girls and boys: Girls base moral reasoning on considering and preserving human relationships, whereas boys base moral decisions on protecting and defending others. Regardless of which theory one ascribes to, it is important to keep in mind that moral reasoning, like cognition, develops gradually, with some overlapping at each stage. A child's moral code is based on his or her parents' teachings and behaviors. Once children internalize a moral code, they use it to judge the actions of others. Box 9.5 gives an example of a moral exercise.

Communication

Language improves so that school-age children are able to communicate more effectively with others. The ability to use language is important and enhances socialization and group belonging. Earlier forms of communication, which may have been more limited to gestures and crying, are now socially

unacceptable. The unacceptability of these forms helps to reinforce language acquisition.

School places an emphasis on building vocabulary, proper grammar, pronunciation, and sentence structure. School-age children can use nouns, verbs, and adjectives in their sentences. For the most part, they use the proper tense in speech. Their sentences describe their feelings, thoughts, and points of view. The use of swear words or slang increases as a result of peer influence. These words help to express their emotions and give them a sense of importance. A secret language is sometimes used by this age group to transmit messages back and forth to one another. Not only does this give children a degree of privacy, but it also enhances their sense of group belonging. Table 9.2 provides a schedule of language development.

NUTRITION

For continued growth of the musculoskeletal system, nutritional requirements during this stage include an

TABLE 9.2 Language Development

Age	Development
6 years	Has vocabulary of 3,000 words, understands meaning of complex sentences, and can read
7 years	Tells time and prints well
8 years	Writes and prints
9 years	Describes objects in detail and writes well
10–11 years	Writes lengthy compositions, begins dictionary skills, and develops good grammar

BOX 9.5 Moral Exercise

Read the following exercise to the class. Ask the children how they would react in similar circumstances. Discuss the responses with the class.

Two brothers are walking home from school and are approached by a classmate, who gives the older boy a joint (marijuana cigarette) to smoke. The younger brother watches his brother accept and begin to smoke the cigarette. Despite his younger brother's protests, the older boy tells him not to tell anyone what he has just seen. He reminds the younger boy that he must keep this to himself or risk losing his (the older brother's) respect and friendship.

What should the younger brother do: keep the information to himself, or share it with his parents and risk upsetting his sibling?

HELPFUL HINTS

Lying

- Parents should set good examples. Do not ask your child to lie on the phone, for example, saying that you are not home when you are but do not feel like talking.
- Give your child permission to tell the truth by listening and not setting excessive punishments.
- Admit your own mistakes.

adequate intake of calories from proteins, carbohydrates, fats, vitamins, and minerals. Calcium is especially important at this time to allow the building of dense bones. Caloric requirements vary from child to child based on body size, activity, and metabolism. In the 1,800-calorie diet recommended by MyPlate for this stage, children need 5 ounces of proteins, 3 cups of dairy, 2½ cups of vegetables, 1½ cups of fruit, and 6 ounces of grains per day. Box 9.6 lists indicators of good nutrition. The child's food preferences result from cultural influences, family preferences, and peer influences. By the time children enter school, their food habits are well established. These habits can be further influenced by increased exposure to different cultures.

Important considerations in planning meals for the school-age child include maintaining weight within normal limits and avoiding a diet high in cholesterol. The recommended daily intake of cholesterol is 300 mg or less per day. Between 3% and 25% of school-age children have rising blood cholesterol levels, increasing their risk for cardiovascular disease. To keep cholesterol intake down, provide a diet that is low in saturated fats—that is, fats from animal sources, such as meat and dairy products. Both blood cholesterol levels and weight should be monitored during the child's routine health checkups.

Breakfast is one of the most important meals of the child's day. It should supply children with one-fourth to one-third of their daily nutritional needs. Children should not be allowed to skip breakfast before going to school. Lunch programs often supply children with the noontime meal. Parents should monitor the school lunch program to make absolutely certain that it meets the standards and nutritional needs of the growing child.

Food fads and new habits begin at this time. Excessive sweets and caffeine should be avoided because they may interfere with concentration and

cause hyperactivity. Children should be encouraged to become involved in shopping for, preparing, and serving food and cleaning up after meals.

Obesity

Obesity is a rapidly growing problem beginning in early childhood. The causes of this problem include poor nutrition, unhealthy eating patterns, social pressures, and genetics. Excessive weight gain contributes to decreased physical abilities, making it more difficult for the child to engage in sports and athletic activities. Prevention and treatment must begin early to ensure successful results.

In some cultures being overweight is not a concern. Research has shown that certain children of Hispanic, African American, or Native American descent may be more likely to condone being overweight than white or non-Hispanic children. Other contributing factors to obesity include family lifestyles, family dynamics, peer pressure, and socioeconomic level. Busy families may use fast foods or prepackaged foods that are calorie dense as a way to save time. Advertisements and commercials precondition children to seek out undesirable foods.

The psychological impact of obesity on the growing child is a concern because it often results in lowering the individual's self-esteem. Children may fear being teased about their weight by their peers. Teasing only furthers the child's feelings of shame and despair. Studies of Western civilization indicate that society generally views obese individuals very negatively. Overweight children have been shown to be more likely to become overweight adults, with an increased risk of developing diabetes, cardiovascular disease, or both.

Strategies for managing obesity should include selecting healthy foods and engaging in an active lifestyle. Lifestyle changes work best when they involve the whole family. Regular meals must be planned ahead of time and should include nutritious foods, and exercise should be incorporated into the daily schedule. Parents should encourage schools to promote healthy meals and snacks for their children to enjoy.

SLEEP AND REST

Sleep routines should be well established by this stage. An average 6-year-old child needs about 12 hours of sleep, whereas an 11-year-old child needs about 10 hours. A 6-year-old child can tire easily and become very irritable. For this reason

B O X
9.6 Signs of Good Nutrition

- An alert, energetic attitude
- Height and weight within the normal range
- Skin is smooth, moist, and has good color
- Hair is shiny
- Eyes are clear, with no circles underneath them
- Teeth are white, bright, straight, and without discoloration
- Good gastrointestinal health, including a good appetite and proper elimination
- Well-developed, firm muscles and good posture
- A good attention span

parents need to supervise activities and incorporate quiet, restful activities to prevent overexhaustion. Some children may even benefit from a short afternoon nap. If children are chronically tired during school hours, their academic performances and social relationships will suffer.

Sleep for some younger children may continue to be restless and interrupted by nightmares. As the child grows older, nightmares usually decrease. They also become less terrifying and less real as the child begins to be able to separate fantasy from reality.

PLAY

The focus of play illustrates the movement that school-age children make from pretending and fantasy toward reality and concrete thinking. School-age children are full of energy and willing to learn new skills. The style of play for this age group permits the use of cooperation and compromise. Many younger children are not yet ready for competitive activities and become upset at losing. Parents must be careful not to push their child into competitive play before he or she is actually ready to handle this kind of demand.

Most 9- to 11-year-old children are involved in many play activities. They are usually very competitive and active. Children are now able to learn and follow rules and regulations. The style of play for this period of development is referred to as team play. Team play usually is with groups of the same sex and may be competitive in nature. Boys are likely to be better than girls at running, jumping, and throwing. This difference may be because girls have fewer opportunities to engage in these activities and are less encouraged to do so. Efforts are now being made to emphasize and fund girls' sports activities to the same degree as boys' sports activities. This may help to enhance girls' sports performance and competitiveness. Much of the play of both sexes is based on group or team activities.

Children are chosen by their peers to participate on a team based on their abilities to excel in the skills required to play the game. Being selected first helps validate the child's self-esteem and worth. By this stage children have learned that practice helps to improve their skills. Skill and motor coordination determine the child's overall performance and acceptance by others. Organized team sports such as Little League or team swimming may appeal to this age group. Competition now serves as a motivating force to practice and improve.

Although most of the play during this stage involves sports and athletic activities, some children prefer sedentary activities such as crafts and board games. Collections of all sorts (cards, little boxes, cars, stickers, dolls, and other items, some of little or no value) are very popular at this stage. Ownership seems to have greater importance than actual monetary value.

SAFETY

The leading cause of accidental deaths for this age group continues to be motor vehicle accidents. State regulations for car safety should be carefully observed. Children should be taught to use seat belts whenever they are passengers in automobiles and school buses.

The increased motor skills of school-age children help contribute to the increased numbers of accidents and injuries they sustain. An additional factor is that most children at this stage are ready to attempt any new skill with or without practice or training. For the most part they are much less fearful than they were during earlier years. To minimize danger from biking accidents, skating, or skateboarding, children should be encouraged to wear helmets and protective gear when engaged in these popular activities.

School-age children should be taught common water safety practices, such as never swimming alone and only diving in water approved for diving. Children should be instructed not to swim in canals, in drainage basins, or in water with unknown currents.

Many bone and muscular injuries occur during this stage because of the child's physiological development and increased participation in sports. During the school-age period, the epiphyseal cartilage, or bone end, is the site for future bone growth. These

---

H E L P F U L   H I N T S

Safety Precautions to Teach Children

- Wear protective equipment.
- Observe traffic signals.
- Practice water safety: Learn to swim, and never swim alone.
- Use the buddy system when walking to and from school.
- Never talk to or accept rides from strangers.
- Always follow your instincts and avoid peer pressure.

points are weak and become potential sites for fractures. Final bone ossification, or hardening, occurs at puberty.

Stranger Danger

Children at this stage of development must be advised to avoid being lured away by strangers. They need to know how to protect themselves by avoiding walking alone in dark, remote areas.

Today parents and teachers must advise children to avoid chat room and Internet sites that child predators frequent. Children must be advised not to divulge any personal information to anyone on the Web. Parents need to make certain that they supervise and monitor their children's computer usage. Software to monitor a child's computer use is available.

School Violence

In recent years the media has brought to our awareness the rapidly increasing incidences of violence in school. School violence can be defined as any harm, whether physical or psychological, that is directed toward schoolchildren and their property. School violence involves those acts not only in the school, but also around the school or on playgrounds. The increase in these incidences has led to parental concerns for the safety of their children and increased school security. Schools around the nation are adopting a zero-tolerance policy toward school violence. To accomplish this, authorities must first understand the causes of violence and the signs of impending trouble.

The two most common factors known to contribute to school violence are a breakdown in communication in the home and school and the easy availability of weapons. Consider that an estimated 1.2 million elementary school children come home every day to a house with a gun and no guardian. Other contributing factors to violence are bullying behavior and stress in the home and school. Children under stress do not have the ability to cope effectively and may resort to violence. When they feel hurt or become angry, some children use revenge to regain control and feel powerful. This is especially true of some boys who are unduly influenced by peer pressure. Male children are often encouraged to be tough and unfeeling, and their expression of power can lead to violence. Good parenting can help decrease violent behavior. Parents and teachers should be diligent in recognizing behaviors that can quickly lead to violence. Such signs include difficulty getting along with peers, outbursts of temper, violence directed toward pets, decreased productivity in the home or at

school, sleeping and eating problems, social isolation, and preoccupation with violent video games and movies. Box 9.7 lists some helpful hints to decrease school violence.

HEALTH PROMOTION

In general, the school-age years are considered a healthier period than earlier years of development. It is common to see a slight increase in the incidence of upper respiratory tract infections when children first enter school, probably because of exposure to many other children. Once their immune systems adjust, children are able to resist many infections. As their organs continue to mature, there is less risk of ear infections, febrile seizures, and dehydration.

School-age children continue to need supervision in hygiene and daily care. There may be a higher incidence of urinary tract infections in girls related to their anatomy and daily toileting practices.

Yearly checkups should also include a urine examination for infection and diabetes mellitus and blood tests for iron-deficiency anemia and cholesterol levels. Blood pressure screening should be instituted at this time. Other routine measurements include continued monitoring of weight, height, and growth. Health promotion must include nutritional guidance. By school age all of the primary immunizations have been completed, and children need to receive boosters to help maintain immunity. They normally receive a tetanus–diphtheria booster every 10 to 14 years, the human papillomavirus immunization, and the meningococcal vaccine. Refer to Appendix B for the complete immunization schedule.

Before beginning school and every year thereafter, children should get their eyes checked by an ophthalmologist. Most visual problems can be corrected with

---

BOX 9.7 Decreasing School Violence

- Spend more family time with children.
- Maintain open communication lines in school and at home.
- Regulate the viewing of violent programs on the Internet and television.
- Store any weapons securely in the house.
- Perform random checks of lockers and school bags.
- Supervise entry and exit points at school.
- Have only one entry or exit to the school.
- Use metal detectors at the school entry.
- Encourage peer counseling.
- Teach conflict resolution in the home and at school.

glasses and retraining exercises. Adequate lighting is important to help maintain proper vision. Regular hearing tests should be scheduled to determine baseline hearing levels. Parents should instruct children about avoiding exposure to excessive noise, which may damage the ears and lead to hearing loss.

School-age children need adequate exercise to help develop strength and muscle endurance. Poor posture can indicate fatigue or a minor skeletal defect. Children should be screened for scoliosis—the abnormal lateral curvature of the spine—by the school nurse and by the doctor during their physical examinations. To examine a child for scoliosis, have him or her bend over, and examine the lumbar thoracic region for unequal curvature. This condi-

tion is seen more frequently in girls than in boys. Early recognition can lead to prompt treatment and correction with exercises or a brace.

Special Health Concern: Substance Abuse

School-age children are easy prey to substance abuse through peer pressure. Some may gravitate toward alcohol, tobacco, or drugs based on a familiarity with such items in their homes. Parents need to model desired behaviors and offer information and guidance to prevent substance abuse in their children. For a complete discussion of substance abuse, see Chapter 10.

SUMMARY

1. The period of development known as school age, the middle years, or late childhood is characterized by slow, consistent growth.

2. This stage begins with entrance into formal school and ends with the onset of puberty.

3. Five important accomplishments occur during this stage: (1) growth becomes slow and steady; (2) children move away from the family and toward peer relationships; (3) children become less self-centered and more goal-directed; (4) deciduous teeth are replaced by permanent teeth; and (5) sexual tranquillity replaces sexual curiosity and preoccupation.

4. The permanent teeth develop in the same order as the deciduous teeth.

5. Initially, school-age children experience an increased number of respiratory infections because of their increased exposure to other children. Once the immune system matures, this becomes a relatively healthy period of development.

6. Heart rate and respiratory rate slow, whereas blood pressure readings increase. Changes in the nervous system permit expanded cognitive processes.

7. There is marked improvement in existing gross and fine motor skills, permitting children more independence.

8. This period is sometimes called latency, a time when sexual energies are dormant. Because

peer relationships at this stage are mainly with children of the same sex, this stage is thought of as a period of "homosexuality."

9. According to Erikson, the task for this stage of development is industry. Children are now capable of focusing on reality, and they gain satisfaction from their accomplishments.

10. Friendships are very important and are the cornerstone of the school-age child's social world. During this stage children are able to develop reciprocal relationships with their peers. It is common for them to establish intimacy with their friends and share their feelings and possessions.

11. Discipline teaches the child boundaries and helps to set limits on behavior. Too much discipline may lead to acting-out behavior; insufficient discipline may lead to insecurity and doubt.

12. Television violence may adversely affect many school-age children. For this reason parents should supervise children's choices of programming.

13. About one-fourth of school-age children are at home alone while parents are at work. These "latchkey" children need special guidelines to follow while alone.

14. According to Piaget, in this stage children move from the preoperational level of cognitive development to concrete operational

thought, which permits organized thinking and the ability to understand and follow rules.

15. School becomes a major focus of the child's environment. Unlike the experience in preschool, when the focus was on protection, play, and nurturing, the emphasis is now on education and learning.

16. According to Kohlberg, school-age children are at the preconventional level of maturity. Reciprocity is the concern for others that school-age children develop. Trust and loyalty are demanded of friends. The child's moral code is based on the teachings and actions of the parents.

17. Language improves, enabling children to communicate more effectively with others.

18. School places emphasis on the development of vocabulary, grammar, pronunciation, and sentence structure.

19. The nutritional requirements during this stage include an adequate diet of nutrients necessary for growth of the musculoskeletal system. Food preferences result from cultural, family, and peer influences. Breakfast is one of the most important meals of the child's day. It should not be skipped and should supply one-fourth to one-third of the daily nutritional needs.

20. The average 6-year-old child needs about 12 hours of sleep, whereas 11-year-old children need only 10 hours of sleep each night.

Inadequate sleep can produce irritability and interfere with the child's academic and social relationships.

21. School-age children play and carry out most self-care activities independently. They learn to write, draw, and dance and develop many other creative hobbies. In the home, children are able to take responsibility for their possessions and like to earn money for small jobs.

22. The style of play for this stage of development is referred to as team play. At this time children are able to learn to follow rules and regulations. Most play occurs in same-sex groups and is competitive in nature.

23. The leading cause of accidental deaths for this age group continues to be motor vehicle accidents. Children should be instructed to use seat belts whenever they are passengers. Other causes of increased injuries are related to the school-age child's natural tendency to attempt new skills without help, supervision, or training.

24. Children of this age need adequate exercise to help develop muscle strength and endurance.

25. School-age children should be screened for abnormal curvature of the spine known as scoliosis. They need to receive booster vaccinations to maintain their immunity.

26. As school-age children's organs continue to mature, they are better able to resist infections and tend to recover more rapidly from illnesses.

CRITICAL THINKING

Exercise #1

Helen Lightbourne is the mother of 7-year-old Heather, her first-born child. Ms. Lightbourne expresses concern to the pediatric nurse that Heather appears to have two loose teeth. Her specific concern is the management of the loose teeth.

1. What information should the nurse plan to share with Ms. Lightbourne about the expected pattern of tooth loss?
2. How would you instruct Ms. Lightbourne to care for Heather's primary teeth?
3. What common complication should she be alerted to as the permanent teeth erupt?

Exercise #2

What advice would you offer to the mother of a 6-year-old who tells you that she found her child playing doctor with another child during a playdate?

MULTIPLE-CHOICE QUESTIONS

1. The change in posture typical of school-age children is due to:
   a. Tightening of the ligaments that support the long bones
   b. Lengthening of the musculoskeletal fibers
   c. A shift in the center of gravity
   d. Flattening and broadening of the rib cage

2. School-age children experience an increase in blood pressure because of:
   a. Decreased cardiac muscle strength
   b. Reduction in the capacity of the atrium
   c. Slightly increased hemoglobin levels
   d. Development of the ventricles

3. Stress experienced by school-age children may be manifested as:
   a. Ritualistic behavior
   b. Magical thinking
   c. School phobia
   d. Egocentric thinking

4. According to Erikson, the psychosocial task for school-age children is known as:
   a. Trust
   b. Industry
   c. Inferiority
   d. Initiative

5. During the school-age period, interest in sexual activity:
   a. Peaks
   b. Is dormant
   c. Directs the child's actions
   d. Involves heterosexual relations

6. The number of hours of sleep that the average 6-year-old child needs is:
   a. 10
   b. 12
   c. 8
   d. 15

7. Two factors that contribute to the increase in school violence are:
   a. Increased interest in sporting and hunting
   b. Lack of education and low income
   c. Breakdown in communication and gun availability
   d. Strict discipline and control

8. Excessive weight gain can result in:
   a. Increased agility
   b. Increased attention span
   c. Decreased physical ability
   d. Decreased potential for infection

9. Which of the following behaviors may contribute to problems with losing weight?
   a. Altered sleep patterns
   b. Vegetarian diet
   c. Following the food pyramid
   d. Snacking between meals

10. Routine medical screening is important at this age for detecting:
    a. Amblyopia
    b. Scoliosis
    c. Acne
    d. Sexual abuse

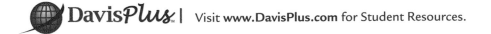 | Visit **www.DavisPlus.com** for Student Resources.

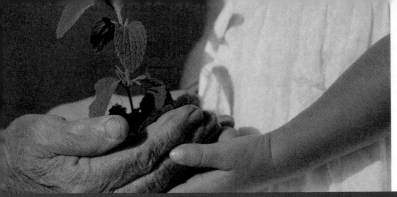

CHAPTER 10

Puberty and Adolescence

Key Words

adenohypophysis

adolescence

ambivalence

anorexia nervosa

apocrine glands

bulimia

depression

ejaculation

emotions

estrogen

gonads

larynx

menarche

ova

ovaries

penis

preadolescence

primary sex characteristics

progesterone

puberty

scrotum

secondary sex
characteristics

sexually transmitted
diseases

sperm

testes

testosterone

Chapter Outline

Learning Objectives

At the end of this chapter, you should be able to:

- List four physical changes occurring in puberty.
- List four physical characteristics of adolescence.
- Describe three developmental milestones of the adolescent period.
- Describe the primary psychosocial task of adolescence as identified by Erikson.
- Describe the cognitive level of functioning during the teenage period of development.
- State how teens develop moral reasoning.
- List three factors that help to promote wellness in the teen.
- Describe three special concerns that may adversely affect adolescent health.

The period known as **puberty,** or **preadolescence,** is a time of rapid growth normally commencing between ages 11 and 14 and taking an average of 2 years to complete. It is marked by the development of **secondary sex characteristics.** Puberty ends (and adolescence begins) with the onset of menses, or menarche, in girls and the production of sperm in boys. The growth patterns affecting the onset of puberty are influenced by factors that include heredity, climate, nutrition, gender, and socioeconomic status (Fig. 10.1).

Four major changes associated with the pubescent period are as follows:

1. Rapid physical growth
2. Changes in body proportions
3. Development of primary sex characteristics (sex organs)
4. Development of secondary sex characteristics

This phase of life witnesses major physical changes and opportunities for success in school, in relationships, and in life. Parents need to understand what children are feeling and struggling with developmentally. Understanding what is normal during this time is reassuring and empowering. Common frustrations include:

• Wishing for independence while needing supervision at home and in school
• Being concerned about appearance while undergoing major body changes

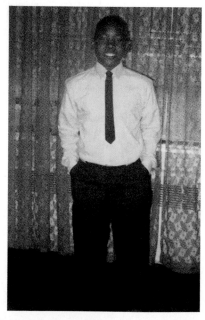

FIGURE 10.1 The age of puberty varies with each individual.

• Seeking peer acceptance while feeling anxious about or frustrated by those same peers
• Struggling to achieve in school while accepting an increasing workload and more responsibility
• Fluctuating between adultlike behavior and childlike impulses
• Maintaining a demanding physical and social schedule while needing increased amounts of rest and sleep

The term **adolescence** is from Latin and means "to grow and mature." It refers to a transitional period that begins with sexual maturity and ends with cessation of growth and the movement toward emotional maturity. This period of development bridges the gap between dependence and independence, or childhood and adulthood. Adolescents need to accomplish the tasks that help prepare them for adulthood. The major characteristics of adolescence include:

• Stormy emotions
• Feelings of insecurity
• Introspection
• Experimentation and learning
• Testing of values and beliefs

PHYSICAL CHARACTERISTICS

Puberty

Height and Weight
Puberty is second to the prenatal period as the phase of most rapid growth. This growth spurt occurs in girls earlier than in boys. The feet are usually the first part of the body that shows the effects of the growth spurt, followed by the legs and trunk. Height increases 20% to 25%. Boys grow 4 to 12 inches (10 to 30 cm) and girls grow 2 to 8 inches (5 to 20 cm) during this period. Increases in weight follow increases in height. These weight changes are related to increases in fat, bone, and muscle tissue. Boys gain between 15 and 65 pounds (7 and 30 kg), and girls gain 15 to 55 pounds (7 to 25 kg). Different parts of the body grow at different rates, making the whole body seem temporarily out of proportion. The bones grow longer and change shape. The trunk begins to broaden at the hips and shoulders.

Development of Sex Characteristics
Primary Sex Characteristics
The **primary sex characteristics** are the **gonads,** or sex glands. The gonads are present at the time of birth but remain functionally inactive until the onset

of puberty. The maturation of these glands is influenced by the adenohypophysis, or anterior lobe of the pituitary gland. The pituitary gland secretes a hormone that stimulates the gonads. In boys, the male gonads, or testes, are located in a sac called the scrotum, found outside of the body. The testes produce male sex cells, or sperm, and the male sex hormone testosterone. Ejaculation, the release of sperm, indicates that the testes are functionally mature. In addition, the penis, or male sex organ, grows in length and circumference.

The female gonads or sex glands are the ovaries, located in the pelvic cavity. Their primary function is to produce the female sex cells (ova, or eggs) needed for reproduction and the female sex hormones estrogen and progesterone. The onset of the menstrual flow, which is called menarche, indicates that a girl is capable of reproduction. The menstrual flow is a monthly discharge of blood, mucus, and tissue from the uterus. It lasts from puberty until menopause. The usual monthly cycle is every 21 to 24 days, with each monthly period or discharge lasting an average of 5 days. Average blood loss with each period is 30 to 60 mL. Some girls and women experience headaches, cramps, swelling, and irritability before and at the onset of their periods.

The whole menstrual process is an emotionally charged event. Attitudes toward menstruation are assimilated from cultural and personal experiences. Education regarding menarche should begin during the school-age period in the home setting. Adequate preparation leads to a more positive initial experience. The primary concerns of young girls are related to hygiene, preventing clothes from getting soiled, and embarrassment. In addition, girls at this stage need to be informed about restrictions, activities, and taboos. If any questions or misconceptions about menstruation exist, they will need to be openly explored with the teen.

Secondary Sex Characteristics

Secondary sex characteristics play no direct role in reproduction but appear at this time. Initially, pubic hair is sparse and lightly pigmented; it then becomes darker, coarse, and curly. In boys, axillary and facial hair appear after the pubic hair growth. Boys' skin thickens, and hair appears on the arms, legs, shoulders, and chest. In boys, the larynx, or voice box, and the vocal cords increase in size, resulting in deepening of the voice.

Changes in the distribution of fat and an increase in the width and roundness of the hip and pelvic bones are secondary sex characteristics occurring in girls. Breast development in girls follows an orderly sequence, resulting in the increase of fatty tissue and the maturation of the mammary glands. Hair also appears in the groin and the axillae.

In both boys and girls, the sebaceous glands produce oil and become larger and more active. This increased activity may be related to the appearance of acne (pimples) seen in many adolescents at this time. The apocrine glands (sweat glands) in the armpits and groin become larger, producing a characteristic odorous secretion.

See Table 10.1 for an overview of the physical and sexual developments of puberty.

Adolescence

Height and Weight

The rate of physical growth slows down after puberty. In girls, growth in height ceases between 16 and 17 years of age. Boys continue to grow in height up to 18 to 20 years of age. During adolescence body proportions are similar to those of the adult.

Muscle and Bone Development

Muscle strength and endurance increase, as does muscle size. Some adolescents complain of muscle

TABLE
10.1   Normal Puberty and Adolescent Development

Boys	Girls
11–12 years: growth of the testes, scrotum, and penis; appearance of pubic hair	10–11 years: rapid growth spurt, breast development, appearance of pubic hair
12–13 years: rapid growth spurt	11–14 years: first menstrual period
13–15 years: growth of underarm, body, and facial hair	12–13 years: appearance of underarm hair
13–14 years: ejaculation 14–15 years: deepening of voice	

soreness and fatigue with increased activity. Adolescents may at first be awkward as a result of the patterns of muscle growth. But by the end of this stage, they should have good muscle development and coordination. Motor capabilities improve with practice and training. Posture may be poor, evidenced by slouching. This may be further complicated by a common condition causing lateral curvature of the spine, known as scoliosis. As discussed in Chapter 9, this is more commonly seen in girls than in boys.

Development of Other Body Systems

The weight and volume of the lungs increase, causing a slowing down in the respiratory rate and an improvement in lung performance. Exercise helps to improve both cardiac and respiratory function.

The stomach and intestines increase in size and capacity. Adolescents have increased appetites and therefore require an increase in their daily food intake. Adequate food intake helps to meet the demands of their bodies. A common observation in adolescents is that they are always hungry and can consume enormous amounts of food at one time. The typical teenager will devour groceries as soon as they are taken out of the shopping bags.

At about 13 years of age, teens gain their second molars, and between 14 and 25 years their third molars, or wisdom teeth, appear. The jaw reaches adult size toward the end of adolescence.

VITAL SIGNS

Normal pulse range for this developmental stage is between 60 and 90 beats per minute. The respiratory rate of an adolescent is about the same as that of an adult. The normal respiratory rate for adolescents should be 16 to 24 breaths per minute. Exercise produces an improved physiological response. The changes in the circulatory system include an increase

---

HELPFUL HINTS

Concerns During Puberty

- Your child appears too thin.
- Your child exhibits sudden outbursts of anger.
- Your child seems preoccupied with family problems.
- Your child's grades are not at the expected level of performance.
- Your child avoids peer interactions.

---

in the size of the heart and in the thickness of the walls of the blood vessels. These changes result in improved pumping ability of the heart. There is also an increase in blood volume. In boys, greater force is needed to help distribute blood to their larger body mass. This force, in turn, causes an increase in blood pressure.

DEVELOPMENTAL MILESTONES

Motor Development

In the beginning of the adolescent stage, teens exhibit some clumsiness as a result of their rapid physical growth. The adolescent's motor functions are comparable to those of the adult. Eye–hand coordination is markedly improved, allowing for good manual dexterity.

Sexual Development

Teens at first gravitate toward individuals of the same sex and ridicule those of the opposite sex. As their bodies undergo the physical changes of puberty, they suffer from heightened emotions, increased worries, and lack of self-confidence (Table 10.2). They are sensitive about the sizes of their body parts and readily compare themselves to their peers. Girls are preoccupied with the size of their breasts, and boys are concerned about the size of their penises. These concerns continue into adolescence. From the time of sexual maturity, the teen can be sexually aroused to orgasm through self-stimulation. Masturbation is a normal part of sexual expression and has no harmful effects, but masturbation can result in feelings of anxiety and guilt if the adolescent is led to believe that it is shameful or unhealthy. Parents should respect adolescents' needs for privacy and knock before entering their rooms.

The extent and age of onset of sexual activity varies from individual to individual. Recent surveys indicate that sexual activity begins early in this country; some children are sexually active at age 10 or 11. Typical sexual behavior in the early dating period includes kissing, necking, and petting. Many teens engage in sexual intercourse. Studies indicate that girls sometimes become sexually active because of pressure or coercion and that the first sexual encounter may be a great disappointment. Boys may also become sexually active because it is expected of them.

TABLE
10.2   Teenagers' Concerns About Their Changing Bodies

Boys	Girls
Penis size. Most boys compare penis size with that of peers. Average length is 5–7 inches (12–17 cm) when erect.	*Breasts* may not be exactly symmetrical. Size varies. Choose a well-fitting bra.
Embarrassing erections may occur at any time. Try to think of something else to help it subside.	*Menstruation* usually begins between 11 and 14 years of age, lasts about 5 days, and occurs every 28 days on average.
Morning erections commonly occur during dreaming.	*Menstrual discomfort* can often be relieved by using heat, taking Advil or Tylenol, and moderating your activity level.
Wet dreams, or ejaculation while sleeping, may occur during dreaming.	*Pregnancy* becomes possible with onset of menstruation.
Voice changes occur as the voice box enlarges, causing the voice to gradually deepen.	*Hygiene* is important especially during menstruation. Regularly bathe or shower.
Perspiration increases because the apocrine sweat glands are highly active. Wash daily and use a deodorant.	Concerns are the same.
Acne and skin blemishes are more common. Cleanse daily. Topical skin-colored creams may help cover small blemishes.	Concerns are the same.

Sexual activity is given high priority at this time in adolescents' lives. Girls traditionally set the limits on sexual interactions. A great deal of pressure to conform to the group's behavioral standards exists. Sexual uncertainties and confusion often arise; many teens give in to peer pressure or lie to their friends about their sexual adventures. By conforming, the individual may find group acceptance. Successful resolution of the search for identity is necessary during the teen years for the young person to find emotional sharing and intimacy.

Research indicates that teenagers acquire most of their information about sex from their peers rather than from more authoritative sources. This may result in transmission of incorrect information. Youngsters should receive sex education before they become teenagers. Young people need to be well informed about reproduction, their bodies, and the responsibilities of sexual behavior. Good sex education, which should include explicit information about the prevention of **sexually transmitted diseases** (STDs) and unwanted pregnancy, enables adolescents to make responsible choices about their own sexuality.

Sexually Transmitted Diseases

The incidence of STDs is increasing in this population. The best means of prevention is information. Every teenager should be taught safe sex practices, whether they choose to be sexually active or not. STDs include chlamydia, trichomoniasis, herpes genitalis, gonorrhea, syphilis, and AIDS. Each of these diseases has its own cause, signs and symptoms, and plan of treatment, but all are spread through vaginal, oral, and rectal intercourse. Table 10.3 summarizes information on STDs.

Teen Pregnancy

Teen pregnancy is both an individual and a social concern. The pregnant adolescent has twice the mortality rate of a nonadolescent pregnant woman. This increase in mortality is related to the fact that the adolescent is still herself growing and will compete with the developing fetus for the needed nutrients. Expected weight gain and the need for additional nutrients should be calculated on an individual basis. Teen pregnancy carries increased risks of complications for both mother and baby. Early recognition and medical supervision may help promote a more

TABLE 10.3 Sexually Transmitted Diseases

Name	Symptoms
Chlamydia	May be asymptomatic or may cause a yellowish vaginal discharge, painful or difficult urination, and spotting between menses or after intercourse; may spread to other pelvic organs
Trichomoniasis	Usually causes thin, frothy, yellow–green vaginal discharge; vaginal itching, tenderness; redness; painful urination and intercourse
Herpes genitalis	Usually causes genital blisters, pain, swollen glands, vaginal discharge and itching
Gonorrhea	May be asymptomatic or may cause a purulent yellow–green vaginal discharge; may cause painful urination and intercourse
Syphilis	Causes painless ulcer (chancre) on genitals, lips, or anus in early stage
AIDS	Causes lethargy, weight loss, skin lesions, and fungal infections

positive outcome. Although teenagers may be physically mature, they may not yet be emotionally mature enough to handle parenthood. Pregnancy and parenthood during the teen years interrupt plans, education, and usual activities. Young teenagers who become pregnant may need additional counseling and time to choose between the various options of abortion, adoption, or parenting. Their decisions may have a serious impact on them for the rest of their lives.

Rape

Adolescent rape appears to be on the increase, and a large number of offenders are themselves adolescents. The exact number of rape cases is not clear because young women are the least likely to report these crimes. Not only are teens at risk for rape by strangers, but they also are at risk for date rape. Education for both male and female teens helps dispel myths about rape and provides preventive strategies.

Psychosocial Development

Psychosocial development is rapid throughout puberty and adolescence. Table 10.4 reviews teenage behavioral issues and offers tips on how parents can deal with them.

Puberty

Several general behavioral characteristics are common during puberty. Individuals enter this stage happy and slowly become negative in their attitudes and interactions. The basis for some of this negativity is growing self-consciousness. This self-doubt

TABLE 10.4 Teenage Behavioral Issues

Behavior	Advice for Parents
Rebelliousness, argumentativeness, or rudeness	Overlook what you can. Avoid confrontation. Be as tolerant as possible. Avoid seeing behavior as a rejection of parental love.
Need for privacy	Make certain that teen has own space. Understand teen's self-conscious behavior. Accept individual's need for some privacy. Offer help, but step back if rejected. Keep lines of communication open.
Dishonesty	Avoid overreaction. Reinforce reality. Maintain consistent principles.
Responsibility	Listen attentively. Expect maturity to be uneven. Encourage decision making and acceptance of responsibility. Set reasonable rules.
Curfews	Allow for unexpected delays. Encourage frequent phone contact.

TABLE
10.4 **Teenage Behavioral Issues—cont'd**

Behavior	Advice for Parents
	Set good examples for teen. Allow social life to center around the home.
Friends	Accept friends without criticism. Try to get to know friends. Avoid showing disapproval.

and worry are related to their changing bodies. Much of the behavior is influenced by an overall negative outlook. Youth at this age tend to spend more time by themselves and in their rooms than they did at earlier ages. Many move away from their earlier friendships and need to find their places in new group settings. Until this happens, they may be isolated and alone.

Social antagonism is demonstrated best by their interactions with family, peers, and society. In the family setting preadolescents are argumentative with their parents and jealous of their siblings. Their desire for independence becomes the root of conflict with authority figures. They resent supervision and directions, viewing both as signs of their weakness and helplessness. This antagonism may extend into heterosexual interactions. Family relationships change dramatically during this stage of development. These changes produce turmoil and conflict. In the struggle for independence, the teen wishes to be free of restrictions and parental control. Chores, curfews, dating, telephone use, money, driving, schoolwork, and friendships are some of the issues that spark disagreements between parent and child. Parents want teens to listen and conform to their regulations. Teens complain about not feeling trusted. A common cry is, "Why can't I go or do like everyone else can?" Teens are often argumentative and critical of their parents' ways. Some teens withdraw and confide less in their parents, leaving the parents feeling shunned and removed. Teens often act as though they are embarrassed to be seen with their parents.

Adolescence

Erikson described the primary psychosocial task for adolescents as the search for identity. The individual must answer the question, "Who am I?" Identity begins with a separation of the individual from the family. As adolescents begin to separate, they start to explore and then incorporate ideals and values that will become part of their own self-concepts. Before they can accomplish this fully, they test out and question these values and beliefs, comparing them to the beliefs of outsiders. Confusion, depression, and discouragement often accompany this period. Marked fluctuations appear in adolescents' moods, ranging from low self-esteem to feelings of grandiosity. They are more likely to experience increased physical symptoms at this time.

This is a difficult time for both adolescents and their families because teens tend to blame their parents for most of their problems. The movement away from the family expresses the teen's need for freedom and independence. Complicating this need is their continuing desire for parental love, support, and guidance. These conflicting needs for independence and dependence create what is known as ambivalent feelings. **Ambivalence** is having two opposing feelings about the same person or object. Adolescents are truly ambivalent about many issues: loving and hating their families, wanting freedom and needing supervision, wanting to be part of a group of peers and wishing to be left alone. Besides feeling ambivalence, teens experience many different, sometimes conflicting emotions. **Emotions** are the expressed feelings that influence a person's behavior. The charged emotions characteristic of this period are caused by both the physical and hormonal changes that are occurring. The increased social pressures placed on this age group further heighten adolescents' emotional responses. Boredom is common during this development period. Individuals give up earlier forms of play activities, fearing that they represent babylike behavior. Daydreaming and fantasizing may occupy a great deal of their time alone. A sense of humor is generally present but often used at the expense of others. Name calling and teasing peers and others seem to give adolescents a sense of satisfaction. Although they are likely to tease others, they are usually not able to handle teasing that is directed toward them.

Emotions cover a wide range of expressed feelings. Some commonly expressed emotions are anger, fear, worry, jealousy, envy, and happiness. *Anger* can be very disruptive and destructive to relationships. It is often expressed when teens are denied privileges. They angrily complain that they "are being treated like children." Anger can also result when they are teased, criticized, or lectured. The manner in which they express anger varies from individual to individual. They may sulk, withdraw, or have an angry outburst. *Fears* may be imaginary or real and are usually related to social situations or inner feelings of inadequacy. *Worries* stem from issues related to school performance, vocational choices, relationships, appearance, and group acceptance. *Jealousy* may arise in their relationships, whereas *envy* is mainly related to social status and material possessions. *Happiness* occurs when the individual succeeds and feels at ease.

Many teens find part-time employment. Work has many benefits for this age group. Work helps the individual develop knowledge and skills that can be applied in adult life. Work gives the adolescent a sense of belonging in the adult world. Furthermore, work teaches responsibility and provides a source of income. This teaches money management and principles of saving.

Ages 13 to 14 Years

Young teenagers may hide their feelings from others and sulk instead of opening up and discussing what is bothering them. They become openly more negative and hostile. Issues are seen mostly from their own points of view. This narrow perspective creates an attitude of intolerance toward others. Compromise is something that 14-year-old children find hard to do. Friends are very important at this time, with teenagers identifying more with their friends than with their families. Boys tend to have small groups of friends, whereas girls usually have one or two best friends. Friendships create a much needed sense of belonging. Experimentation with clothing and hairstyles begins at this time. Door slamming and harsh verbal outbursts are typical ways in which a 14-year-old teenager deals with stress. Sense of

humor for most teens is based on their negative outlooks. They readily insult or tease parents and siblings and may show disrespect to their teachers.

Ages 15 to 16 Years

By this age teenagers are less self-absorbed and better at compromising. They are now more tolerant of others' views. They can now think more independently and make more of their own decisions. Their curiosity and interests increase, allowing them to further develop specific skills relating to math, science, music, or sports. Thinking is abstract, and they can more readily discuss and debate issues. They are likely to continue to experiment with clothing, hairstyles, and attitudes. This experimentation helps them to shape their self-image.

Teens at this age often test their boundaries, pushing them to the limit. Risks are taken because they see themselves as impervious to danger. In fact, some teenagers believe that they are immortal. Socially, many teens are less shy and more adventurous. Many show an interest in traveling with clubs or other organizations.

Dating begins around 15 to 16 years of age. "Crushes" are typical of the early dating period. Crushes are distinguished by strong feelings of attachment and what the individual believes to be love. These crushes usually last 1 to 6 months. Physical attraction to an individual of the opposite sex is the immediate factor that draws the teen's attention. Dating is the major source of fun and recreation for the teenager. It helps establish social status and recognition within the peer group. It also provides the individual with personal and social growth. Teens who begin dating later than others or who are less popular often feel pressure that leads to feelings of inadequacy and rejection. Depression or a profound feeling of unworthiness may result and must be closely monitored. At first, dating may be characterized by short-lived sexual relationships. Some teens are secretive about their dating and feelings, whereas others share their innermost thoughts with their closest friends.

Ages 17 to 19 Years

At this point in development a sense of seriousness becomes more evident. Teens are now very involved with their own activities in school, at work, or with friends. Regardless of which activities they choose, the one common denominator is that the activity is based outside the home, keeping them away from family for longer periods of time. At 17 to 19 years, teens are idealistic. They like to work for a cause and follow the ideals they hold important and right.

Stress increases for this age group, related to the many uncertainties about the future. As the stress level increases, so do temper outbursts. Difficulties continue between the teenager and parents. Usually teens believe that they know more and are more in touch with the real world than are their parents. This leads to frequent discord and disharmony. By this age many teens have established more stable sexual relationships. They may have one serious boyfriend or girlfriend with whom they spend a great deal of time. Usually at this age, teenagers focus relationships on deeper traits such as honesty, reliability, and a sense of humor. Sexual behavior varies with individuals based on earlier teachings and peer pressures.

Peer relationships are very important at this stage. Peers share the same age, feelings, experiences, goals, and doubts in ways that parents can't. Friendships tend to develop among those of similar social classes and with similar interests. Peers offer social and emotional fulfillment. Teens wish to have their peers recognized and accepted by their parents. Development of a self-concept is further influenced by teenagers comparing their own perceived appearances to those of their peers. Real or imagined differences threaten self-esteem. The significance of a slight blemish or defect will be magnified and weaken confidence. Box 10.1 offers suggestions for ways parents can promote self-esteem in their adolescent children.

Socialization further develops through peer relationships. The social behavior of the adolescent changes from earlier patterns to resemble those of the *social group* to which he or she belongs. The influence of the group on individuals depends on the amount of shared intimacy and contact. Teens may form cliques, crowds, and gangs. An important feature of these groups is that the individual must conform to the patterns or rules determined to be socially acceptable by the group. One of the strongest needs for a teen is to feel accepted by the group members. Perceived acceptance or the lack of it will influence the teen's behavior and attitude. Different personality traits emerge at this stage. The popular teenager feels secure, happy, and confident. The unpopular teen feels alienated, resentful, and antagonistic. The role of a leader falls to the person having the most admired qualities.

Many demands are placed on adolescents at this stage of development. Society expects them to select vocations and think seriously about their futures. Impending graduation from high school causes teens to wonder if they should continue with their schooling or begin jobs (Fig. 10.2). This question is of great magnitude for teenagers, who are often unable to simply decide what to wear in the morning or whether to go out on a date or with a group of friends. Those who are unable to select a career may develop fear and self-doubt.

Other demands placed on this age group include development of a value system and demonstration of socially responsible behavior. At the end of this stage the individual should have moved toward becoming more economically independent. Toward the end of this stage many adolescents are able to bridge the generation gap by establishing close relationships with their grandparents (Fig. 10.3).

B O X **Promoting Positive Self-Esteem**
10.1 **in Adolescents**

- Be positive.
- Recognize achievements.
- Be genuinely interested.
- Be sensitive.
- Encourage self-expression.
- Value opinions.
- Avoid belittling.
- Show respect.
- Encourage decision making.

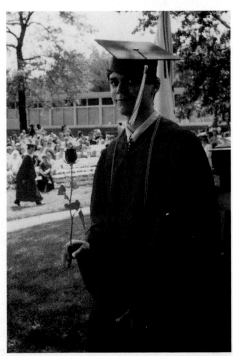

FIGURE 10.2 Graduation from high school is a key event.

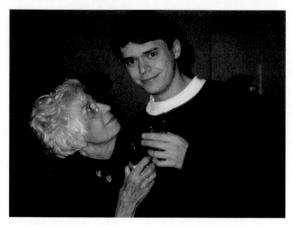

FIGURE 10.3 Adolescents and older adults bridge the generation gap.

Discipline

Discipline during adolescence is important. Many of the conflicts between parents and teens are based on choice of friends and issues surrounding dating. Different family patterns and parenting styles have different effects on the developing teenager (discussed in Chapter 3). The democratic style of parenting encourages youth to make decisions. Parents always have the right to approve or disapprove of expressed beliefs. This style of parenting best supports the child's developing sense of self. In the autocratic style of parenting, the youth is not permitted free expression of feelings or views. Parents make decisions based on their own feelings and judgments. The teen is then expected to follow along with what the parents decide for him or her with little input from the teen. This style of discipline may hinder or slow the teen's growth process and moral development. In the laissez-faire parenting style, the adolescent is left to decide what he or she wants or believes is best. Although most teens say that they want most to be free to decide, in this set of circumstances they feel ignored and unloved. It appears that feelings of independence and strength come easiest to adolescents whose parents listen, explain, and make clear what is expected of them.

The use of "grounding" is appropriate for serious offenses by adolescents. This technique provides them with an opportunity to learn the consequences of their behavior. When a child or teenager is grounded, parents should give specific jobs or household chores to be completed within a certain time frame. Parents must evaluate and praise the completed tasks. Grounding is effective when a teen generally follows the rules and shows an understanding of the consequences of the offenses.

Cognitive Development

During adolescence, maturation of the central nervous system may lead to a shift from a concrete thinking style to formal operational thought processes. Training and studies help the adolescent progress from concrete thinking to more formal ways of reasoning. However, without proper training or motivation, adolescents may not move beyond the level of concrete thinking.

Formal operational thinking is conducted in a more logical manner than concrete thinking. Some scientific reasoning and problem solving can be mastered at this point. Individuals are capable of looking at all possibilities. They can think abstractly beyond the present and imagine a sequence of events that might occur and the consequences of those events (or of their actions). This operational thinking does not guarantee that a teenager will make the right choices, however. Other factors such as peer pressure, the need to be accepted by the group, or the desire to look cool often have a greater impact than reason and judgment. Adolescents are able to analyze a problem, set up a hypothesis, collect evidence, and come up with possible solutions. In addition, they are conversant on many topics. Topics that hold their interest include politics, religion, justice, and other social issues.

School is at the center of teens' development. Most of their time is spent at school or in activities related to their schooling. Social skills, friendships, and peer interactions are of utmost importance to teenagers. Currently, the law in most states requires teens to remain in school until the age of 16. Transition from middle school to high school may be both exciting and stressful for the teenager. Several factors complicate the stress of high school. Teens must come to terms with their changing appearance and developing self-image. Self-doubt may serve to complicate their ability to enter new relationships. New friends are sought out, and many new groups and clubs may be joined. In high school teens are expected to be more independent and responsible for the learning process. This places more challenges and demands on them. Instead of having only one teacher for all subjects, they now have a teacher for each subject.

Many differences exist in the performances and academic achievements of today's teenagers. Several factors may determine an individual's success in high school, including socioeconomic background, family relationships, and peer and social pressures. Life after high school may include college near home or away, work, marriage and parenting, or some combination of these.

Moral Development

Cognitive development is a prerequisite for moral reasoning. Moral judgment is based on earlier learned principles of right and wrong. Parents directly and indirectly influence the moral judgments of their children. Positive listening and empathy enable families to foster moral development. Teenagers must learn to make decisions for themselves and guide their own behavior according to learned standards. Society has determined that adolescents can no longer expect adults to guide all of their decisions.

During early adolescence teens are usually at the conventional level of moral development. They can follow rules and show concern for others. They express a strong wish to be trusted by their parents. Following this stage of development, they progress to the transitional phase of moral development—that is, they begin to question everything and everyone. This questioning places them in direct conflict with any person of authority, but it also helps them to gain autonomy from adults and begin to substitute and try out their own codes of ethics. Teens look at rules, see many injustices, and feel that they have the right to change these rules. They believe that they can make a difference, and they often want to get involved in social issues. They are usually ready to take a stand on what they believe. Slowly, they gain responsibility and show an understanding of duty and obligation.

Adolescents are further developing their spiritual awareness. They begin to question and compare religions. They can philosophize and think logically about religious doctrines. They speculate, search, and think about conflicting ideologies. During this period of awakening, they may reject formal or traditional religious practices in favor of their own styles of practice. Some move completely away from their family practices and may gravitate toward other, less traditional ideologies. A small number of teens may gravitate toward certain groups or cults.

Communication

Language skills and vocabulary increase during adolescence. Verbal communication is the means by which adolescents make their thoughts and beliefs known. They verbally argue or defend their ideas. Adults need to encourage their free expression and should listen to and exchange opinions with them. This give-and-take type of relationship helps to foster a teen's growth and sense of self.

In peer settings adolescents frequently develop a common language typical of their groups, times, and cultures. Having their own slang creates a sense of belonging for teens and sets them apart from others.

The lives of today's adolescents revolve around the use of media and technology. Cell phones, tablets, computers, and the Web are part of every aspect of their lives, and the amount of time adolescents spend using technology has increased in the last decade (Fig. 10.4). Technology can be a powerful educational tool, expanding knowledge and bringing education to their fingertips. However, technology can also be used as a powerful social tool for adolescents. Teens are now multitasking: watching TV, texting, or using cell phones while eating, driving, or doing other tasks. The use of cell phones while driving has increased the number of motor vehicle accidents and deaths. Television has a great impact on individuals, and its highly persuasive effect can be educational or potentially detrimental depending upon the program and amount of viewing.

Other interests include social platforms like Facebook, messaging, chat rooms, Twitter, and photo streaming. These are just a few of the technological media forms popular with today's teenager. Parents must be aware of their teen's use of all technology and social media. The sites should be carefully monitored for appropriateness, and time spent using this technology should be closely monitored.

NUTRITION

Because of the rapid growth that occurs during the adolescent period, teens need an increase in calories, protein, minerals, and vitamins. The average caloric need for teenage girls is 2,600 calories per day; for teenage boys it is 3,600 calories per day. These

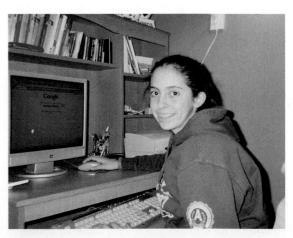

FIGURE 10.4 Technology drives the teen's activities.

needs are easily filled because the teen's appetite increases, allowing increased intake of food. Boys never seem to get enough food to keep them from feeling hungry. This age group also seems to enjoy food more than they did as children. The teenager's protein intake should be between 12% and 16% of the daily dietary intake. The increased need for calcium is necessary for skeletal and muscle growth and for the increased amount of total blood volume. Iron intake must be monitored after menarche because girls at that time may be more susceptible to iron-deficiency anemia.

The American Academy of Pediatrics recommends that adolescents with a family history of high cholesterol be tested and screened for high blood pressure. Dietary management may be instituted for those individuals with familial hypercholesterolemia, elevated test results, or hypertension.

Eating habits are affected by time, pressures, and peer influence. Fruits and vegetables are often passed over for other favorites such as meats and potatoes. Snacks are generally chosen for their accessibility and taste with little regard for nutritional value. Some youth favor milk, and others move away from it toward carbonated drinks. Teens are likely to consume large amounts of soda or carbonated beverages. Some favor regular colas with high caffeine and sugar contents. Diet colas are not any healthier because they contain artificial sweeteners, which have been the subject of much medical controversy. Studies have shown that large consumption of sugary sodas can lead to both obesity and dental caries.

In comparison to previous generations, there may be a slight increase in the number of teens who are vegetarians. Some teenagers choose a vegetarian diet for moral or health reasons; others give little reason for their decisions. The practice of vegetarianism varies greatly. Some individuals simply eliminate meat from their diets; others avoid all animal products, including dairy. Vegetarians need to include cereals, legumes, and vegetables in their daily diets. These substances are needed to provide the essential amino acids for growth and tissue repair.

Dieting has become a national pastime. Hundreds of fads and quick weight-loss gimmicks are advertised. Current fashion trends may have added to the increased number of eating disorders. **Anorexia nervosa**, which affects a large number of adolescent girls and an increasing number of boys, is willful starvation that can result in weight loss of as much as 25% or more of a teen's body weight. The average age for the onset of anorexia used to be 13 to 17 years; now it is 9 to 12 years. This is more than an eating disorder: it is a complex emotional disorder that requires immediate medical attention. Anorexia accounts for a large number of deaths among adolescent girls. **Bulimia**, another eating disorder, is characterized by a series of eating binges followed by periods of purging or self-induced vomiting. This condition also warrants intense medical treatment. Obesity may also be listed as an eating disorder. Some teens are unable to maintain their desired weight and are in need of nutritional supervision to promote healthy weight loss.

Many teenagers today have unhealthy eating habits or unhealthy concepts of dieting. Studies have indicated that 42% of young children wish they were thinner. A majority of children in early school years state that they feel they should be on a diet. These trends highlight how media and commercialism affect young peoples' beliefs and choices.

SLEEP AND REST

The growth spurt that occurs during puberty and early adolescence causes an increased need for sleep. Adequate sleep and rest are needed to help maintain optimal health during this stage of development. In this stage a teen requires about 8 hours of sleep to be fully rested. Teens have a tendency to stay up late to watch television, send text messages, or talk on the telephone. Staying up late causes them to be too tired to wake up in the morning or, when awakened, to be irritable. There also seems to be a direct correlation between lack of sleep and poor performance in school. Some teens are merely too tired during school to concentrate and learn (Fig. 10.5).

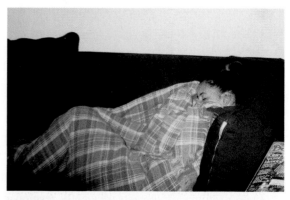

FIGURE 10.5 Naps allow the teen to catch up on lost sleep.

EXERCISE AND LEISURE

Exercise is another important factor in helping teens maintain good health. It is one area in which many teens actively participate without much prodding. A teen's ability to perform skillfully and compete determines popularity and group acceptance. Some teens choose not to participate in sporting activities. Their reasons for avoiding these activities are either lacking skills or having sedentary natures and personalities. The activities that they may be interested in often challenge thinking rather than muscle coordination and skill. The patterns of exercise established during adolescence are likely to continue into the adult years.

Many teens take on part-time jobs in addition to school and extracurricular activities. These teens must learn to balance their time and other activities. Part-time employment offers an adolescent spending money and exposure to the work world.

Adolescents involved in athletics must increase their caloric intake of carbohydrates and proteins. In addition, they need to make certain that they drink enough fluid to maintain hydration before, during, and after engaging in strenuous exercise.

SAFETY

The leading cause of death in adolescence is accidents related to teens' increased motor abilities and strength, combined with lack of judgment. This combination puts them at great risk for harm.

Although driving represents independence for the adolescent now (Fig. 10.6), motor vehicle accidents are responsible for a majority of deaths during this developmental stage. Poor judgment, lack of driving skills, failure to follow rules and use seat belts, and texting while driving contribute to the high number of motor vehicle accidents involving teens. Driver education courses and defensive driving programs can help reduce the number of accidents.

Teens must be strongly encouraged not to drink and drive. Those who drink must be told to appoint a designated driver. Parents need to model proper behavior to help instill these values in their teens.

The second leading cause of death among all adolescents and young adults is homicide. Risk factors include race and socioeconomic status. Half of all homicides are associated with alcohol use. Both alcohol and drug use have further complicated vehicle-related injuries and deaths.

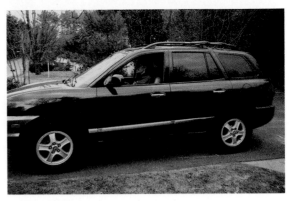

FIGURE 10.6 Driving is an important milestone.

Sporting activities also account for many injuries during this stage. Teens often exercise little caution when competing in athletic activities. Proper physical examinations must be done before a teen engages in any sporting event. Teens must adhere to the use of proper protective equipment when participating in contact sports. It has been shown that protective clothing can reduce the number of sporting injuries. Boys tend to have more injuries related to contact sports such as football and hockey, whereas girls have more injuries related to gymnastics. Some sport injuries have a seasonal pattern.

The incidence of injuries and deaths related to firearms is steadily on the increase for children and adolescents in this country. Many of these accidents could be prevented with proper storage of and training in the use of firearms. An alarming number of the accidents involving firearms occur in or around the home. Parents need to take responsibility for proper education about and supervision of firearms. Some toy items have been found to cause injuries and lethal damage in the hands of children and teens. Many manufacturers have stopped producing toy guns that may be mistaken for real firearms and could result in devastation and harm.

HEALTH PROMOTION

In general, a teen's state of health is reflective of his or her habits and nutritional patterns. The number of acute illnesses decreases during this stage of development. A yearly medical checkup is suggested for this age group. The examination should include vision and hearing screening. Problems with eyesight should be promptly corrected with glasses or contact lenses. Teens must be instructed to avoid using stereo headphones at high volume, as frequent exposure to excessively loud noise has been proven to cause nerve damage and lead to hearing loss. Some teens have even shown significant hearing loss as a result of frequent attendance at loud concerts. Weight and height measurements and nutritional guidance should be a part of each health visit. Dental examinations must be scheduled every 6 months or more frequently if there is dental decay or problems with malocclusion.

Blood pressure recordings must be monitored during the teen years to help detect any signs of abnormalities so that preventive measures and treatment may be promptly instituted. Blood cholesterol levels are examined and dietary interventions are offered to those individuals who appear to be candidates for high blood cholesterol. Girls are prone to anemia; therefore, a complete blood cell count should be done at least yearly or more often. Symptoms such as fatigue, weakness, or excessive menstrual flow may be indicative of anemia.

Generally teenagers have high resistance to early childhood illnesses. The well-functioning immune system still needs the support of booster immunizations at ages 14 through 16 years for the prevention of diphtheria and tetanus. Proper nutrition and other healthy living practices help determine the teenager's overall health.

Teenagers should continue to be assessed for any signs of spinal abnormalities such as scoliosis, discussed in Chapter 9. Many teens need reminders about the importance of good posture to prevent musculoskeletal pain and deformity in later years.

Teens also have many concerns and questions about skin care and hygiene. Teens are generally very sensitive about the appearance and the condition of their skin, so much so that even the appearance of a small blemish will cause them to become distressed (Fig. 10.7). They should be instructed in the basics of proper skin care. If they develop an acute case of acne, further medical treatment is necessary.

Depression

Depression, a prolonged feeling of sadness and unworthiness, is a serious problem affecting many teens. Stress from school, family, and personal relationships may overwhelm a teenager and lead to this mood disorder. Teens are more prone to this condition because they spend more time in self-reflection, which may lead them to disappointment and despair. Signs of depression may go unnoticed by family and friends. The risk of suicide increases for depressed persons. Suicide is the third leading cause of death in the 15- to 24-year-old age group.

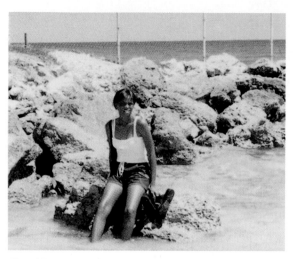

FIGURE 10.7 Appearance is very important at this stage.

Young men are the most affected by violence and suicide. Many factors may contribute to adolescent suicide. Depression, low self-esteem, poor impulse control, substance abuse, and emotional isolation are some of the common contributing factors leading to suicide. The common signs of depression are listed in Box 10.2.

Health care workers should assess depressed persons for possible clues to impending suicide. They should listen carefully and try to understand the person's feelings in addition to the actual words spoken. Be sure not to undervalue what emotions the person is expressing. It is important to openly ask if the individual is contemplating suicide. Individuals with suicidal plans are at great risk for carrying out their plans. Be sure to report any suggestion or suicidal inclinations to others so that necessary preventative measures may be instituted. Constant close supervision helps maintain the individual's safety until other interventions reduce the threat of self-destruction.

BOX 10.2 Signs of Depression and Suicidal Thoughts

- Crying spells
- Insomnia
- Eating disorders
- Social isolation or withdrawal
- Acting-out behaviors: school phobias, underachievement, truancy, temper outbursts, substance abuse
- Feelings of hopelessness
- Unexplained physical symptoms
- Loss of interest in appearance
- Giving away of possessions

Substance Abuse

Substance abuse refers to out-of-control use of tobacco, alcohol, and other drugs. The need to be accepted often causes teenagers to smoke cigarettes. Even with the current legislation curtailing the sale of tobacco to minors, many easily obtain cigarettes. Antismoking campaigns have been instituted with minimal success. The need for early parental education and positive role modeling may be the best deterrent to the use of tobacco.

Experimentation with alcohol is considered to be another teenage rite of passage. Most teens begin drinking before the legal age. Drinking may occur at home, in school, or in other social settings. Some teens may feel that drinking helps them to deal with their feelings or avoid facing certain realities. Both tobacco and alcohol are used in the movies as a prop to portray sexuality. This greatly influences children and adolescents. Alcohol abuse occurs when the intake of alcohol interferes with day-to-day activities. Intense counseling and support groups may help the teen who has a substance problem.

Drug experimentation can begin at any age but most often occurs during adolescence. Any drug, prescription or nonprescription, may be abused. Research indicates that the most common offender is marijuana. Starting with occasional use, some teens may become habitual users. This behavior may then extend to the use of other drugs. Drug use has been shown to lead to other social problems, including sexual promiscuity, diseases, and pregnancy. Refer to Box 10.3 for signs of possible drug use.

B O X
10.3 Signs of Drug Abuse

- Altered sleep patterns: drowsiness, sleepiness, lethargy, or hyperactivity
- Mood swings
- Change in appetite
- Marked irritability
- Loss of interest in friends, school, and other activities
- Secretiveness
- Loss of property or money
- Impaired judgment
- Change in hygiene or appearance

SUMMARY

1. Puberty or preadolescence is a period of rapid growth ending with reproductive maturity. In girls puberty ends with the onset of menarche; in boys puberty ends with the production of sperm.

2. The major changes associated with puberty include rapid physical growth, changes in body proportions, and the development of primary and secondary sex characteristics.

3. Primary sex characteristics affect the growth and maturation of the gonads, or sex glands.

4. The male gonads are the testes, which, when mature, produce sperm and the male sex hormone. The release of sperm, known as ejaculation, indicates functional maturity.

5. The female gonads are the ovaries. The production of ova and female hormones signals maturity.

6. Menarche is the first menstrual period. Menstruation will occur monthly from puberty until menopause.

7. Secondary sex characteristics refer to all the changes that have no direct role in reproduction. These changes include hair growth, increased activity of the sweat glands, voice changes in boys, and widening of the hips and pelvis in girls.

8. Youth of this age tend to spend more time by themselves and move away from earlier friendships. In many settings teens are argumentative, causing their family relationships to change.

9. Adolescence is a transitional period that begins with sexual maturity and ends with physical maturity. This stage bridges the gap between dependence and independence, childhood and adulthood.

10. Dating begins at about 15 to 16 years of age. It helps establish social status and recognition and provides a means of recreation with the peer group.

11. Sex is given high priority at this time. Teens usually experience a great deal of pressure to

conform to the group's standards. Many teens engage in sexual intercourse during the adolescent period.

12. Sex education must be provided in the home and further reinforced in school.

13. Masturbation is considered to be a normal part of sexual expression.

14. Sex education needs to be provided before the teenage period of development. Teens continue to need advice about prevention of STDs and pregnancy.

15. The major characteristics of adolescence include stormy emotions, feelings of insecurity, introspection, interest in experimentation and learning, and testing of values and beliefs.

16. According to Erikson, the psychosocial task for this stage is the search for identity. Identity begins with the separation of the individual from the family. The movement away from the family expresses the teen's need for freedom and independence.

17. Adolescents are ambivalent about many issues, including loving and hating their families, wanting freedom and needing supervision, or wanting to be part of a group and wishing to be alone. Some of the commonly expressed emotions are anger, fear, worry, jealousy, envy, and happiness.

18. Peer relationships are very important at this stage. Peers share the same age, feelings, experiences, goals, and doubts in ways that parents cannot.

19. Teens form cliques, groups, and gangs. They have strong needs to be accepted by the members of these groups. Group acceptance helps them to feel happy and confident; nonacceptance leads to feelings of alienation and resentment.

20. Society places many demands on teenagers. They are expected to select vocations and think about their futures.

21. Maturation of the central nervous system causes a shift from concrete thinking to formal operational thought processes. This thinking style is more logical. Teens can think abstractly and reason scientifically. School is the center of activity for the teenager. Success in school depends largely on socioeconomic background, family relationships, peer influence, and social pressures.

22. Moral judgment is based on the learned principles of right and wrong.

23. Adolescents also develop spiritual awareness. They question, philosophize, and compare religions.

24. Discipline during adolescence is very important. Many of the conflicts between parents and teens are based on the choices of friends and issues of dating.

25. The rapid growth that occurs during adolescence calls for an increase in nutritional requirements. Eating habits change during adolescence; meats and potatoes are favored over fruits and vegetables. Snacks are chosen for accessibility and taste.

26. In early adolescence teens have an increased need for additional sleep. About 8 hours are needed for teens to be fully rested. A tendency to stay up late causes the teen to be tired and irritable in the morning. Lack of enough sleep appears to relate to poor school performance.

27. Exercise is important to help maintain the teen's state of health.

28. The leading cause of death during adolescence is accidents.

29. A teenager's general state of health is reflective of habits and nutritional practices. Teens require yearly medical checkups. Proper nutrition and other healthy practices help contribute to an overall healthy lifestyle.

CRITICAL THINKING

Exercise #1

Anna Avery, 14 years of age, arrives at the walk-in clinic seeking advice. She tells the health care provider that she has had sexual intercourse once with her boyfriend. She admits that she will continue to be sexually active. She expresses a concern about not wanting to become pregnant or infected with an STD. Anna feels that she cannot discuss these concerns with her parents.

1. Outline a simple teaching plan to present to Anna.
2. List the major functions of dating in adolescence.
3. Suicide prevention is an important safety issue when dealing with teenagers. Explain how this should be added to your preventative health plan for Anna.
4. Experimentation with alcohol, drugs, and tobacco is common during this stage of development. Teens often engage in these unhealthy practices to gain acceptance from their peers. How will you educate Anna about the risks of these unhealthy practices?

Exercise #2

How do you think one's self-esteem may relate to one's career choices? Explain your answer.

What are the major sources of conflict between adolescents and their parents? Explain.

MULTIPLE-CHOICE QUESTIONS

1. Usually, the first part of the body to show a growth spurt during puberty is:
   a. Arms
   b. Legs
   c. Feet
   d. Head

2. The major psychosocial task of adolescence, according to Erikson, is:
   a. Autonomy
   b. Identity
   c. Intimacy
   d. Trust

3. Menarche is best defined as:
   a. The development of body hair
   b. The onset and release of female hormones
   c. The first menstrual flow
   d. The development of breasts

4. Which of the following physical changes usually occurs during adolescence?
   a. A decline in male hormone production
   b. A decrease in blood volume
   c. A decrease in sebaceous secretions
   d. An increase in muscle strength and endurance

5. Bulimia is characterized by:
   a. Periods of starvation
   b. Periods of binge eating
   c. Gradual increases in weight
   d. Gradual loss of bone mass

6. Moral development in the beginning of adolescence is demonstrated by:
   a. Acceptance of society's rules and standards
   b. Questioning of existing rules and standards
   c. More self-centered behavior
   d. Strong individual moral codes

7. One of the objectives fulfilled by dating is:
   a. Establishing adult behaviors
   b. Reinforcing principles of justice
   c. Fulfilling personal and social status
   d. Helping to promote independence

8. Assessing a person for suicidal risk can best be done by:
   a. Establishing a close relationship with the person
   b. Confirming the positive aspects of life
   c. Asking if the person has suicidal plans
   d. Allowing the person time alone to figure out his or her goals

9. Which comment best describes Erikson's task for the adolescent?
   a. I hope to build equity for the future.
   b. I want to share my life with my soulmate.
   c. I hope to complete my education and become a lawyer.
   d. I'll probably live forever.

10. The guiding force driving the teen's food choices is based on:
    a. Nutritional needs
    b. Health promotion
    c. Peer pressure
    d. Cost of meals

11. One advantage of the technology available to adolescents today is that it:
    a. Supports violence
    b. Provides education
    c. Supports self-esteem
    d. Fosters adjustment to changing body image

12. One of the current causes of motor vehicle accidents in adolescents is:
    a. Photo streaming on social media
    b. Time spent on social media
    c. Exposure to violent games
    d. Use of cell phones while driving

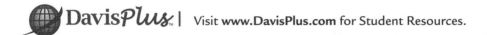 DavisPlus | Visit www.DavisPlus.com for Student Resources.

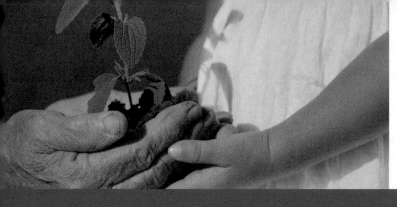

Key Words

aerobic exercise

basal metabolic rate

carcinogens

cholesterol

compatibility

free radicals

gingivitis

hypertension

insomnia

intimacy

introspection

mammography

Mantoux skin test

obesity

occult blood

osteoporosis

Papanicolaou test

presbyopia

proximity

reaction time

reciprocity

resistance exercise

respectability

saturated fats

sexuality

sun protection factor

trans fats

unsaturated fats

vital capacity

Learning Objectives

At the end of this chapter, you should be able to:

- List four goals for the early adult period of development.
- Describe three physiological changes that occur during early adulthood.
- Describe the psychosocial task as identified by Erikson for the early adulthood period.
- Name three nutritional concerns for young adults.
- Describe two health screening tests important for women in the early adult period of development.

Early adulthood covers the period from age 20 through the early 40s. This stage of development is generally described as a stable time of growth. Gradual biological and social changes are expected at this stage. As some body systems grow and develop, others begin to show the effects of aging. All early events, experiences, and patterns of growth help shape and prepare individuals for adulthood.

Adulthood is a period that most adolescents have anticipated and strived for. Entrance into this stage is usually accompanied by positive feelings, dreams, and aspirations. The goals for this time include choosing and establishing careers, fulfilling sexual needs, establishing homes and families, expanding social circles, and developing maturity. Toward the completion of this stage, adults begin to compare their early dreams with their accomplishments. As this occurs, they must reconcile the differences and accept the reality or institute changes.

PHYSICAL CHARACTERISTICS

Height and Weight

Physical growth is completed in adulthood. Men continue to show growth in the vertebrae until age 30. This growth adds about 3 to 5 mm in height. Women usually attain their full statures before their 20s.

Bone and Muscle Development

Peak bone mass is attained by age 35. There is a gradual loss of bone mass after this age in women. Although bone growth stops, bone cells are replaced at the site of any injury. Exercise helps to increase endurance, strength, and muscle tone. Actual muscle mass differs in men and women based on nutrition, exercise, and amounts of the hormone testosterone; for this reason, men usually have more muscle mass than women. Increase in muscle mass is not dependent on an increase in the number of muscle cells. Muscle capacity for sports varies with age. The ability to engage in vigorous sports such as tennis and football declines after the first half of adulthood; therefore, interest in other sports such as golf may first begin in the later part of adulthood. Capacity and maximum work rate without fatigue begin to decline after age 35. Injury occurring during this stage best responds to rest and immobilization.

Dentition

Wisdom teeth erupt toward the end of adolescence or in the early 20s (see Chapter 10). Failure of these teeth to erupt may lead to pain and overcrowding and may require surgery. Gum disease, or gingivitis, affects many adults and is considered preventable. It is the major cause of tooth loss in the adult years. The need for proper care of the teeth and gums cannot be overemphasized. Proper care includes regular brushing, flossing, and limiting excessive consumption of sweets. Good oral health care includes visits to the dentist every 6 months.

Development of Other Body Systems

All organs and body systems are fully developed and matured by this age. Changes in body shape, growth of body hair, and muscle development slowly continue through the 20s.

Maximum cardiac output is reached between ages 20 and 30; after that, cardiac output gradually declines. During the adult years the heart muscles thicken, with fat deposits in the blood vessels producing a decrease in blood flow. Certain practices, including using alcohol and tobacco and eating foods high in cholesterol content, may increase an individual's risk for cardiovascular disease. The heart and vessels become less elastic with advancing age. This rigidity may contribute to the decreased cardiac output and increased blood pressure commonly seen in later adulthood.

The ability of the lungs to move air in and out is known as vital capacity. Vital capacity decreases between ages 20 and 40. Peak respiratory function is age 25 for men and age 20 for women. This gradually declines owing to loss of elasticity in the lungs. Adults who smoke tend to lose elasticity more rapidly than nonsmokers. This loss of elasticity also leaves the individual more susceptible to respiratory infections. Exercise can maintain and maximize lung capacity.

Appetite remains unchanged in this stage. After age 30 the gastric secretions and digestive juices diminish significantly. Poor eating habits lead to common gastric discomforts and indigestion. The basal metabolic rate, which is the amount of energy that an individual uses at rest, decreases with advancing age. This change may result in an increase in weight even when dietary habits remain unchanged. Adults need to try to maintain normal bowel elimination with a diet containing roughage or fiber and adequate fluids. A balance of diet and exercise and regular patterns of elimination promote normal bowel functioning. Individuals should report any change in their normal patterns of elimination to their physician so that that proper medical investigation and treatment can be instituted.

Skin cells undergo some changes as a result of exposure to the sun and pollutants in the environment. Excessive exposure to ultraviolet rays may produce skin cancer, particularly in light-skinned individuals. (See "Exposure to Carcinogens" in this chapter.) Adolescent acne usually clears up by adulthood. For the few cases that do not, a number of different treatment regimens can be offered.

Both the number of cells in the nervous system and the size of the brain decrease after puberty. Changes in sensation and perception can be recognized during this stage. However, speed and accuracy of these perceptions are not yet affected. Reaction time, the speed at which a person responds to a stimulus, increases noticeably between ages 20 and 30. Visual acuity may decline after age 25 owing to decreased elasticity and increased opacity of the lens. By age 40 there is often a decreased ability to see objects at close distance. This condition, known as presbyopia, advances with age. Corrective lenses can correct vision in the person suffering from this condition. Hearing ability is best at age 20; after that there is a gradual hearing loss, particularly for high-frequency tones. Hearing loss occurring at this point usually has little effect on the individual's activities of daily living. Excessive exposure to loud noise from music or work may accelerate hearing loss. Most adults learn to compensate for the minor losses.

The body system that is actually functioning at peak capacity is the reproductive system. In women, the menstrual cycle is well established. Women should report irregular patterns of menstruation or serious discomfort to their physicians. Generally, men are free of reproductive problems at this stage. One concern that may threaten the couple's sexuality and emotional well-being is infertility. Approximately 14% of couples experience the inability to conceive. Couples who are experiencing difficulty conceiving should seek counseling and medical supervision. These couples usually experience tremendous stress and anxiety, and often they blame themselves or each other. Those who decide to undergo fertility testing and evaluation frequently encounter expensive medical bills. For some couples infertility treatment may not be successful. These couples need support and time to consider other options. Suggestions to assist in conception include the following:

- Determine time of ovulation (using basal temperature measurements or with commercial kits).
- Plan intercourse for every other day during fertile period.
- Practice deep vaginal penetration using the male superior position.
- Avoid using any lubricants or douches.
- Have the female remain lying on her back for 20 minutes following intercourse.

VITAL SIGNS

The normal resting heart rate for the adult ranges from 60 to 90 beats per minute. The normal respiratory rate ranges from 18 to 24 breaths per minute. Normal blood pressure readings range from 110 to 130 systolic and 70 to 90 diastolic.

DEVELOPMENTAL MILESTONES

The major developmental milestones for this age group include choosing and establishing careers, fulfilling sexual needs, establishing homes and families, expanding social circles, and developing maturity.

Motor Development

Most individuals have reached peak physical efficiency during this period of development. Muscle strength and coordination peak in the 20s and 30s and then decline gradually between ages 30 and 60. The muscles of greatest strength include those of the back, arms, and legs.

Sexual Development

Adults must first come to terms with themselves as sexual beings and then become comfortable with their own sexuality. Sexuality is a broad term that includes anatomy; gender roles; relationships; and thoughts, feelings, and attitudes about sex. Many factors influence the development of sexuality: biological development, personality traits, cultural and social influences, and religious and ethical values. Education expands the adult's knowledge and understanding of sexual behavior, permitting the development of positive feelings. This helps promote communication and openness in intimate relationships. The goal is to enable people to achieve pleasure and sexual satisfaction in their relationships.

Part of fulfilling sexual needs is the adult's ability to experience and share love. Romantic love is a deep emotional experience, with mutual sharing of warm and tender feelings. Unlike many individuals at earlier stages of development, mature adults have the basis for establishing these intense relationships. Romantic love incorporates intimacy and passion. Love is reciprocal and allows for giving and sharing with one another. The mutuality of sharing and the bonds of commitment foster a sense of security between individuals. Love brings people together and is more than just a sexual experience.

For most men and women, sexual concerns are usually stable during this stage of development. Most adults by their mid-20s have already established comfortable patterns of sexual behavior, and most feel comfortable with their masculinity or femininity.

Many studies have been done on human sexual response. Although feelings and attitudes vary greatly among individuals, basic responses to sexual arousal have common features. The best-known study was by Masters and Johnson, who described the cycle of human sexual response by dividing the response into four distinct stages: excitement, plateau, orgasm, and resolution. The *excitement phase* begins with feelings and sensations that produce muscle tension and vasocongestion in the reproductive organs. A state of heightened excitement occurs during the *plateau phase* just before orgasm. During the *orgasmic phase*, there are rhythmic contractions in the vagina and penis and, in the male, ejaculation (release of semen). The other physiological responses to sexual arousal include increases in blood pressure, respiration rate, heart rate, and muscle tension and engorgement or swelling of the genital tissues. These responses add to the overall arousal state. During the *resolution phase*, the reproductive organs return to their unaroused state. Men have a brief refractory period during which they cannot have a repeated orgasm. It is possible for women, if they are stimulated and desirous, to have repeated orgasms, one following another. Most recent research in the area of sexual behavior focuses on the importance of integrating the mind and body to achieve a satisfying, healthy sexual experience.

Psychosocial Development

By the time adults have reached their 20s, they should have developed strong senses of identity. Ego identity or sense of who one is allows adults to accomplish the next task—intimacy—as described by Erikson. Erikson broadly described intimacy as not only sexual intimacy, but also emotional intimacy between lovers, between parents and children, and

between friends. This definition of intimacy involves warmth, love, and affection. Individuals must be capable of giving of themselves in an emotional relationship. Introspection, or self-reflection, is the tool that is needed to permit the sharing of innermost thoughts. The individual must learn to be truly open and capable of trust. Intimacy is not just sex, but who we are and how we express ourselves in our male or female roles. These roles are affected by culture and time. A radical change has taken place in the female role since the early 19th century. Today's women may share with a partner or manage alone the many responsibilities in the home, workplace, and community. Similarly, the male role has changed to encompass not only breadwinner but, in some cases, also homemaker and caregiver.

Adults who are uncertain of their identities often shy away from meaningful relationships and enter casual interactions that lack interrelatedness. This may lead to isolation and self-absorption. Without trust and commitment, these relationships are usually unfulfilled and doomed to failure.

Choosing and Establishing a Career

It is necessary to understand work roles and their meanings to better understand adult life. Events such as being hired, promoted, fired, and retired are considered critical milestones in the work cycle of an adult. Work is one of the major social roles of adulthood. Most adults work. Work makes possible personal, social, cultural, and financial survival. Work roles affect the individual's sense of identity because in our society people are often judged by what they do for a living and how much they earn. Work has different meanings for different people. For some, it represents prestige and social recognition; for others, it is a source of disappointment. Work may enhance self-worth, respect, and creativity. Work also may represent service to others.

Both men and women enter the workforce with hopes of upward mobility—a better job, an increase in salary, or a promotion. Some young adults may seek continuing education or vocational training to succeed and maximize the available economic opportunities (Fig. 11.1). Wages, promotions, and the ability to accumulate expensive possessions are used as measurements of work-role success. Internal and external pressure is placed on all individuals to succeed in their occupations.

Unemployment
Job security is a concern for many adults in the workforce today. Large companies have been forced to downsize and trim staff at all levels from

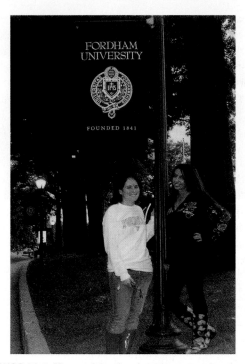

FIGURE 11.1 Young adults place importance on education.

management to entry-level positions. The escalating costs of retirement plans, salaries, and health care have forced corporations to save money by laying off workers who otherwise would have remained until their later years. This has caused a sense of insecurity and unrest among young adults.

Global economic instability also causes great stress for the adult population. Many of the world's economies have recently endured one of the worst financial crises since World War II. This crisis began in 2008 and was caused by the collapse of the biggest mortgage lenders. A lack of adequate government oversight has been blamed for the collapse. Regardless of the cause, the collapse has resulted in high unemployment numbers.

Periods of unwanted unemployment create increased stress for individuals, their families, and their support systems. Prolonged joblessness can cause serious psychological and social problems. Whether it is a permanent or temporary job loss through downsizing, restructuring, or otherwise, the individual suffers from a loss of steady income and, often, a loss of self-worth. Lengthy unemployment may eventually lead to depression and social isolation.

Women in the Workforce

The experience for women in the workforce may be different from that of men. Women are faced with pressures of family, self, and work. The demands of an occupation may have to be balanced with the demands of marriage, childbearing, and parenting. These conflicts may lead to career obstacles and undue stress. For some women, work allows economic independence and may create less pressure to marry. Many choose marriage for reasons other than economic security.

Women's occupations are also changing. In a recent study, college women indicated that they were pursuing careers in law, business, medicine, and engineering. These careers are no longer dominated by men. The changing roles of women have meant that men need to adjust to women as coworkers and bosses in the workforce and as family providers.

Women in the workplace encounter sexual harassment or inequities more frequently than do men. Sexism, like other prejudicial stereotyping, has an adverse effect on society. *Sexism* refers to all the attitudes, beliefs, laws, and actions that discriminate on the basis of gender and lead to stereotyping and unequal treatment of individuals. One consequence of negative stereotyping is that victims may believe that the portrayal is true; as a result, they may undervalue or further degrade themselves. Box 11.1 lists signs of sexual harassment. Sexism is still evident in the employment status of women. For example, there is still a significant earnings gap between men and women: The U.S. Bureau of Labor Statistics has stated that earnings differ based on race, ethnicity, and gender. In 2013, pay for women was 82.2% of the median weekly earnings of men. There have been attempts to make the public more aware of these issues, and workers and management more sensitive to people's rights and feelings.

Establishing a Home and Family

For many, early adulthood is the time to establish a home and family. Families are becoming more diverse both in format and structure. Many young adults choose to leave their families of origin and start homes of their own after their adolescent years. Finding a place to live and call one's own is an

BOX
11.1 Signs of Sexual Harassment

- Continual or repeated verbal abuse of a sexual nature
- Graphic sexual comments, gestures, or postures
- Display of sexually suggestive objects
- Sexual propositions, threats, or insinuations suggesting that if the person refuses to submit sexually, his or her employment, wages, or status will be adversely affected

important step for young adults. Where they settle down largely depends on available jobs and income. Some young adults want to remain close to their families of origin. A major decision for an adult is whether to choose a mate or to remain single. In the United States, although the number of marriages is high, many young adults postpone marriage or choose to live alone. In addition there has been a significant increase in the number of unmarried couples living together. Unlike three or four decades ago when couples had three, four, or more children, today's couples often have only one or two. Today's couples often delay pregnancy and childbearing until their careers and financial security are achieved.

Relationships may be long lasting or short lived, depending in part on each individual's goals and needs (Fig. 11.2). Adults who have not resolved the conflict of identity usually experience the most difficulty in their close relationships. Adults who are involved in a relationship must establish clearly defined roles to minimize conflicts. The decision to start a family and raise children is an individual choice (Fig. 11.3). Some adults become involved in their careers and delay parenting. Others make the choice to remain childless. Still others choose to raise children as single parents. Chapter 3 has additional readings on family styles and arrangements.

Expanding Social Circles

Adults tend to select friends on the basis of similarity of life stage, such as age of children, duration of

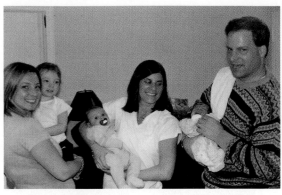

FIGURE 11.3 The decision to start a family frequently occurs at this stage.

marriage, occupational status, or community interests. Adult friendships often last over long periods and survive separation. Young adults share feelings, experiences, and confidences with their friends. Friendships may be either acquaintances or intimate relationships. Characteristics of intimate friendships include reciprocity, compatibility, respectability, and proximity. Reciprocity refers to mutual helping and supporting between friends that allow them the freedom to rely on one another. The central theme of reciprocity is giving and receiving. Compatibility describes the feeling tone of the relationships. The components of compatibility are comfort, ease of the relationship, and friendship. Respectability emphasizes role modeling and valuing. Proximity describes the frequency of interaction and the duration of the relationship; these two factors are more important than geographic location. Adult friendships occur in a variety of settings including the home, work, and community. These relationships are necessary because they provide individuals with emotional support and stability.

Developing Maturity

Mature adults have developed both internal and external systems of controls and restraints. These allow them to behave in acceptable manners. Mature adults have established philosophies of life that incorporate their beliefs and ethical values and help them make decisions and choices and maintain their senses of individuality. Mature adults have broad perspectives and are open to suggestions but not overly influenced by others. They are capable of living, sharing, caring, and respecting others. Another sign of maturity is an individual's ability to develop an interest in the community's needs. Mature adults are able to take responsibility for their actions. They are able to deal with problems or setbacks without losing sight of their goals.

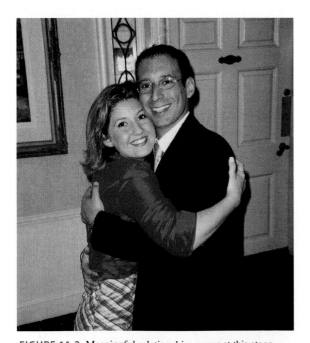

FIGURE 11.2 Meaningful relationships occur at this stage.

Cognitive Development

Unlike persons in earlier stages of development, the adult is no longer primarily egocentric. Adults are therefore capable of being objective and looking at issues from wider perspectives. Cognitive ability draws on an individual's ability to solve problems and use information. It determines the how and why of knowledge. Most adults are at the level of formal operational cognitive functioning. This permits them to attain an increased amount of learning or function at their peak intellectual levels. Injury or insult to physical or emotional health may adversely affect cognitive development and learning. By drawing on their past experiences, adults have increased abilities to reason, solve problems, and set priorities.

Intelligence is a measurement of what a person knows. Most intelligence is measured by testing. Tests usually ask for the recall of a body of knowledge acquired during schooling. People from lower socioeconomic levels may have lower intelligence scores; research has shown that they would score higher if they were given the same learning opportunities as people in higher socioeconomic levels.

Approximately 35% of young adults attend colleges or vocational schools. School helps adults to organize their time, expand their awareness, and sharpen their understanding of the world.

Some older adults return to school after many years and find that it takes them a little longer to adjust to the learning environment. One adult learning theorist suggested that the best climate for adult learners is one of mutual respect, trust, support, and caring. Adults learn at different rates because of individual differences. They usually have more than one reason for learning. They are motivated by things that have personal meaning and importance to them. *Reinforcement* is the force that helps them continue their learning processes. Positive reinforcers for the adult learner include praise, social approval, and recognition. These positive reinforcers are stronger motivators than coercion and force.

Moral Development

Most adults are in the postconventional stage of moral development. They have the capacity to choose the principles and rules by which they live. For many individuals moral issues are not a matter of absolute right or wrong but need to be viewed in the context in which they occur. For example, adults may know that killing is wrong, yet during war they are able to report to active duty and perform the duties of soldiers and kill if necessary. Under the circumstances of a war, these actions would be considered honorable and moral acts.

Highly moral individuals respect the rights of others. Morality is not just a rule but a code of behavior to guide one's actions. Some views on morality extend beyond love, ethics, and justice to a state in which one finds mutual satisfaction. A true understanding of oneself and others leads to mutual satisfaction. This interpretation of moral development is sometimes described as a feminist perspective of morality. As with other developmental issues, morality is a highly individual matter.

Many adults exhibit a strong interest in religion, sometimes returning to the religious teachings of their own upbringing to teach religion to their offspring. In most families the mother's religious values and beliefs are more likely to be practiced than those of the father.

NUTRITION

One goal of *Healthy People 2020* is to promote health and decrease chronic disease through healthy diet and weight. Nutrition and one's eating habits play an important role in physical and mental health and development. A sound diet is crucial to a person's general state of health at any age. Dietary needs in the adult years differ little from those in adolescence. Caloric requirements are based on the adult's age, body size, amount of physical activity, and gender. Men generally need between 2,700 and 3,000 calories per day, whereas women need only 1,600 to 2,100 calories per day. Each individual must adjust his or her caloric intake based on lifestyle (active versus sedentary) to help maintain a desired body weight.

Protein

It is recommended that 15% of an adult's daily caloric intake be in the form of protein. Protein sources include dairy products, meat and fish, legumes, soy products, and nuts. Recent research has shown that adults who consume fish as a part of their diets are at lower risk for heart disease. Certain types of fish, such as salmon, trout, mackerel, and bluefish, are especially recommended because they contain omega-3 fatty acids, which help to lower total serum cholesterol levels. Currently, scientists may recommend fish oil supplements as long as the individual takes the recommended dose and is under medical supervision. Excessive amounts may be harmful. For vegetarians, flaxseed oil may be used as a supplemental source of omega-3 fatty acids.

Types of Fat

Only a very small amount of fat is needed in the diet to maintain good health. Extra fat only serves to add additional calories and contributes to obesity. A diet high in fat also raises blood cholesterol levels. Cholesterol is a part of many foods in our diets. The liver manufactures and filters out excess cholesterol. Cholesterol is an essential component of cells in the brain, nerves, blood, and hormones. However, an increase in serum cholesterol is considered the major cause of coronary artery disease. People with cholesterol levels less than 200 mg are at least risk for coronary artery disease, whereas those with levels more than 240 mg are at greatest risk. To maintain healthy cholesterol levels, an adult requires only about 30% of total caloric intake from fat. The American Heart Association recommends that women eat no more than 6 ounces of meat per day and that men eat no more than 7 ounces of meat per day. Table 11.1 offers a summary of different types of fats.

Trans fats are made by adding hydrogen to vegetable oil, which helps retard food spoilage while enhancing its taste. The U.S. government has begun restricting the use of trans fats in food preparation, as scientific research has directly linked their use to coronary heart disease.

Saturated fats, which become solid at room temperature, are found in meat, poultry, and dairy products (butter, cream, whole milk) and in palm oil and cocoa butter. Foods high in saturated fats should be kept to a minimum. Different cuts of meats vary in their saturated fat contents. Meats with visible fat usually have higher saturated fat contents. Trimming the visible fat from the meats and removing the skin from poultry can help reduce the total saturated fat content. Eggs and organ meats (liver, heart, and kidney) are very high in saturated fat and therefore should be used sparingly. Baking and broiling are preferable to frying and sautéing because they render the fat from meat without adding extra oil.

Unsaturated fats are likely to be liquid at room temperatures. These fats are derived from plant sources such as corn, cottonseed, safflower, and soybeans. The terms *monounsaturated* and *polyunsaturated* refer to the compound's specific chemical composition. Recent research indicates that a diet low in saturated fat and high in monounsaturated fat decreases the risk of colon and rectal cancers.

Carbohydrates

The daily caloric intake for adults should contain 50% to 60% carbohydrates. Complex carbohydrates, such as grains (wheat, rice, corn, and oats), peas and beans, and starchy vegetables (potatoes and yams), are rich in vitamins and minerals and high in fiber content. Fiber promotes bowel elimination.

Vitamins and Minerals

Daily vitamin supplements can be taken but should never be used as a substitute for natural food sources or taken in therapeutic doses unless prescribed by a physician.

The young adult must safeguard against rapid bone loss and the development of osteoporosis. Osteoporosis is a disorder characterized by decreased bone mass resulting from the loss of minerals from the bones. This disorder primarily affects women beginning in the fourth decade. There are two main reasons for the high incidence of osteoporosis: (1) Women have proportionately less bone mass than men; and (2) as menopause approaches, women's estrogen levels decline, causing the rate of mineral resorption to exceed the rate of bone formation. Adequate calcium intake, regular

TABLE 11.1 Types of Fat in Different Foods

Type of Fat	Foods Where Found
Saturated fats (high in cholesterol)	Liver, kidneys; eggs; shrimp, lobster, oysters; coconut and palm oils; whole milk, butter, cheese; red meat
Monounsaturated fats	Canola, olive, and peanut oil; avocados; olives; almonds, cashews, and hazelnuts
Polyunsaturated fats	Corn, cottonseed, safflower, sunflower, sesame, and soybean oils
Omega-3 fatty acids	Halibut, mackerel, herring, salmon, sardines, fresh tuna, trout, and whitefish; flaxseed oil

exercise, and hormone replacement therapy may help decrease the risk of osteoporosis.

Calcium and vitamin D are essential for the maintenance of strong bones and teeth. Most women consume far less calcium than the recommended 1,000 to 1,500 milligrams per day. Good sources of calcium and vitamin D include milk and dairy products, meats, dark green vegetables, canned salmon, sardines, and tofu.

Free radicals are chemical substances produced during metabolism; it is suspected that they play a role in cellular aging. Vitamins C and E have been identified as antioxidants, or substances that can interfere with the formation of free radicals. Vitamin E can be found in vegetable oils, wheat germ, nuts, legumes, and green leafy vegetables. Vitamin C is found in fruits and vegetables. Vitamin C is not stored in the body and must therefore be supplied daily.

Sodium

Hypertension, or high blood pressure, is a condition that places an individual at greater risk for heart disease and stroke. It affects many adults. For reasons that are not understood, African Americans have a higher incidence of hypertension than do other ethnic groups. Some studies indicate that foods high in sodium may cause elevated blood pressure. Individuals with a history of hypertension should limit or avoid excessive intake of sodium-rich foods. Sodium is found in many prepared foods, including prepared or cured meats and fish, soups, sauces, condiments, and certain snack foods.

SLEEP AND REST

Adults need an average of 7 to 9 hours of sleep each night. Adequate sleep helps the adult function with maximum productivity. Some individuals may complain of **insomnia,** or inability to sleep. Manifestations of insomnia include taking a long time to fall asleep, awakening frequently during the night or too early in the morning, and feeling tired and unrested on awakening. Diet, stress, fatigue, and poor physical health may be contributing factors. Sleep difficulties are sometimes a side effect of medication. The excessive use of caffeine, alcohol, nicotine, sleeping pills, and other drugs can further disturb the body's natural sleeping patterns. Insomnia that persists beyond a couple of weeks may indicate a medical problem that warrants further attention.

HELPFUL HINTS

Steps to Promote Better Sleep

- Avoid eating large meals before bedtime.
- Plan regular exercise in the early afternoon.
- Follow a bedtime routine.
- Practice relaxation before bedtime.
- Use the bed only for sleep, not for reading or watching TV.
- Establish a schedule to awaken each day at about the same time.

EXERCISE AND LEISURE

Physical fitness can improve at any age with regular participation in exercise (Fig. 11.4). **Aerobic exercise** works the large body muscles, elevating cardiac output and metabolic rate. Aerobic exercises help to develop muscle fitness, endurance, power, and flexibility. Aerobic exercise is the best form of exercise for burning calories. Brisk walking, cycling, and running are some examples of aerobic exercises. **Resistance exercise,** such as weightlifting, burns fewer calories but builds muscle mass and maintains metabolic rate.

To improve cardiovascular health, it is recommended that an adult exercise 3 to 5 times a week for at least 30 minutes at each session. After several weeks of training, the person will have achieved maximum cardiac output, thereby increasing speed of oxygen delivery to the tissues. Lack of proper exercise can produce fatigue, headache, backache, and complaints of joint pain. Exercise should be incorporated into the adult's daily routine. Many social experiences can be built around the adult's exercise program

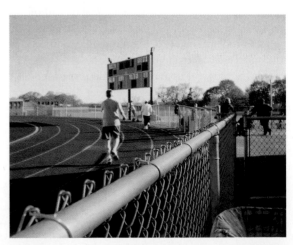

FIGURE 11.4 Young adults should engage in regular exercise.

SAFETY

Safety concerns for young adults include care handling firearms and motor vehicle accidents. These concerns are similar to those for the adolescent years, as described in Chapter 10. Adults now need to expand their safety concerns beyond themselves to those of their children and other family members. Safety in the home must always be emphasized and practiced. Fire safety and prevention in the home must be addressed, including the use of fire extinguishers and smoke detectors and proper storage of flammable materials. Batteries in smoke detectors should be changed twice a year to ensure proper functioning. Each family member must be aware of a plan for escape in the event of fire in the home. Adults can best teach safety measures by setting good examples for their children to observe and follow.

HEALTH PROMOTION

Health assessment during the adult years should consist of a yearly physical examination. As part of the examination a complete blood analysis should be performed so that any early problems or abnormalities can be identified and corrected. Because of the increase in tuberculosis (TB) cases in the United States, adults should receive a **Mantoux skin test** to screen for TB. The increase in the number of cases has been linked to the development of drug-resistant strains of bacteria and the increasing numbers of immunosuppressed individuals. A follow-up chest x-ray must be done if the results are positive. A yearly electrocardiogram (ECG) is useful to provide a baseline cardiac picture. Blood pressure screening and weight assessment must be part of the adult's yearly health assessment. Early detection of health problems can lead to prompt intervention and ultimately protect against future illness.

Gynecological concerns include problems with conception, infertility, and menstrual discomfort or disorders. The **Papanicolaou test** (also called *Pap smear*) is used to screen for cancer of the cervix. There are five levels of test results: class 1, the absence of abnormal cells; class 2, atypical but nonmalignant cells; class 3, abnormal cells; class 4, cells that are possibly but not definitively malignant; and class 5, conclusive for cancer. All women should have a yearly Pap smear. If there is a familial history of cervical cancer, this test should be instituted as early as adolescence.

All women older than 20 should be familiar with the correct method for performing breast self-examination (BSE). BSE has been shown to be the single most important examination used to detect early breast disease. It should be performed once a month about 1 week (7 days) after the end of the menstrual period. Box 11.2 outlines the steps in BSE. The test begins in front of the mirror with an inspection of the breasts for gross irregularities. Palpation for lumps or indiscretions can then be done standing up (for example, in the shower) or in a supine position (for example, while lying in bed). Although breast cancer is rare in men, it can occur; therefore, men and women should examine their breasts and report any unusual lumps or growths to their physicians. **Mammography,** or breast x-ray, should be initiated at age 40 and performed every other year until age 50 and yearly thereafter. If the woman has a family history of breast disease, a mammogram is suggested as early as in her 20s, with a yearly mammogram follow-up.

In men, health screenings should include monthly examination of the testicles for early detection of

---

BOX 11.2 Breast Self-Examination (Monthly)

While standing in front of the mirror:

1. Keep your arms at your side and then raise them above your head.
2. Look carefully at the size, shape, and contour of each breast.
3. Look for puckering, dimpling, or changes in the skin texture.
4. Note if there is any nipple discharge.

While lying down on your right side:

1. With a pillow under your right shoulder, place your right hand behind your head.
2. With the fingers of your left hand, press gently in a circular motion, starting at the outside of your breast and spiraling toward the nipple. Gently feel for any lump or thickening.
3. Examine your underarm and the area below your breast.
4. Repeat for your left breast.

While standing in the shower:

1. Raise your right arm and use your left hand to examine your right breast.
2. Using a circular motion, start from the outer area and proceed inward.
3. Gently feel for any lump or thickening.
4. Repeat for the left breast.

tumors or other growths. Box 11.3 describes testicular self-examination.

All adults, men and women, should have an annual rectal examination that includes a simple test for occult blood (hidden blood) in the stool. The presence of occult blood may indicate any one of several gastrointestinal diseases.

Adults should have a tetanus booster every 10 years and yearly influenza pneumococcal immunization. Additional immunizations may be needed for those who are traveling outside the country or who are in classroom and dormitory settings. Information on needed immunizations may be obtained at the physician's office or at the local health department.

A person's state of health and life practices may contribute to the development of heart disease. The risk factors that contribute to heart disease include lack of physical exercise, smoking, and elevated blood cholesterol and blood pressure levels. To control these risk factors, individuals must engage in moderate activity, avoid cigarette smoking, manage weight through appropriate diet, and comply with their prescribed medication regimens. Recent statistics have shown a decline in the number of deaths from heart disease in populations with healthier lifestyle practices.

Exposure to Carcinogens

The National Cancer Institute estimates that about 80% of all cancer cases are related to lifestyle practices. Many cancers can be prevented by avoiding carcinogens (cancer-producing agents) and following healthy practices. Tobacco usage is associated with a number of cancers of the mouth, throat, and respiratory system. Overall mortality among both men and women who smoke in the United States is about three times higher than mortality among similar people who never smoked. Recently, much attention has been given to the harmful effects of secondary exposure to smoking. Exposure to

secondhand smoke causes nearly 42,000 deaths each year among adults in the United States. Many states, as a result, have implemented legislation to limit or ban smoking in public places. Box 11.4 offers suggestions for quitting smoking.

Many carcinogens are found in foods, especially those that are pickled, smoked, or cured. Pesticide residues left on fruits and vegetables or in meats may further place an individual at risk for developing cancer. Fat in the diet may act as a cancer promoter, causing cancer of the breast and colon. Fiber is the indigestible material contained in certain foods. It has been shown that a high-fiber diet may help prevent cancer of the colon or rectum. Fiber is found in whole grains, breads, cereals, and vegetables. Excessive alcohol use has been implicated in cancer of the throat, esophagus, mouth, and liver.

Viruses may also act as carcinogens. Some of these viruses are spread through sexual contact. Safe sexual practices, including the regular use of condoms, help prevent the spread of these viruses in addition to HIV and human papilloma virus (HPV).

Other forms of cancer may be attributed to carcinogens present in today's industrial society. Many regulatory agencies have worked to help reduce the amounts of toxic materials present in the environment. Household and garden products are two of the groups of substances that must be used just as the manufacturer specifies to avoid undue harm. There are safe, inexpensive, nontoxic substances that can be substituted for common toxic cleaning and insect-control products (for example, boric acid instead of commercial insecticides; baking soda and vinegar products instead of commercial drain cleaners, oven cleaners, and so forth).

More than 500,000 Americans develop skin cancer during their lives. The main cause of skin

---

BOX 11.3 Testicular Self-Examination (Monthly)

1. Stand in front of the mirror.
2. Look at the appearance of the scrotum.
3. Examine each testicle using both hands.
4. Rotate each testicle between the thumbs and forefingers.
5. Report any dull pain in the groin, change in appearance, firmness, lumps, or irregularity to your physician.

BOX 11.4 Suggestions for Quitting Smoking

- Behavior modification
- Hypnosis
- Cold turkey
- Individual counseling
- Nicotine patches
- Smoking cessation medications, such as buproprion or varenicline
- Acupuncture
- Commercial filters that gradually reduce tar and nicotine content
- Gradual withdrawal
- Support groups

damage and cancer is the ultraviolet rays of the sun. Everyone, especially those who are light skinned, should avoid excessive exposure to ultraviolet light. Clothing and sun-blocking agents offer the best form of outdoor protection. A sunscreen with a sun protection factor (SPF) of 15 or more is generally recommended. The SPF rating is the time in minutes that a person can stay exposed to sunlight without burning. Those planning to be outside for longer than 15 minutes need to use a sunscreen with a higher SPF.

Sensory Impairment Caused by Accidents

Young adults often take their sensory functions for granted, but lack of care and accidents can lead to sensory losses. For example, 90% of all eye injuries occurring in the workplace could be avoided with the use of protective eyewear. Individuals should wear protective eyewear when doing chores and repairs around the home (for example, trimming hedges, using power tools or chemicals) or engaging in certain sports (for example, baseball, racquetball, tennis). Eye injuries can result from chemical splashes, flying debris, or a ball traveling at high speed.

Hearing loss resulting from excessive noise exposure continues to be a concern for young adults both in the home and at work. The same preventive measures are recommended for adults as for adolescents (see Chapter 10).

Routine eye and ear examinations can help detect cataracts, glaucoma, and hearing loss. Early detection and prompt intervention can reduce further loss of function.

Obesity

Approximately 30% of the adult American population is obese. Obesity is defined as having 20% to 30% excess weight. Studies have shown a direct relationship between obesity and mortality. Furthermore, obesity increases the likelihood of developing hypertension, diabetes mellitus type 2 (non–insulin-dependent diabetes), and high cholesterol levels. High cholesterol may contribute to the onset of heart disease and strokes. Obesity has also been implicated in other conditions, such as gallbladder disease, cirrhosis of the liver, kidney disease, and some cancers. Excessive weight adds stress to the weight-bearing joints and may lead to osteoarthritis and back problems. Regular-paced exercise can improve cardiovascular function, promote weight loss, and reduce stress.

Weight loss may be accomplished through diet and exercise. Certain foods contain more calories than others: 1 g of fat yields 9 kcal; 1 g of protein or carbohydrate yields 4 kcal. Therefore, people trying to lose weight may benefit from a low-fat diet. Crash diets or very-low-calorie diets are not only ineffective, but also may be harmful to one's health. Diets of this sort do little to permanently change a person's eating behaviors. Pounds lost on a crash diet are usually quickly regained. Crash diets may lead to food cravings and bingeing and set the stage for the onset of eating disorders. Crash dieting may lead to *weight cycling*—large fluctuations in weight. Recent research has shown that weight cycling often leads to a gradual increase in weight over time. Successful weight control programs are based on helping people develop lifelong behavior changes and good eating habits.

Stress

Common causes of adult stress include work, marital problems, child care concerns, and money worries. Stress reactions are highly individual and develop over years. Adults may develop certain health problems related to stress on the job, in their relationships, or in their lifestyles. Sometimes as people search for career advancement and social acceptance, they may neglect health-promoting activities. Many adults pay too little attention to nutrition and diet. Others "party" and engage in risky behaviors. Unhealthy practices during the adult years can have a direct effect on health in the later years.

Stress-management workshops can help individuals learn how to better handle or reduce stress. Most stress-reduction programs are designed to help adults learn how to manage time effectively, say no, and deal directly with the sources of their stress. A sense of humor and the ability to practice relaxation techniques like yoga are helpful in managing stress (see Fig. 11.4). (Refer to Chapter 1 for other stress-reducing exercises.)

Family Planning

Reproductive planning includes decisions about having children. Thanks to modern science and research, many contraceptive choices are available to the individual. Nevertheless, family planning and contraception are controversial subjects in the

United States today. The high numbers of unwanted pregnancies and elective abortions point to the need for better education and reproductive counseling services. Through education and counseling, individuals are better able to make responsible decisions that are right for them and will result in happiness. Contraceptive methods should be based on an individual's values and beliefs along with knowledge of a given contraceptive product's reliability, side effects, and impact on sexual satisfaction.

The ideal form of birth control is one that is safe, effective, affordable, and acceptable to the parties using it. The common methods of contraception used today include hormonal methods (oral contraception commonly referred to as "the pill" and subcutaneous implants), intrauterine devices, and chemical and barrier methods (condoms, diaphragms, spermicides, and cervical caps). For religious or other reasons, many people choose not to use any birth control devices but instead rely on a natural method of pregnancy prevention called the *rhythm method*. This method requires that the woman monitor her basal body temperature (resting temperature upon waking) for fertile and infertile periods and that the parties refrain from sexual intercourse on the days of the menstrual cycle when the woman is most likely to conceive. A summary of the common birth control methods and devices is listed in Table 11.2. Sterilization via tubal ligation for women and vasectomy for men are irreversible forms of birth control that should be undertaken only by those individuals who have been counseled and fully understand the permanence of their decisions.

TABLE
11.2 **Birth Control Methods**

Method	Advantages	Disadvantages
Natural, calendar, or rhythm method: monitoring basal body temperature, checking cervical mucus for fertile and infertile times; practicing coitus interruptus (withdrawal before ejaculation)	Is free, safe, and acceptable to most religions	Requires abstinence for 5 days during fertile period; is not very reliable
Hormonal: oral contraceptive, implant, or morning-after pill	Is almost 100% effective when used properly	Can cause weight gain; can cause irregular menses; may cause hypertension, increased risk for strokes, heart disease, and breast cancer
Mechanical barrier: condom, diaphragm, cervical cap, sponge	Is inexpensive; may prevent transmission of sexually transmitted diseases	May tear or dislodge; decreases sensation; increases risk of toxic shock syndrome
Chemical barrier: spermicidal cream, jelly, foam, and vaginal suppositories	Is easily obtained	Is messy; may cause local irritation
Intrauterine device: intrauterine progesterone contraceptive, intrauterine copper contraceptive	Doesn't affect hormonal cycle or interrupt sex act	May cause infection, hemorrhage, perforation, spotting

SUMMARY

1. Early adulthood covers the period from age 20 through the early 40s. This is generally described as a stable period of growth.

2. Physical growth is completed. Most individuals have reached peak efficiency during the early portion of this stage.

3. Muscular strength and coordination peak in the 20s and 30s and then slowly decline between ages 40 and 60.

4. Gingivitis affects many adults and is considered preventable. Wisdom teeth make their appearance from late adolescence through early adulthood.

5. Early changes may be noticed in sensation and perception. After age 40, there may be a decreased ability to see objects at close distance. This condition is known as presbyopia and is treated with corrective lenses. An adult may detect some loss of high-frequency hearing.

6. The reproductive organs are functioning at peak efficiency during this stage. In women the menstrual cycle is usually well established. Women with irregular cycles or menstrual discomfort should seek medical advice. Generally, men are free of reproductive problems during this stage of life. If problems with infertility arise, the couple should be referred to a physician for testing and guidance.

7. Cardiac changes include a gradual decline in cardiac output and loss of elasticity in the muscles and vessels. These changes may contribute to an increase in blood pressure. Respiratory function peaks during the 20s.

8. The major developmental milestones for this age group include choosing and establishing careers, fulfilling sexual needs, establishing homes and families, expanding social circles, and developing maturity.

9. Erikson viewed the psychosocial task for the adult as intimacy. He described a broader meaning of intimacy between lovers, between parent and child, or between friends.

10. Formal operational cognitive functioning develops further during the adult period. Adults are capable of being objective and of looking at issues from a wider perspective.

11. Adults are at the postconventional stage of moral development. As with other developmental issues, moral development progresses at a highly individualized rate.

12. Diet is crucial to health. Caloric intake is based on the adult's age, body size, amount of physical activity, and gender. Men generally need between 2,700 and 3,000 calories per day, whereas women need 1,600 to 2,100 calories per day.

13. On average, an adult needs 7 to 9 hours of sleep each night. Many factors may contribute to the problem of insomnia, including stress, diet, fatigue, and poor health.

14. Physical fitness can improve at any age with regular participation in exercise.

15. Accident prevention continues throughout the adult years. Improper use or care of the sensory organs can lead to disease or injury. Protection against injury during sports includes training and the use of protective clothing and gear.

16. Young adults are concerned about not only their own safety, but also that of their children and family members.

17. Yearly visits to the physician are recommended.

18. Cancer prevention is important. Many cancers can be prevented by avoiding carcinogens in the environment and by practicing healthy living. Excessive exposure to ultraviolet rays, especially by light-skinned persons, may produce skin cancer. Using sunblock and wearing protective clothing when outdoors may prevent skin cancer.

19. Weight management is important because obesity can lead to many disorders such as diabetes, heart disease, and stroke. The best approach to weight control is through education that leads to a change in lifetime diet and exercise patterns.

20. Stress management can help people learn how to handle stress more effectively through time management, saying no, and dealing directly with the stress.

CRITICAL THINKING

Exercise #1

Bob and Sue are a married couple in their 30s. They have been married for 4½ years and have decided to start their family. They have been trying to become pregnant for 8 months and have not been successful. Each blames the other person and thinks that they are too stressed for it to happen. They have made an appointment with Sue's physician for an evaluation.

1. What questions should be asked to better understand this couple's problem?
2. Could relaxation help aid in conception?
3. Should they consider alternatives to pregnancy and childbirth?

Exercise #2

Vivian Andrews is your next-door neighbor. Vivian is 30 years old and is 5 feet, 4 inches tall and weighs about 180 pounds. She works part-time as a receptionist in an office. Her job is located about half a mile from her home; however, she rides the bus to and from work. She confides in you, a licensed vocational nurse, about her history of obesity. She shares with you a weight-reduction diet that she has cut out of the newspaper. The diet consists of fruits and vegetables and only one protein food source each week. She has read that this will guarantee a weight loss of 10 to 15 pounds in 1 week's time.

1. What would you advise Vivian about this diet? Give reasons to support your advice.
2. Outline a diet for Vivian that would be conducive to healthy weight loss.
3. List several lifestyle changes or modifications that would promote Vivian's health.

MULTIPLE-CHOICE QUESTIONS

1. Cynthia Beckford is a healthy 30-year-old woman. Which of the following are normal age-related physical changes that you would expect her to be experiencing?
   a. An increase in bone cells
   b. A decrease in muscle cells
   c. An increase in new brain cells
   d. A loss of some elasticity in the lung

2. The major cause of tooth loss in individuals older than 35 years is:
   a. Tooth density
   b. Dental caries
   c. Gingivitis
   d. Stomatitis

3. Andrew Previs, age 40, is having his annual eye examination. He has noted a decline in his visual acuity. The most likely cause of this symptom at this age is:
   a. Widening of the iris
   b. Eyestrain
   c. Opacity of the lens
   d. Loss of corneal cells

4. The psychosocial task for the young adult is:
   a. Identity
   b. Intimacy
   c. Introspection
   d. Egocentrism

5. The psychological outcome of prolonged unemployment is often:
   a. Job phobia
   b. Social isolation
   c. Regressive behavior
   d. Selflessness

6. A sign of maturity in adulthood is the individual's ability to:
   a. Exert excessive self-restraint
   b. Develop an interest in community activities
   c. Make life choices based on the advice of others
   d. Frequently change jobs

7. The best time to perform breast self-exams is:
   a. 1 week after menses
   b. 1 week before menses
   c. At any time during the month
   d. On or about the 10th day of the month

8. Foods that contain omega-3 fatty acids include:
   a. Salmon, trout, and bluefish
   b. Milk, butter, and cheese
   c. Shrimp, clams, and lobster
   d. Eggs, liver, and kidneys

9. Which of the following substances have been identified as a cause of heat disease?
   a. Proteins
   b. Carbohydrates
   c. Omega 3 fish oils
   d. Trans fats

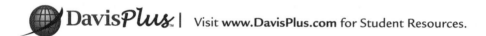 **DavisPlus** | Visit **www.DavisPlus.com** for Student Resources.

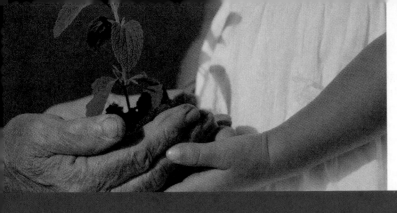

CHAPTER 12

Middle Adulthood

Key Words

benign prostatic hypertrophy

cataracts

climacteric

coitus

dermis

dyspareunia

empty-nest syndrome

fibrocystic breast disease

generativity

glaucoma

hormone replacement therapy

hot flashes

menopause

presbycusis

procreation

stagnation

Chapter Outline

Learning Objectives

At the end of this chapter, you should be able to:

- List three physiological changes that occur during middle age.
- Describe the psychosocial task that Erikson identified for this stage.
- List three goals unique to this stage of development.
- Describe three areas of health concern for the middle-aged adult.

Middle adulthood, or middle age, covers the period from the mid-40s through the early 60s. In the past, middle adulthood was defined as the period of development after traditional childbearing roles were completed. Today, however, many women are entering the workforce and delaying marriage and childbearing to advance their careers. For this reason the more current definition of middle adulthood is a transitional period of development after the early adult years but prior to the retirement years.

Images and perceptions about the meaning of middle age are conflicting. Some describe this stage as the peak of life; middle-aged individuals are often considered to be powerful, wise, and in control. Conversely, others believe that life goes downhill after 40 and middle age is a time when there is a decrease in energy and physical attractiveness, along with an unhappy home life.

Our belief is that middle age is a natural consequence of development and should be viewed as a time of growth and progression rather than one of decline and regression. During this stage of development, adults should reach their peak performance and maturity level if they maintain a healthy lifestyle.

Several goals have been identified for this stage, including establishing and adjusting to new family roles, securing economic stability for the present and future, maintaining a positive self-image, and evaluating or redesigning career options (Fig. 12.1).

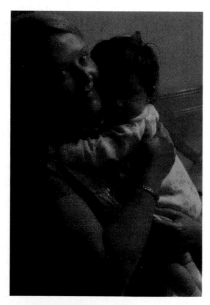

FIGURE 12.1 Family ties are important.

In addition, adults must maintain healthy lifestyles and physical well-being.

PHYSICAL CHARACTERISTICS

Height and Weight

As individuals age, they may gradually lose 1 to 4 inches of height. Body contour changes because of an increase in fat deposits in the trunk region. Middle-aged adults also note that, even without gaining weight, they may require a larger clothing size because their body weight becomes redistributed. Proper exercise and diet can help slow the effects of aging on the body.

Muscle and Bone Development

Most physiological changes associated with this stage appear gradually and at different times for different persons. A noticeable change during this stage is related to loss of muscle tone and elasticity in the connective tissues. The loss of muscle tone gives the skin a flabby, less firm appearance in the face, abdomen, and buttocks. As muscle tone decreases, muscle strength also gradually decreases. Wear and tear in joints makes individuals prone to degenerative joint diseases. Exercise, weight control, and diet may help maintain normal joint function.

Bone mass peaks at age 35, slowly declines, and then accelerates after menopause. Bones lose mass as a result of demineralization. This results in more porous, brittle bones, producing a condition known as osteoporosis. This condition affects more females than males. Genetics, smoking, alcohol and caffeine consumption, sedentary lifestyle, and poor nutrition are some of the major contributing factors leading to this condition. There is a higher incidence of osteoporosis in white and Asian individuals. Preventive measures are aimed at the modifiable factors, which include exercise, diet, exposure to sunlight, hormone replacement, and adequate calcium intake.

Dentition

Some adults complete their dentition, whereas others may not have room for their third molars (wisdom teeth) to fully erupt. If these impacted wisdom teeth cause pain and problems, surgery may be required. Periodontal disease can be prevented with proper mouth care and maintenance (see Chapter 11). Regular checkups and proper brushing and flossing have been shown to help maintain healthy teeth and gums.

Development of Other Body Systems

The muscles of the heart and lungs lose elasticity, and there is a slight decrease in maximum efficiency—that is, blood pressure increases slightly and efficiency of air exchange decreases somewhat. In general, all muscles show a slight decreased capacity to perform work and require a longer time to recover after exertion.

Many changes are noticed in the skin. The cells of the dermis (inner layer) become less elastic, resulting in wrinkling and sagging of the skin. The most obvious changes appear on the face as laugh lines around the mouth, lines around the eyes, and loose skin under the chin. Marked weight loss can further exaggerate these changes. Noticeable hair changes for some individuals include graying, thinning, and slowed growth. Race, genes, and gender all influence patterns of hair growth.

There is a decline in both visual and aural acuity (see Chapter 11). The optic lens becomes thicker and more opaque, leading to decreased peripheral vision. The eyes have a decreased ability to focus on near objects (presbyopia) and are less able to adjust to changes from dark to light. Most of the visual changes can be successfully managed with the use of corrective lenses. Laser surgery can correct some of these defects, and recovery is rapid. Many people develop a degree of presbycusis, or loss of hearing acuity. This is related to thickening in the capillary walls of the ear. Lack of proper care and excessive exposure to loud noise can further exaggerate these losses.

During the middle years adults may begin to notice a gradual loss of taste discrimination. This usually is a minor change that does not affect appetite or food selection. The general condition of the mouth and teeth will have a more noticeable effect on diet.

VITAL SIGNS

There should be no significant changes in the healthy middle-aged adult's vital signs as compared to those of a younger adult. (See Chapter 11 for normal adult ranges.)

DEVELOPMENTAL MILESTONES

Sexual Development

People continue to live as sexual beings throughout their entire lives. However, advancing age may change a person's options, opportunities, and means of sexual expression. Many myths still exist with regard to middle-aged sexuality and performance. The middle years are often depicted as a period of decreased sexual activity, pleasure, and interest. Some even portray middle-aged marriage as a loveless, sexless relationship. For many people today, middle age is a time when both partners are actively engaged in the workforce, seeking financial and career rewards. This may leave little time to nurture intimacy in sexual relationships. Many couples complain that they have little time or energy for their sexual relationships.

The loss of reproductive capacity, either naturally or surgically, is no cause for the loss of *libido* (sexual drive) and sexual pleasure. Very often women are at their peak sexual capacities, desires, and pleasures during this period. Sexual concerns for men relate to changing roles, reduced levels of testosterone, and anxieties over sexual performance. Other psychosocial factors, including work-related stress and a general lack of physical fitness or health, may cause men to note diminished sexual responsiveness.

The change of life that occurs in both men and women is scientifically referred to as the climacteric. In women this change of life is most commonly known as menopause, the cessation of menses, which results from a progressive decrease in the production of estrogen and progesterone. The completion of menopause results in the end of reproductive ability. There appears to be a strong genetic influence affecting the onset and duration of menopause. A daughter can generally predict the course of her change of life by looking at her mother's menstrual history. Menopause usually begins between 45 and 55 years of age, with the average age of onset being 51.

Menopause usually begins with noticeable changes in a woman's menstrual cycle. The cycle may become irregular and shorter in duration, with longer intervals between periods. Some women experience spotting between periods. The amount of blood flow may increase or decrease (normal blood loss during menses is between 30 and 60 mL), or the menses may come to a sudden stop. Internally, the ovaries, fallopian tubes, and uterus decrease in size. The ovaries no longer secrete reproductive hormones and ova. The vagina may lose some elasticity and become drier. These changes may lead to itching and discomfort (**dyspareunia**) during **coitus** (intercourse). Using a lubricant during sexual intercourse will reduce the discomfort caused by increased vaginal dryness.

Menopausal women frequently experience **hot flashes,** which are caused by vasodilatation of the capillaries and a sudden rush of blood to the skin surface. During the hot flash the body becomes very warm; this is followed by excessive perspiration, vasoconstriction, and chilling. The hot flash involves mostly the head and neck region and may be visible to the onlooker. It may last for a few seconds or up to a few minutes and may recur any number of times a day. Frequently the individual also may complain of other symptoms, including night sweats, insomnia, and a general feeling of anxiety. Table 12.1 summarizes menopausal signs and suggested interventions.

Hormone replacement therapy (HRT) is an effective treatment for reducing menopausal symptoms. HRT is not recommended for women with a family history of breast disease or cancer. HRT has been reported to reduce the risks of heart disease and osteoporosis when used under proper medical supervision.

Some women view menopause as a natural event that will culminate in new freedom and beginnings. Others may view menopause more negatively—as an end to their reproductive years. Education and an exploration of their feelings can help women gain insight into and understanding of their bodies and the changes that they experience at this stage.

There is no significant physiological change of life for males. During middle age there may or may not be lower levels of testosterone with fewer numbers of viable sperm. Men with low testosterone levels and symptoms such as lethargy or low sex drive may benefit from testosterone replacement. Men remain capable of producing sperm and of **procreation** (reproduction) well into their 80s. The main change that men experience during middle age relates to their thinking patterns and self-image. As they notice some of the physical changes associated with middle age, some men try to look and act younger. Problems with male sexual functioning are usually caused by disease or related to mental outlook. Middle-aged men who are threatened by the aging process may find that they are also having difficulties functioning sexually. Some may even attempt to prove their sexual appeal by taking younger sexual partners. This is sometimes referred to as a *mid-life crisis.*

Some individuals at this stage begin to experience a stressful period triggered by many factors that might cause a midlife crisis. Others feel free and fulfilled, are content, and are able to master and enjoy multiple roles.

Psychosocial Development

According to Erikson, the primary task of middle adulthood is **generativity,** which refers to an

TABLE
12.1   **Menopausal Signs and Suggested Interventions**

Signs	Interventions
Hot flashes followed by chills	Dress in layers. Avoid high necklines. Wear cotton.
Palpitations, nervousness, headache	Have routine physical examination to rule out medical problems. Decrease stress.
Loss of muscle strength	Exercise regularly.
Decreased elasticity of the skin	Limit exposure to the sun.
Increased facial hair	Remove with electrolysis or waxing.
Decreased vaginal lubrication	Use water-soluble lubricants before coitus.
Sleep disturbances, fatigue	Follow relaxing routines at bedtime.

individual's desire and ability to serve the larger community. For many adults, generativity also includes having a positive influence on their own children. However, as Erikson points out, an adult does not have to have children to be generative. With or without children, many middle-aged adults are more self-confident about the skills and knowledge they have acquired over the years. Thus, they may feel more able to expand their nurturing beyond their immediate family circles. They often demonstrate a concern for their communities and look to what they can do to make improvements that will benefit future generations. Examples of generativity include volunteer work in the church, school, hospital, or community. Achievement of their lifelong goals and of larger generative goals usually results in satisfaction about themselves and their lives.

Failure to achieve generativity results in self-absorption and stagnation. Stagnant individuals are preoccupied with themselves and refuse to accept life as it is or to change those things with which they are dissatisfied. Immaturity and self-absorption may lead to depression and acting-out behavior.

Establishing and Adjusting to New Family Roles

Role changes are a part of middle adulthood, as they are in other life stages. For many, time is no longer primarily spent on child-centered activities but on couple-centered activities. The couple may find more leisure time to devote to pursuing their own interests. Partners who have completed their early-parenting roles may find that they now have to reacquaint themselves with each other and redefine their new roles and responsibilities.

The development of true intimacy is critical to the survival of close relationships. Intimacy promotes trust and mutual caring. The deepening of intimate bonds can allow partners to share their joys and defeats in a mutually supportive, enabling manner. To successfully make the transition required by new roles, each partner needs to appreciate the other's growth, individuality, and needs. Both individuals in a relationship must be flexible and ready to support each other's struggle to adapt to new roles. Although respect for the partner's individuality is needed at any stage in a couple's relationship, marriages in middle age often show signs of stress caused by earlier unresolved conflicts. These conflicts may be related to finances, role divisions, or intimacy. Problems that resurface, and new problems that may arise, must be discussed and resolved to preserve the relationship. Some couples may seek marriage counseling if they need additional outside help in resolving conflicts. Today, an increasing number of divorces occur in the middle and older years. After many years of marital discontent, men and women finally choose to divorce. For most, these are not impulse divorces but have been contemplated for years.

Another adjustment that may be particularly stressful for some couples occurs when the last child leaves home. The empty-nest syndrome, or launching children, occurs when children move on with their lives, leaving the parents to live alone. As a result, parents have a difficult time adjusting to a home without children. This is sometimes especially difficult for women. This phenomenon is less common today than it was in earlier generations because more women manage dual roles in the home and in the workplace. Many middle-aged women find that after their children leave home, they have less stress and more time to pursue their own goals and ambitions.

Others may have postponed marriage and childbearing and now, in their middle years, still have young children at home. One result of this trend to postpone childbearing is a decrease in the average number of children per family—the longer marriage is postponed, the fewer children the couple is likely to have after marrying. Parenting at this stage may place additional stress on the parents because their energy levels may not be quite as high as when they were younger. However, young children may bring a new youthfulness and spurt of energy to the lives of middle-aged parents.

Many people become grandparents in midlife. Today's grandparents are different from those of the past. No longer is this role associated solely with advanced age and infirmity. Many of today's grandparents are youthful in their appearance and outlook. Some are still actively working or fulfilling lifelong dreams. Others assume the child care role, allowing their grown children, the parents, to work or complete their educations. A few grandparents are placed as primary caregiver when their grown child can no longer provide adequate parenting. Still others find pleasure and joy in the role of grandparenting and leave the act of primary care to the child's parents.

Grandparenting may take on different styles, described as formal, informal/spoiler, surrogate, wisdom provider, and distant figure (refer to Chapter 11). The formal grandparent allows the parents to discipline their children while maintaining a close interest in the children. The informal/spoiler grandparent attempts to establish a close, somewhat indulgent relationship with the grandchildren. The surrogate style is assumed by grandparents who tend to most of the child-rearing activities while the parents are at work. Surrogate grandparents may be in the position to make many of the parenting decisions. The wisdom figure role is bestowed by family beliefs and customs that imply that the older person is one of high esteem and regard. Family members look to the grandparent for knowledge and guidance. The distant grandparent role is one in which the grandparents have limited contact with their children and grandchildren. The role may be the result of living arrangements that prevent frequent visits, or it may be the result of earlier family conflicts. Many grandchildren appear to have strong bonds of attachment and affection toward their grandparents (Fig. 12.2). Regardless of the grandparents' style, their role is important to children of all ages.

Just as middle-aged individuals' relationships with their children change, so do their relationships with their parents. Most middle-aged adults have close relationships with their parents and maintain regular, frequent contact. Some continue to have mutually nurturing relationships, whereas others maintain relationships based on duty and obligation.

Middle-aged adults may find that they need to adjust to the role of parenting their parents. During middle age some adults realize that they can no longer rely on their parents for support; instead, their parents now need them for support. Economic problems or failing health may result in the need for a change in roles. Caring for elderly parents can cause added stress on a family. If elderly parents need care, more often the daughter assumes this role. For many middle-aged adults, caring for elderly parents is a major challenge. Sometimes decisions need to be made about helping parents to move to retirement centers or nursing homes or to make their homes with their middle-aged children. All feelings accompanying these changes must be acknowledged. Individuals caring for elderly parents need to arrange for outside support so that they, too, get respite from caregiving. Caregivers need a strong support network to help assist them with the many daily stressors. See Box 12.1 for hints on caring for aging parents.

Establishing Economic Security for the Present and Future

By middle age, most people are at their peak earning capability and job status. Plans for economic security best begin when people first enter the job market. It is not sufficient to wait until middle age to start to save toward retirement.

Economic security may be strained when middle-aged parents are paying or helping to pay for their children's college education. College has a major impact on many middle-aged parents' financial security plans. If parents have delayed having children, the need to finance their children's higher education bills may come when their own earning capacity is beyond its peak. Economic security also becomes a special challenge for middle-aged adults who need to help their own parents financially.

Maintaining a Positive Self-Image

Middle-aged adults need to accept the visible age-related changes of this stage without losing self-esteem. In our youth-oriented society, so much emphasis is placed on the importance of looks and staying young that individuals may feel threatened by the aging process. Many resort to surgery, cosmetics, dieting, and exercise to preserve their youthful appearances. A balance of mental and

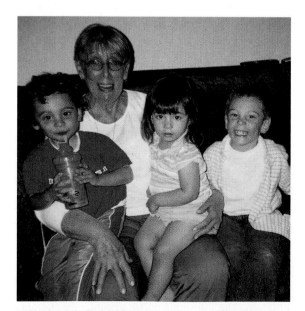

FIGURE 12.2 Grandchildren are important at this time.

B O X
12.1   Caring for Aging Parents

- Recognize and respect older parents' feelings.
- Expect ambivalent feelings in oneself—both a sense of responsibility and a sense of resentment.
- Maintain open lines of communication between siblings and other family members.
- Establish limits and delegate tasks whenever possible. Include pleasurable activities in your daily activities.
- Seek out support services, support groups, home health care, respite care, and senior-citizen centers.

physical health and positive social interactions will allow the individual to maintain a healthy sexuality and positive self-esteem.

Evaluating and Redesigning Career Options

Adults hope to reach their peak career goals by middle age. Those persons who have not done so must come to terms with their accomplishments. This may result in the decision to change careers or go back to school. The concept of a single job or career may be a thing of the past. Most adults today work more than one job to meet the rising costs of living. Some women enter the workforce for the first time when their children are grown and more independent. Others find that they are forced to make job changes because of changes in technology and the job market. Job loss, retraining, and relocation all have an impact on today's middle-aged workers.

Cognitive Development

Mental ability and memory remain at peak performance, as in the earlier adult period. Middle-aged adults are capable of thinking in a pragmatic and concrete manner. They display a unique potential to integrate objective and rational modes of thinking, which is a sign of true maturity. Many middle-aged adults are enrolled in courses to help further their job-related knowledge or fulfill personal areas of interest. Individuals returning to school at this time may encounter some difficulty in adjusting to the learning environment. For example, they may have difficulty setting up study schedules, memorizing, and just being in a classroom situation. Once enrolled, adult learners go through a brief period of adjustment but, providing they do not get discouraged and quit, they quickly acclimate to the demands of learning. They may need more time to learn and complete tasks but often do so with much more accuracy than the young learner. Motivation to learn is often greater and is enhanced by life experiences and needs. Box 12.2 has some suggestions for the adult learner.

Moral Development

Middle age is a time in which many individuals look inside themselves and reassess their values and beliefs. Spirituality may become more important during this stage and may guide the person in making moral decisions. A commitment to improving the welfare of others enhances the individual's own moral growth. At this stage of development, most people have a clear understanding of what constitutes personal needs, moral duties, and society's demands.

B O X
12.2 Suggestions for the Adult Learner

- If several years have lapsed since you were last in school, it may take a few weeks to get back into the routine.
- Motivation and perseverance are important keys to success in learning.
- Keep up with the reading assignments; ask yourself if you understand what you have read.
- Try to meet the learning objectives in the text.
- Look up words that you don't understand.
- Study the illustrations and tables given in the text.
- Summarize what you read.
- Complete any end-of-chapter questions and exercises.
- Prepare for your examination from the first day of class.
- Review your test after it is scored to figure out what you missed. Use these errors as clues to what you must review for future exams.

NUTRITION

The dietary needs of middle-aged adults are similar to those of adults in their 20s and 30s. All middle-aged adults should limit their intake of sodium, caffeine, and fats. The basal metabolic rate gradually slows down during the middle years, possibly affecting weight. It is not unusual to gain 5 to 10 pounds or need a larger clothing size without increasing food intake. This is related not only to the slower metabolism but also to the redistribution of weight. In females redistribution of weight refers to an increase in the waist and hips, while in men weight is redistributed to show an increase in abdominal girth and a decrease in muscle mass in the lower body. To compensate for these changes, middle-aged adults must decrease their caloric intake and increase their amount of physical activity. Healthy eating patterns should continue throughout this stage. Adequate calcium intake is needed and can be achieved by ingesting two or more servings of calcium-rich foods per day. A minimum of 1,500 mg of calcium is needed daily. Calcium is needed to maintain bone mass and muscle contraction and to regulate blood pressure. (See Chapter 11 for specific dietary guidelines.)

SLEEP AND REST

Sleep requirements for middle-aged adults are less than for people in earlier stages. Many individuals state that they experience more difficulty falling asleep or staying asleep. Stress, poor health, or lack of exercise may contribute to sleep problems. Many middle-aged adults notice that they no longer have an abundance of energy. They may tire more easily and need rest periods following strenuous exercises. (See Chapter 11 for ways to promote sleep.)

EXERCISE AND LEISURE

Some middle-aged adults are sedentary and need to be reminded of the benefits of exercise, whereas others actively engage in regular exercise. Chapter 11 outlines different types of exercise. Middle-aged adults should engage in regular exercise for at least 30 minutes at least three times a week. Before beginning any exercise program individuals should check with their health care provider. Regular exercise has been shown to increase one's life expectancy and improve the quality of life. Regular exercise is also helpful in weight control. Suggested types of exercise include brisk walking, swimming, bicycling, and other forms of aerobic exercise.

Choice of hobbies varies greatly among individuals. For many adults, leisure activities may center around the home. Travel, gardening, art, and music are just a few of the areas of interest for some in this age group (Fig. 12.3). Some adults develop new interests or talents, whereas others now have the time to nurture old interests. Many people find pleasure

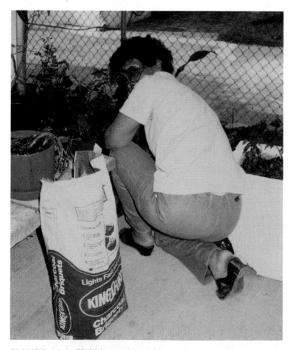

FIGURE 12.3 Hobbies and activities promote wellness.

in devoting time and service to others in their communities. Volunteering at local hospitals and schools benefits both the doer and the recipients. Filling leisure time with rewarding, pleasurable activities is important in preparing for retirement. When the leisure activities of midlife are continued into the later years, there is a smoother transition into old age.

SAFETY

Accident prevention is a concern for all ages. Motor vehicle accidents continue to contribute to many injuries and deaths in this age group. Identifying safety issues and reducing risk factors in the workplace help to decrease the number of job-related injuries and accidents. The Occupational Safety and Health Act of 1970 was passed to increase the health and safety of all working men and women. Continuous surveillance and identification of individuals at high risk for injury helps promote preventative strategies.

HEALTH PROMOTION

It is possible for a person to maintain sound health throughout the middle years despite the general slowing down of body processes. Weight control, healthy lifestyles, and avoidance of accidents help to promote wellness into the later years.

Many of today's middle-aged adults are concerned with appearance and physical fitness. Much media attention has been devoted to diet and health care, making many members of this age group very conscious of wellness and healthy lifestyles. The skin reflects one's general state of health and age, and recent interest has focused on cosmetic creams, lotions, and injections of a neurotoxin known as Botox. The success of these products is limited. Some individuals attempt to correct the effect of time by undergoing expensive cosmetic surgery.

To maintain health and wellness, the middle-aged adult must have a yearly physical examination. Weight management should be a goal for this age group. Middle-aged adults should be screened for blood cholesterol levels. Elevated serum cholesterol has been associated with cardiovascular and coronary artery diseases. An elevated high-density lipoprotein (HDL) level is desired, whereas a low-density lipoprotein (LDL) level increases the risk for cardiovascular diseases. For some, diet and exercise may maintain desirable blood cholesterol levels. Others may need to combine diet and exercise with cholesterol-lowering medications.

Middle-aged adults should also have eye screening tests for glaucoma and cataracts. Glaucoma is a condition that frequently begins in middle adulthood. It is caused by the buildup of fluid in the chambers of the eye. This increased pressure may go unnoticed until irreparable damage has been done to the person's vision. A routine noninvasive eye examination may help detect the onset of glaucoma. Medications or corrective surgery can help prevent further loss of vision. Cataracts result in a cloudy formation on the lens of the eye. Cataracts form gradually and eventually inhibit the passage of light through the lens. They are common after age 60 and may be caused by the presence of other chronic conditions. Once detected, cataracts can be surgically corrected with excellent results.

Cancer of the colon is more frequent in middle adulthood than in earlier ages. Much attention has been given to diet and its relationship to colon cancer. A diet high in fiber and low in fat is recommended to decrease the risk of both colon cancer and heart disease. It is now recommended that both men and women have a colonoscopy yearly after age 50 as screening for colon cancer. Early examinations may be recommended for adults with a family history of colon disease.

Fibrocystic breast disease, a benign condition, may begin in the 30s and continue until menopause. Ninety percent of women develop some degree of this disease, which is characterized by large, sometimes uncomfortable cysts in the breast tissue. Estrogen has been implicated in contributing to the development of this disease. It is thought that estrogen helps to cause engorgement and swelling of the cells lining the mammary ducts. After menopause, with the decrease in estrogen levels, there appears to be a decrease in tissue swelling and cyst formation. At this time there is no known correlation between the development of fibrocystic disease and the onset of breast cancer. However, all irregularities and lumps found in breast tissue should be investigated thoroughly by a trained examiner. Women older than age 50 should have annual mammograms and Pap screenings. HPV testing should be done every 3 years to age 65. Women with a high risk for cervical cancer may be screened more often.

Men older than age 50 frequently develop an enlarged prostate gland. This condition, called benign prostatic hypertrophy (BPH), is common and should be distinguished from cancer of the prostate gland. Early signs of this condition include difficulty voiding, diminished urine stream, dribbling, and frequent need to urinate. A yearly rectal examination after age 40 will help detect an increase in the size of the gland. Blood testing can help detect prostate-specific antigens (PSAs) found at early stages of prostate malignancies. Early detection and prompt treatment can improve the outcome of both BPH and prostate cancer.

Heart disease and cancer continue to be the causes of most deaths at this stage of development. The leading chronic conditions affecting middle-aged men include heart disease, back problems, visual impairments, and asthma. The leading chronic conditions affecting women include arthritis, hypertension without heart involvement, and depression.

SUMMARY

1. Middle adulthood or middle age covers the period from the mid-40s through the early 60s.

2. Today many women in the workforce delay marriage and childbearing to enhance their careers. Thus, many middle-age adults are still active parents at this stage.

3. Middle age is a natural consequence of development and a time of growth and progression rather than decline and regression.

4. During this stage adults reach peak performance and maturity.

5. Most physiological changes appear gradually and at different times for different persons.

6. Loss of muscle tone and elasticity in the connective tissues occur. Demineralization causes the bones to become porous and brittle.

7. Periodontal disease is common and can be prevented with proper mouth care and maintenance.

8. The skin loses elasticity and becomes wrinkled.

9. Hair growth slows; thinning and graying of the hair occur.

10. The eyes lose accommodation and the ability to focus on near objects. A loss of hearing acuity is noticeable at this stage.

11. Goals at this stage include establishing and adjusting to new family roles, securing economic stability for the present and future, maintaining a positive self-image, and evaluating or redesigning career options.

12. The major challenges and opportunities that middle-aged adults experience include a renewed focus on themselves as a couple, the empty-nest syndrome, grandparenting, and parenting the parent. Adults hope to establish economic security and reach peak job status during middle age.

13. Menopause indicates the cessation of menses and loss of reproductive ability. Menopause usually begins between the ages of 45 and 55 years.

14. There is no significant physiological change of life for men. Men remain capable of producing sperm well into their 80s. The main change that men experience is in their thinking patterns and self-image.

15. According to Erikson, the task of middle age is generativity. This means that individuals demonstrate concern for and interest in their communities. Nonachievement of generativity results in self-absorption and stagnation.

16. Mental ability and memory remain at peak levels of performance. Middle age is a time when adults look inside themselves and reassess their values and beliefs.

17. Middle-aged adults have a clear understanding of what constitutes personal needs, moral duties, and society's demands.

18. The nutritional needs of middle-aged adults remain similar to those of young adults. This age group must pay close attention to diet, exercise, and healthy lifestyles. Weight gain may occur.

19. Middle-aged adults require less sleep than those who are younger. Some adults experience difficulty falling or staying asleep.

20. Leisure-time activities vary and are important in preparing for retirement.

21. Heart disease and cancer continue to be the leading causes of death for this age group. Thorough physical examinations and health screenings must be performed yearly to help detect and treat any existing medical problems.

CRITICAL THINKING

Exercise #1

Bill and Sue have been married for 35 years. They both have been working throughout their marriage, with Bill in finance and Sue in early childhood education. They have three children and five grandchildren all living nearby. Bill has been talking about retiring and moving to Virginia. Sue is concerned about retiring and moving away from the family. Bill told Sue that she has 6 more months to get used to the idea and then he wants to move and start living again.

1. Discuss what factors may promote a successful retirement.
2. Discuss the differences between men's and women's views on retirement.
3. What might help Sue adjust to retirement?

CRITICAL THINKING (continued)

Exercise #2

Mary Jo Frazer, a 52-year-old postal clerk, is having her yearly physical examination. She tells the nurse that during her last menstrual period she noted that she had 2 days of increased blood flow and 2 to 3 days of increased spotting before her period ended. She also complained about having increased anxiety and night sweats.

1. How should the nurse respond to Ms. Frazer's concerns?
2. What screening test is mandatory for this patient?
3. What patient teaching is indicated at this time?

Exercise #3

Mary and Brady have 4 children ranging in age from 8 to 18. Mary's father, a widower, is suffering from memory problems, confusion, and impaired judgment. He has recently moved into the couple's home. He is unable to prepare his meals, and he needs assistance with activities of daily living. The couple want him to be cared for within the family setting. Mary is responsible for the care of the children, home, and her dad. She has no time for all of the tasks that she once took for granted.

1. What interaction should you consider?
2. What community resources would you consider for Mary?

MULTIPLE-CHOICE QUESTIONS

1. Wrinkling of the skin in late middle age is a result of:
  a. Increased water and decreased fat in the skin cells
  b. Loss of elasticity in the dermis
  c. Increased muscle mass and stretching of fibrous tissue
  d. Rapid loss of cells from within the dermis and epidermis

2. Which of the following are characteristics of middle age?
  a. Women are capable of giving birth well into their 60s.
  b. Men are incapable of producing sperm after the age of 70.
  c. Sexual needs and desires cease.
  d. Sexual functioning and sexuality continue throughout this stage.

3. Hot flashes are caused by:
  a. Nervous system excitement
  b. Hormonal influx
  c. Vasodilatation and constriction
  d. Decreased contractility in the blood vessels

4. The psychosocial task of generativity refers to:
  a. How one chooses to achieve economic stability
  b. The task of procreation
  c. Accomplishing one's career and ambitions
  d. Assisting and guiding the next generation

5. Successful coping with midlife changes is best achieved when the individual:
  a. Has children of his or her own
  b. Is married
  c. Has a career
  d. Has a good support system

6. Cynthia Fox is a 55-year-old woman who has recently been diagnosed with fibrocystic breast disease. She asks the licensed vocational nurse (LVN) if this disease has occurred because she didn't breastfeed her two children. The LVN's best response is:
  a. "Don't worry. Nothing you could have done would result in this disease."
  b. "There is nothing that you can do at this time to halt the course of this condition."
  c. "This disease results from hormonal stimulation of the breast tissue."
  d. "Breastfeeding your children usually will decrease the risk of this disease."

7. Adequate calcium is needed in the diet during middle age to:
   a. Build and repair tissue
   b. Strengthen nerve conduction
   c. Maintain bone mass
   d. Improve eyesight

8. Which of the following best represents the dietary recommendations for the middle-aged adult?
   a. High carbohydrates, low fat
   b. High fiber, low fat and sodium
   c. High protein, calories, and fats
   d. Follow Atkins, South Beach, or Jenny Craig diets

9. The LPN recognizes that _____ is known as the "good" cholesterol.

10. Normal physiological changes common in middle age include:
   a. Increased cardiac output
   b. Increased bone density
   c. Improved glomerular function
   d. Thinning of vertebral disks

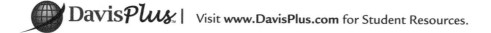 **DavisPlus** | Visit **www.DavisPlus.com** for Student Resources.

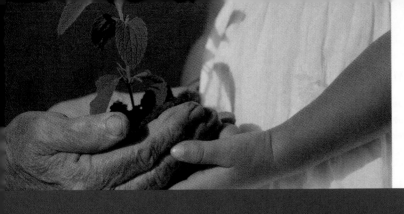

Key Words

activity theory

ageism

aging

antioxidants

atrophy

autoimmune theory

cerumen

clockwork theory

continuity-developmental
theory

delirium

dementia

demographics

disengagement theory

dysphagia

ego integrity

free-radical theory

gerontology

health care proxy

homeostasis

immune-system-failure
theory

integumentary system

keratosis

kyphosis

lacrimal ducts

life expectancy

life span

lipofuscin

living will

lumen

melanocytes

key terms continue on page 200

Chapter Outline

Learning Objectives

At the end of this chapter, you should be able to:

- Describe three demographic changes affecting the older population.
- Contrast the biological and psychosocial theories of aging.
- List four normal, physical, age-related changes that occur during this stage of development.

objectives continue on page 200

Learning Objectives (continued)

- Describe two developmental milestones associated with aging.
- Describe Erikson's psychosocial task for this period of development.
- List three dietary changes important for old age.
- List two health-promoting activities important for old age.

"Old age," as defined by the U.S. government and Social Security Administration, includes all people aged 65 and older. The statistical characteristics, or demographics, of the older population are constantly changing. Old age is best divided into three periods: the young old, ages 65 to 74; the old, ages 75 to 90; and the very old, ages 90 and older.

As with earlier life stages, not everyone older than 65 is the same. Some 80-year-old adults lead active, productive lives, whereas others are unable to be active or independent because of illness. Chronological age is usually an unreliable indicator of mental, physical, and social well-being.

Elderly people comprise the fastest-growing group in the United States today. In 2011 the number of persons 65 years and older totaled 41.4 million, and this number is projected to double to 92 million by 2060. This age group represented 13.3% of the U.S. population, or about one in every eight Americans. Since 2000 the elderly population has increased by 18%, as compared to a 9.4% increase in the population younger than 65.

A dramatic shift in the ethnic composition of the elderly population is expected in the 21st century as a result of immigration patterns. Racial and ethnic minority elderly populations have increased from 5.7 million in 2000 to 8.5 million in 2011 and are projected to increase to 20.2 million by 2030. Of all of the ethnic groups, Asians have the longest life expectancy, followed by whites, Hispanics, African

Americans, and Native Americans. There are several important health care implications based on these ethnic population projections. Language barriers are one of the major complications for our older, ethnically diverse population. Ethnic diversity also influences an individual's decisions about his or her health care, course of treatments, and views on disease prevention.

Many people remain living in their homes, with or without their spouses, or with their families until advanced age. In 2012 more than half (57%) of noninstitutionalized persons lived at home with their spouses. Only 28% of all noninstitutionalized older persons lived alone in the year 2012. The percentage of persons living alone increases with advanced age. In 2011 a total of about 2 million people lived in a household with a grandchild present. Of the population 65 and older in 2011, only 1.5 million (or 3.6%) lived in institutional settings. The percentage increases with age to 11% for persons 85 and older.

In 2011 over half (51%) of persons 65 or older lived in 9 states: California, New York, Florida, Pennsylvania, Texas, Ohio, Illinois, Michigan, and North Carolina. Pennsylvania and Texas each have 2 million or more elderly residents, while Ohio, Illinois, Michigan, and North Carolina are each home to more than 1 million elderly adults. Older people are less likely to change their residences than are younger adults. Those who do usually move within a short distance from their present homes.

Cost of health care is still another factor that influences older individuals and their health care choices. The major source of income for older couples and individuals in 2010 was Social Security followed by income from assets, then pensions, and then earnings. The median income in 2011 was $27,707 for men and $15,362 for women. In 2011, 3.6 million elderly persons (about 8.7%) were living below the poverty level. In 2011, 2.4 million elderly persons were poor or "near poor." Of these, 18.7% were Hispanic, 17.3% were African American, 11.7% were Asian, and 6.7% were white.

Life expectancy refers to the average number of years that a person is likely to live. The most accurate predictors of life expectancy are the ages of one's biological parents. In 2011 the average life expectancy for persons up to age 65 had increased by 19.2 years (compared to previous years). This translates to an additional 20.4 years for women and 17.8 years for men. A person born in the year 2011 could expect to live 78.7 years, or about 30 years longer than an individual born in 1900. This increase in life expectancy since 1900 is largely a result of reduced death rates for children and young adults. In 1900 mortality was primarily from infectious diseases that affected infant and maternal mortality. In contrast, the leading causes of death in 2010 were cancer and heart disease, which commonly appear in older populations. Dietary practices during a person's lifetime may also affect life expectancy. Obesity, smoking, and sedentary lifestyle practices increase the risk of early death.

The goals of *Healthy People 2020* are to improve the health, function, and quality of life. For the population of older adults in the United States, preventative health services are important for maintaining health care quality and patient wellness.

THEORIES OF AGING

Life span is best defined as the maximum number of years that a species is capable of surviving. Life span for humans is 120 years and has remained essentially unchanged for the past 100,000 years.

The aging process begins at conception. This process leads to physiological impairment and eventual death. Aging is a normal, inevitable, progressive process that produces irreversible changes over an extended time. It is important to note that although all persons age, they do so at individualized rates. The symptoms of normal aging are referred to as senescence. Many myths and misconceptions still exist with regard to the aging process. See Box 13.1 for a list of common myths about aging.

The study of aging is called gerontology. No one concept completely explains the aging process or why we age. Many different theories have been developed to attempt to explain the mysteries of aging. Most provide guidelines for assessing a person's adjustment to aging. Understanding aging helps nurses assess, implement, and evaluate care for elderly people.

Biological Theories

Biological theories attempt to explain the physical changes that accompany aging.

Clockwork Theory

Laboratory studies have revealed marked differences in cell reproduction in different species. Cells in species known to have longer life spans reproduce more times than cells of species having shorter life spans. According to the clockwork theory, connective-tissue cells have an internal clock that is genetically programmed to stop cell reproduction after so many reproductions. This "clock" determines the length of one's life.

Free-Radical Theory

The free-radical theory is based on the idea that highly unstable molecules may result from cellular metabolism or substances found in the atmosphere. These particles are very reactive and may combine with proteins, lipids, or cell organelles. Free radicals are believed to cause mutations in the chromosomes, thereby changing cellular functions. According to this theory, these free radicals then cause the breakdowns in the aging process. Antioxidants, such as vitamins C and E, are thought to prevent the formation of free radicals and are therefore considered important

BOX
13.1   Common Myths About Aging

Most old people:

- Are senile
- Live alone, isolated from their families
- Are ill
- Are victims of crime
- Live in institutional settings
- Are set in their ways and cannot learn new skills
- Are unhappy
- Are less productive than younger workers
- Have no interest in sex
- Live at or below the poverty level

dietary substances. The exact role that antioxidants play in the aging process remains unclear, however.

Wear-and-Tear Theory

The wear-and-tear theory suggests that after repeated injury, cells wear out and cease to function. According to this theory, metabolic waste products accumulate over time. These waste products deprive cells of their nutrition and cause them to malfunction.

Immune-System-Failure Theory

The immune system provides the body with antibodies and defenses against foreign invaders. The immune response declines with advancing age. The older body loses lymphoid tissue from specific locations in the body, including the thymus gland, spleen, lymph nodes, and bone marrow. The immune-system-failure theory hypothesizes that the decline in the immune functions causes the body to slow its response to foreign invaders, making elderly people more susceptible to both major and minor infections.

Autoimmune Theory

The autoimmune theory suggests that aging is related to the body's weakening immune system, which fails to recognize its own tissues and may destroy itself. The immune system is programmed to recognize and differentiate its own proteins from foreign invaders. As an individual ages, the immune system appears to lose this ability. As a result, the body begins to attack and destroy its own cells—the autoimmune response. During old age there is an increase in the body's autoimmune response. This is evidenced by a greater incidence of autoimmune diseases such as rheumatoid arthritis and possibly cancer.

Psychosocial Theories

Psychosocial theories attempt to explain how aging affects socialization and life satisfaction.

Disengagement Theory

The disengagement theory suggests that society and the individual gradually withdraw or disengage from each other. Proponents of this theory believe that disengagement provides a means for an orderly transfer of power from the old to the young and that this process is mutually satisfying for both groups. Elderly people are relieved of their societal responsibilities and pressures, and younger people assume leadership. Critics of this theory,

however, believe that as older people's levels of engagement decrease, their levels of contentment also decrease.

Activity Theory

The activity theory suggests that individuals achieve satisfaction from life by maintaining a high level of social activity and involvement. Supporters of the activity theory advise older individuals to find rewarding, pleasurable substitutes for earlier activities. They recommend that older adults remain active in a wide variety of pursuits. If activities must be given up because of age-related changes, replacements must be found. Failure to replace old activities or roles causes people to feel that they have no purpose or social importance. The activities that are most rewarding are those that involve close personal contact. By remaining active, an individual's morale and personal adjustments are higher than those of people who are less active and involved, which may add to their life satisfaction (Fig. 13.1).

Continuity-Developmental Theory

The continuity-developmental theory views each person as a unique individual with a distinct personality. Continuity development refers to the belief that a person's personality and pattern of coping remain unchanged with aging. The aging process is seen as a part of the life cycle, not as a separate terminal stage. Personality patterns are developed over a long time and help to determine whether the person remains active or inactive and engaged or disengaged from society. Knowledge of personality type may be helpful in predicting a person's response to aging. The individual's state of health will also determine how long he or she will remain active and satisfied. Illness may lead to retirement, social isolation, and decreased self-esteem.

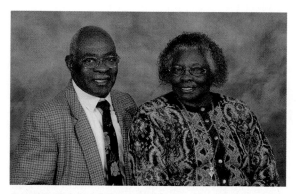

FIGURE 13.1 Couple relationships provide love and companionship.

Natural Remedies Thought to Delay the Aging Process

The following herbs and dietary supplements are used to treat or prevent diseases. Scientific studies have not yet confirmed their benefits or risks. Patients interested in using any natural remedy should check with their physician before taking any of these drugs. All of these substances should be used with caution and reserved optimism.

- Ginkgo (*Ginkgo biloba*) is used to improve circulation and blood flow to the brain.
- Saw palmetto (*Serenoa repens*) is used to prevent or treat prostate enlargement by helping to shrink the prostate gland.
- St John's wort (*Hypericum perforatum*) is recommended for relief of stress, anxiety, and depression.
- Evening primrose (*Oenothera biennis*) is recommended to treat signs and symptoms of menopause and dry skin.
- Black cohosh (*Cimicifuga racemosa*) is used to reduce signs and symptoms of menopause.
- Chondroitin sulfate and glucosamine are currently used by many people to help maintain cartilage.
- Celery seed (*Apium graveolens*) is used to treat gout and arthritis.
- Garlic (*Allium sativum*) is recommended to reduce blood pressure and cholesterol and to prevent blood clots.
- Vitamin E is recommended to help prevent heart attacks and may prevent dementia.
- Vitamin C has long been touted for its usefulness in reducing the severity of colds.

PHYSICAL CHARACTERISTICS

Quality of life is not determined by age but largely by a person's ability to independently perform activities of daily living such as dressing, bathing, toileting, and eating. Health problems should not be viewed as inevitable because many can be prevented or controlled.

Height and Weight

Many signs of aging are evident in both the conformation and composition of the body (Fig. 13.2). Trunk length decreases as spinal curvature increases and the intervertebral disks become compact. This process actually begins much earlier: On average, adults lose 1 centimeter per decade

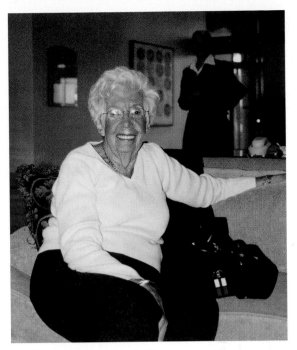

FIGURE 13.2 Physical signs of aging vary with each person.

after age 30. There is also a decrease in shoulder width in both sexes as a result of the loss of muscle mass in the deltoids. There is a slight increase in chest circumference resulting from the loss of elasticity in the lungs and in the thorax. The circumference of the head decreases, and the nose and ears lengthen. Body weight decreases slowly after age 55. Other changes include a loss of body surface area and of active cell mass. Older adults have 30% fewer cells than younger adults. There is atrophy (shrinking) of body fat, giving a bony appearance and a deepening of body areas in the axillae, rib cage, and orbital cavity surrounding the eyes. These changes in body composition are vitally important in helping to understand drug metabolism and nursing interventions for this age group. Decreased body surface area and body fat affect the dosage and rate of drug absorption. To accommodate these physiological changes, lower dosages of medication are used for older persons.

Musculoskeletal System

Postmenopausal women lose bone mass at a faster rate than do men, putting them at greater risk for osteoporosis. The typical person at risk for osteoporosis is the aging, thin, white, menopausal woman, although osteoporosis is now being investigated as a health risk for men also. Box 13.2 offers suggestions for reducing the risks for osteoporosis. Women

Genetic factors:

• Female, fair skin, small body frame, family history, early menopause

Nutritional factors:

• Low body weight, low calcium intake, high caffeine intake, high alcohol consumption

Lifestyle factors:

• Smoking, lack of exercise

Interventions:

• Avoid tobacco use.
• Limit caffeine intake.
• Limit alcohol consumption.
• Increase calcium intake.
• Get regular exercise.
• Take hormone replacement therapy.

older than age 80 have a 1 in 5 chance of sustaining a fracture of the femur. Regular active or passive exercise can minimize discomfort and loss of bone mass. Postural changes also occur, resulting in kyphosis, an exaggerated curvature of the spine, or the typical "dowager's hump." The resultant tilting of the head and flexion of the hips and knees cause the center of gravity to shift. In addition to a loss of bone mass, there is decreased muscle mass accompanied by decreased muscle strength and tone.

These changes affect balance and further increase the risk of falls. Each year 1 out of 3 older adults falls. Falls often lead to severe disability, increased hospitalization and related costs, and an increased number of deaths. Fear of repeated falls may lead to sedentary behavior, impaired function, and lower quality of life.

The attachments known as *ligaments* and *tendons* are less elastic in elderly people, resulting in muscle spasms and decreased flexibility. Pronounced stiffness and diminished range of motion are more noticeable in the morning or following periods of disuse. Complaints of muscle weakness are most frequently caused not by age-related changes but by inactivity.

Cardiovascular System

Normally there is no significant decrease in heart size with advancing age. Heart valves become thicker and more rigid. Lipofuscin, a pigmented metabolic waste product, has been found in greater amounts in various organs of the aged body. Loss of

elasticity in blood vessels, combined with the accumulation of collagen and lipofuscin, results in narrowing of the vessel lumen (diameter), causing a subsequent increase in blood pressure. It is not unusual to have a slight increase in the systolic pressure while the diastolic pressure remains the same. Significant increase in blood pressure is more likely to be the consequence of environmental factors (diet, weight, and stress levels) rather than of age. A decrease in cardiac output of 1% per year occurs between ages 20 and 80 and is a result of the loss of cardiac muscle strength and contractility. This change may be evidenced by a slower heart rate. The older heart needs more rest between beats. Regular exercise can increase cardiac performance and prevent complications. The best type of exercise for maximizing cardiac function is walking. The older person's veins also become more visible and tortuous. Increased pressure on weak vessel walls leads to the increased incidence of varicosities in the lower extremities and rectum.

Respiratory System

The respiratory system is subjected to a great deal of abuse during one's lifetime. The age-related changes are subtle and occur gradually. Several structural changes in the chest diminish respiratory function. Calcification of the rib cage and costal cartilage makes the chest wall more rigid and less compliant. These changes in the thoracic walls make the respiratory muscles work harder. Lung tissue gradually loses elasticity. Vital capacity decreases, and more muscular work is needed to move air in and out of the lungs. Between ages 20 and 60 about 1 liter of vital capacity is lost. Lungs exhale less efficiently, causing an increase in the residual volume. The residual volume refers to the amount of air remaining in the lungs after forceful exhalation. Coughing is less effective. All of these changes make the older person more susceptible to respiratory infections.

Gastrointestinal System

The numerous changes in the gastrointestinal system cause discomfort but are usually not serious enough to place a person at health risk. The amount of saliva decreases, resulting in xerostomia (dry mouth) and dysphagia (difficulty swallowing). A diminished gag reflex places the older person at risk for choking while eating. To decrease the chance of choking, older persons should eat slowly and in an upright sitting position.

Because of the decrease in peristalsis, the muscle movement that propels food through the gastrointestinal system, it takes longer in older adults for the esophagus, stomach, and lower intestine to empty. In the esophagus, this slower emptying increases the risk of aspiration. For this reason, older people should not only eat in an upright position but also maintain this position for an hour after eating. In the stomach, peristalsis—together with decreased gastric secretions—may result in indigestion. The total stomach capacity is also decreased, causing diminished hunger and appetite. Changes in the intestines include decreased absorption of nutrients. Individuals who use laxatives on a regular basis may be at further risk for vitamin and nutrient deficiencies. As the liver ages, enzyme production decreases, which may adversely affect metabolism of both food and drugs.

In the lower intestine, the reduction in peristalsis slows the movement of waste, often producing constipation and increased flatus. To maintain normal bowel functioning, older people need to intake adequate fluid and roughage, or fiber. Regular toileting habits and exercise will further enhance normal bowel functioning. Bowel movements may also be affected by decreased nerve sensations and a delayed signal to defecate. These changes, along with weakening of the external sphincter in the rectum, may sometimes cause bowel incontinence.

Dentition

Tooth loss is not a consequence of the aging process but a result of poor care leading to disease. With proper care, older persons can retain their teeth through their entire lives. As they age, teeth show natural signs of wear and tear, including loss of some enamel, lengthening of the tooth, and decreased ability to cut and chew efficiently. These changes have significant implications for both safety and digestion. Chewing ability and the condition of the mouth and teeth should be considered when preparing foods for elderly people. Soft or pureed foods can be substituted for foods of regular consistency if indicated.

Integumentary System

The integumentary system consists of the skin, hair, nails, and oil and sweat glands. The skin helps the body maintain a state of homeostasis (internal balance). It protects the body from changes in temperature, pressure, and moisture and from invading organisms. Normal aging may compromise the skin's ability to maintain homeostasis. The skin loses some elasticity and becomes wrinkled. As aging progresses,

the skin gets thinner, drier, and more fragile. These changes make the older person more prone to skin breakdown following minor bruising or injury. Normal circulatory changes may delay wound healing.

Older people lose subcutaneous adipose tissue, causing a decrease in their ability to sustain changes in temperature. Further complicating the problem is a normal decrease in the number and function of the sweat glands as a person ages. Older persons perspire less and chill easily. They commonly complain of being chilly if they are seated near a window or draft. A sweater or light cover usually helps increase comfort. Elderly people are also more apt to suffer from heat stroke as a result of reduced perspiration. In warm weather they should avoid overexertion and maintain adequate hydration.

Skin, as it ages, shows irregular pigmentation—senile lentigo—as a result of an uneven distribution of melanocytes (pigmented cells). The actual number of melanocytes in the skin decreases as much as 80% between ages 27 and 65. Extensive repeated exposure to the sun and ultraviolet rays can further exaggerate the normal aging effects on the skin. Many age-related skin changes place elderly people more at risk for skin disorders, such as infections, pruritus (itching), keratosis (thickening), pressure sores, and skin cancer.

Nail growth gradually slows, and nails become more brittle, appearing dull and yellow. Toenails may become thicker and should be trimmed by a podiatrist regularly. Fingernails require special attention, including frequent cleaning and trimming.

In 50% of the population, hair grays by age 50. Hair loss is a common occurrence beginning in the 30s in men and after menopause in women. Hair loss is not confined to the head but occurs elsewhere, including in the axillary and pubic areas. Men show an increase in hair growth in the eyebrows, nose, and ears. Women may note some unwanted hair on the face and chin.

Nervous System

As people age, the number of neurons, or nerve cells, decreases: 5% to 10% of neurons atrophy by age 70; after age 70, the rate of atrophy increases. The result is a decrease in the nervous system's capacity to transmit messages to and from the brain. Brain weight peaks at age 20, and the brain loses 100 grams, or 7% of its weight, by age 80. Cerebral blood flow decreases because of changes in the vessels of the circulatory system. However, problems with memory and learning result not from these normal changes of aging, but from specific diseases that affect the system's ability to function. Other neural changes include slowed motor responses. Reaction time is as much as 30% longer in older individuals. Elderly people must be assessed individually to determine their response time and ability to drive safely.

Sensory System

Normal age-related changes in the sensory system may cause problems with daily functioning and general well-being. The five senses—taste, sight, hearing, touch, and smell—all become less efficient, placing the older person at greater risk for injury. The vision changes that begin in middle age continue during this stage. Presbyopia, the loss of the eye's ability to focus, and opacity (clouding) of the lens progress. The incidence of cataracts and glaucoma increases. Peripheral vision diminishes, and sensitivity to glare increases. Color vision changes with aging: Red and yellow are seen best, whereas the ability to discriminate between green and blue colors diminishes. For safety reasons, bright colors such as yellow and orange are best used to mark curbs and steps.

Blockage of the lacrimal ducts (tear ducts) may cause the eyes to water excessively. Certain medications, vitamins, and diseases can cause eye dryness. Using artificial tears helps to alleviate the discomfort and protect the cornea from drying.

About one-third of persons older than age 65 have sufficient presbycusis (age-related hearing loss) to affect their everyday lives. At age 10 a person can hear frequencies as high as 20 kHz; by age 50, the maximum level is 13 kHz; and by age 60, there is little hearing over 5 kHz. It is best to address older people in low-pitched, moderately loud tones to compensate for the loss of high-frequency hearing. Small insults and injuries or certain diseases may contribute to hearing loss. Changes in the middle ear of elderly adults include thickening of the tympanic membrane and calcification of the bones. The accumulation of cerumen (ear wax) may interfere with the passage of sound vibrations through the external canal to the middle ear and inner ear. Symptoms of this type of hearing loss include fullness, itching, and tinnitus (ringing) in the ears. Conductive hearing may show marked improvement after the removal of accumulated wax. Conductive hearing loss results from the obstruction or reduction in the passage of sound in the inner ear. Other types of hearing loss may be related to nerve atrophy and circulatory changes. Box 13.3 offers suggestions for improving verbal communication with individuals who are hearing impaired.

BOX 13.3 Improving Verbal Communication for Individuals Who Are Hearing Impaired

- Speak clearly and distinctly in low tones.
- Rephrase words as needed.
- Face the listener.
- Use facial expressions and gestures to help clarify your message.
- Communicate in well-lit areas, placing lighting behind the listener.
- Minimize outside distractions.
- Encourage lip reading.

A loss in number of taste buds causes a resulting loss in taste discrimination, first for sweet and later for other tastes. These changes are not solely age related; environmental factors may also contribute. There is little research about age-related changes to the sense of smell. It is believed that the sense of smell declines with normal aging in part because of olfactory degeneration, but loss of smell creates a safety issue because older people living alone may not be able to detect subtle gas leaks or smoke. For this reason the use of warning detectors in the home is most important. Significant changes in tactile sensation are thought to be more related to disease than to aging.

Genitourinary System

After menopause the ovaries, uterus, and fallopian tubes atrophy. The vaginal walls become thinner and less elastic, and lubrication and vaginal secretions decrease. These changes may result in discomfort during intercourse. Vaginal secretions normally protect the vagina from bacterial invaders. This protective function diminishes, making older women at greater risk for vaginal infections.

Approximately 2.5% of the body's calcium may be lost in the first few years after menopause, resulting in bone loss. After this initial period, however, the rate of bone loss slows down. It is believed that estrogen has an antiatherosclerotic effect, protecting women from heart disease. As estrogen levels decline, the incidence of heart disease in postmenopausal women increases to equal that in men. Other common changes occurring after menopause include deepening of the voice, thinning of the pubic hair, and atrophy of the breast tissue. Hormone replacement therapy (HRT) may be considered (see Chapter 12).

After age 50, men experience a gradual decline in testicular mass. It takes longer for older men to achieve an erection, and less semen is released at ejaculation. Testosterone and sperm levels decrease gradually, but healthy men retain fertility well into their older years. Hypertrophy of the prostate gland may cause difficulty in voiding. The prostate gland should be checked during physical examinations. It is separated from the rectum by connective tissue, making its posterior surface easily palpable on a digital rectal examination.

Normal age-related changes affecting the urinary system occur gradually. The kidneys decrease in size and lose some of their functional units, or nephrons, resulting in a one-third to two-third reduction in filtration rate. This can cause a decreased ability to filter, concentrate, or dilute urine. However, even with these age-related changes, the aging kidneys should continue to maintain homeostasis.

The bladder walls lose elasticity, and bladder volume decreases from 250 to 200 mL. Women with a history of multiple pregnancies are at greater risk for further weakening of the pelvic floor muscles, leading to stress incontinence. The signal indicating a need to void may be delayed, making an older person prone to accidents.

Endocrine System

As individuals age, secretory cells of the endocrine system are replaced with connective tissue, thereby decreasing hormone levels. All body tissues and organs are affected by these age-related changes of the endocrine system. Diabetes mellitus and thyroid dysfunction are the two main endocrine and metabolic disorders affecting elderly patients. Table 13.1 summarizes age-related changes in the older person.

TABLE
13.1 **Summary of Age-Related Changes**

Age-Related Changes	Suggestions for Optimal Functioning
Cardiovascular System Blood vessels narrow with the accumulation of fat and scar tissue.	Exercise. Control weight. Follow a diet low in saturated fat with a variety of foods from the food pyramid or MyPlate chart.
Skin and Hair Skin becomes thin and less elastic. Hair may gray.	Limit exposure to sunlight. Use sunblock. Examine skin frequently for damage or changes.
Teeth Gums recede and tooth enamel wears away.	Practice good dental hygiene. Floss and brush frequently. Schedule dental visits every 6 months.
Eyes Changes in the lens cause poor near vision. Lens may start to cloud, forming the beginning of cataracts.	Schedule annual eye examinations and wear corrective lenses as needed. Eat a diet rich in dark-green vegetables.
Ears Some nerve cells are lost, but hearing remains unchanged until age 60 and older.	Avoid exposure to noise pollution.
Brain and Nerves Some brain shrinkage is noted with fewer nerve cells present.	Remain active and involved to stimulate thinking and memory.
Muscles Muscle mass and strength decrease.	Exercise daily to strengthen muscles.

Continued

TABLE

13.1   Summary of Age-Related Changes—cont'd

Age-Related Changes	Suggestions for Optimal Functioning
Bones	
Bone density declines after age 50. Joint flexibility decreases.	Exercise after proper stretching. Maintain a healthy diet. Avoid obesity.
Lungs	
Lungs lose elasticity. Chest wall stiffens.	Avoid smoking and exposure to secondhand smoke. Exercise aerobically on a regular basis.
Digestive	
Levels of enzymes and digestive juices decrease. Less mobility causes constipation.	Eat foods containing fiber. Drink plenty of water. Exercise regularly. Maintain regular toileting habits.
Urinary System	
Kidneys become less efficient, and bladder muscles weaken. Men: Prostate gland enlarges.	Perform pelvic exercises. Drink plenty of fluids. Men: Have yearly prostate exams.
Reproductive System	
Men: Desire usually remains unchanged. *Women:* Hormonal changes with menopause cause less elasticity and lubrication. Interest in sex varies with individual.	*Men:* Avoid alcohol and smoking. Exercise regularly. Maintain normal blood pressure and cardiovascular fitness. *Women:* Use hormone replacement therapy if suggested by physician. Use water-soluble lubricants.

HOMEOSTASIS

Homeostasis is best defined as a balance or equilibrium between the internal and external environment. As an individual ages, the common age-related changes in the body systems make it more difficult for the individual to maintain homeostasis. Changes in thermoregulatory responses that help detect changes in temperature may lead to greater risk of developing hypothermia or hyperthermia in older persons. Normal body temperature in older persons is slightly lower than in younger persons. A temperature reading of 97°F (36°C) may be normal in the older adult. If unaware of this, health care workers may misinterpret a temperature elevation of 99°F as a normal finding in the older individual when in fact it may be a 2-degree elevation and signify the presence of a possible infection. Older individuals are also extremely sensitive to changes in room temperature. The ideal room temperature for older persons is 75°F. Older persons may experience discomfort or chilling, which can lead to hypothermia when exposed to cold temperatures. Exposure to extremely high temperatures may place the older individual at risk for hyperthermia and possible brain damage.

Decreased cardiac reserve that occurs with advancing age may place the person at risk for several problems. Normally during strenuous activity, cardiac output increases to compensate for the individual's increased needs. This is known as cardiac reserve and it is adversely affected by several aging heart conditions. Older persons are susceptible to fluid overload and have difficulty regulating body fluids. The older person's reduced awareness of thirst only further complicates matters.

Additional homeostatic responses include a decreased ability for aged eyes to accommodate to darkness. This makes it more difficult to drive at night or to adjust from light to dark environments.

VITAL SIGNS

Normal age-related cardiovascular changes cause a moderate increase in systolic blood pressure. *Hypertension* is defined as systolic blood pressure greater than 130 mm Hg and diastolic pressure of 90 mm Hg or more. Resting heart rate usually remains unchanged or slows slightly. There is little or no change in the older person's resting respiratory rate. However, more muscle work is needed to move air in and out of the lungs.

DEVELOPMENTAL MILESTONES

Motor Development

Changes in both the musculoskeletal and nervous systems cause movements to slow down with advancing age. Both gross and fine motor skills may be affected by stiffened ligaments and joints. Gait speed and step height decrease. Postural and balance changes further affect mobility.

Sexual Development

Contrary to popular belief, elderly people are capable of enjoying satisfying sexual relationships. Affection and pleasure-seeking behaviors are important and may be expressed differently as individuals age and opportunities arise. Men need more stimulation to reach erection. Women can use estrogen creams or other lubrication to prevent discomfort caused by drying of vaginal tissues. Respect for the individual's privacy in all settings helps promote dignity and a positive self-image.

Psychosocial Development

Successful resolution of the first seven stages of Erikson's psychosocial development prepares the older person for the task of ego integrity. **Ego integrity** is similar to a life puzzle in which all the pieces fit nicely together. Each stage of development completes the integration of the person, adding meaning to his or her life. Those who develop a sense of ego integrity usually feel satisfied with their accomplishments. They may look back over their lives and admit to certain failures and disappointments, but generally they feel that they have been successful. Ego integrity allows them to proceed with a sense of calm toward death, confident of having left a legacy for future generations.

Wisdom acquired throughout a life of experience is a common characteristic associated with a sense of ego integrity. The process of **reminiscence,** or life review, reassures older people about their accomplishments and worth. Reminiscing allows an elderly person to weave his or her life together, giving events and memories meaning and order. It facilitates an understanding of the past, puts the past in context, and allows the person to make peace with disappointments and face the future with optimism.

People who feel that their lives have no meaning or that they have made the wrong decisions develop despair. This produces helplessness and lack of control over their lives. Despair is also associated with fear of death and anxiety about the future.

As with Erikson's other tasks, developing ego integrity is also affected by one's family and other socialization experiences. All of these experiences combine to help shape one's attitude toward aging. If old age is seen as a time of decline and nonproductiveness, these negative expectations are more likely to be fulfilled. **Ageism,** or prejudice against older people, contributes to negative perceptions of the aging process. Educational programs help combat ageism and foster positive attitudes toward older individuals. Furthermore, if young children have good role models, they are more likely to have positive attitudes toward aging throughout their lives and thus be helped to establish ego integrity themselves.

Achieving ego integrity also involves adjusting to changes in body image, family roles, work and leisure, and sexuality, and facing the inevitability of death.

Changes in Body Image

How we view aging will ultimately affect how we cope with our changing bodies. Physical appearance has a strong impact on a person's self-concept. Most of the visible changes of aging occur gradually, giving older persons time to adjust to their new images (Fig. 13.3). An individual whose identity is based solely on physical attractiveness continues to see life from that perspective and may become depressed.

Changes in Family Roles

As couples grow old together, they must make several adjustments. Physical or emotional illness of either spouse may frequently cause role changes in older marriages. One spouse may become the nurse or caregiver. This may cause anger, resentment, and depression in either the giver or receiver of care. Patterns of dominance may shift from the man to the

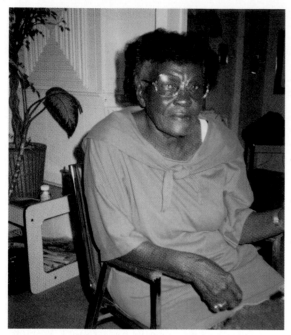

FIGURE 13.3 Older people need to accept their change in body image.

woman or vice versa. Roles may also change with retirement, placing new limitations and stresses on both parties. Husbands may spend more time at home than ever before, causing conflicts if they try to assume the in-charge role in the home. Other men may find that their roles have changed to that of homemakers while their wives continue to work. Any one of these role changes requires a period of adjustment.

Death of a spouse produces a role change and adds stress to the remaining individual and other family members. The loss of a spouse is a highly significant life event. Studies indicate that married elderly individuals are generally healthier than unmarried persons. Married persons have a lower incidence of chronic diseases and institutionalization than single, widowed, and divorced individuals. In addition, studies indicate that mortality rates are higher among recently widowed men (6 months) and women (2 years). Married women older than age 65 are more likely to be the surviving spouses than are married men in the same age group.

Two problems common to widowhood are loneliness and decline in income. Frequently, a widow finds that she is unprepared to be the decision maker and financial overseer. Former relationships and activities may disappear, forcing her to pursue new activities. Given time and support, many women lead independent, well-adjusted lives after the death of their spouse. Many elders seek new

relationships for companionship. Past marital experiences, good health, adequate income, and the attitudes of grown children are factors important to successful relationships.

Some widowed or divorced elders seek remarriage as an option. For a long time elders were forced to give up their former spouse's Social Security benefits when they remarried, but Congress has since passed legislation that allows the surviving spouse to choose between the benefits of a former spouse and those of a new spouse, whichever are greater.

Older people may lose friends because of death or relocation. Some older individuals on fixed incomes find it necessary to move to new communities, giving up old friends and neighbors.

The divorce rate of older persons has been increasing as individuals live longer. Debilitating illnesses, disabilities, and marital distress are the main reasons cited for divorce in this age group. Anger and guilt both have an adverse effect on widowed and divorced individuals. Divorce also places individuals at risk for economic difficulties. A nursing assessment of the emotional and social support systems of those who are widowed or divorced can help identify their risk factors and specific needs. Once these factors are known, referrals and counseling may be offered.

Elderly people fear loss of independence more than any other loss, commonly expressing the feeling that they do not want to become a burden to their families. Illness or disability may result in loss of independence. If this happens, every effort should be made to help the affected individual maximize his or her capabilities and independence for as long as possible. This enhances self-esteem and increases feelings of usefulness.

One role that helps decrease feelings of isolation for many individuals is grandparenting (Fig. 13.4). Most elders have regular, frequent contact with their grandchildren. Most children have strong feelings of affection for their grandparents. Age and state of health will help to determine the amount of interaction and style of grandparenting they share. Many individuals live long enough to assume the role of great-grandparent.

Changes in Work and Leisure

Work gives many people identity and self-esteem in addition to financial rewards. Many older people continue to work after age 65. In 2012, 26.8% of older persons were in the workforce. The projected number of people ages 65 to 74 in the workforce

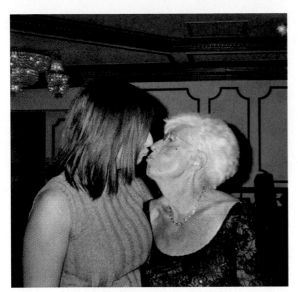

FIGURE 13.4 Grandparenting often provides satisfaction.

by 2022 is 31.9%. Older workers place more significance on social aspects of a job, whereas younger workers usually value income most. Job studies have shown that older employees have higher job satisfaction, lower absenteeism rates, and lower job turnover numbers. Despite these positive factors, subtle age discrimination still exists against older workers. Older persons have great difficulty finding and keeping jobs. The job market today continues to show preference toward young workers, who are often hired over older, more skilled people.

Many older adults continue to work to postpone retirement because the discontinuation of one's work role causes a change in lifelong habits. Many people's self-worth is directly tied to their work roles. Although they may have dreamed about having more leisure when they were young, they may find retirement to be less appealing as the time approaches. Some men who have been in the workforce for many years may still look forward to retirement. For many years retirement was basically experienced by men. Today, with more women in the labor force, retirement issues affect women as much as men. Women who retire at age 65 can expect to live another 19.2 years, which is 3 years longer than men retiring at the same age. Many individuals delay retirement planning because proper planning includes many decisions. How much money to save, where to save the money, and what to invest in are just some of the financial planning concerns. Currently, it is believed that one will need between 70% and 90% of preretirement income to

retire and maintain the same standard of living in retirement (Box 13.4).

The state of an older adult's health is the most important factor contributing to the adjustment to retirement. Prior work and leisure habits may also influence the adjustment. Factors that help promote positive feelings toward retirement include adequate income, social support, and a strong self-concept. These factors are important in helping today's older adults adjust to the increased length of retirement. Someone who retires today at age 65 may be retired for 20 years or longer. Of course, the best time to plan for retirement is when an individual first enters the workforce. Appropriate planning can help a person look forward to a peaceful retirement and allow him or her to continue to grow mentally and emotionally and be satisfied.

Even with preparation and planning, retirement is an evolving process with phases of reaction and development. Researchers have identified seven phases. The *remote phase* is a period of denial in which the individual has prepared little for the process. During the *near phase* the person may participate in some planning. The *honeymoon period* is characterized by a time of euphoria; during this stage people try to do all the activities that they have not had time for in the past. A sense of *disenchantment* sometimes occurs as reality sets in, and individuals may strive to come to terms with their expectations. During the *reorientation phase* individuals must reestablish goals and change their lifestyles. Adjustment to reality is part of the *stability phase*. If the person resumes work or becomes ill or disabled, the retirement role *terminates*.

Although much of our society is work oriented, many individuals derive satisfaction from the leisure that comes after a productive work life, feeling that they have earned the time to pursue other interests.

BOX 13.4   **Things You Should Know About Financial Preparations for Retirement**

- Know your personal retirement needs.
- Determine your Social Security benefits.
- Look into employer's pension plans or profit sharing.
- Contribute to a tax-sheltered savings plan.
- Put money into an individual retirement account (IRA) if applicable.
- Do not touch savings.
- Start early.
- Know where your money is invested.
- Ask questions from qualified individuals.
- Avoid "too good to be true" investments.

Leisure, too, can be viewed as "productive" in the sense that it enhances one's sense of well-being and may include activities that also benefit others in the community. The activities that people pursue vary greatly according to individual interests.

Changes in Sexuality

Unfortunately, one of society's misconceptions is that older adults cannot and should not be sexually active. Older people, despite all the myths, continue to have the capacity to enjoy sex well into late life. Sexual expression during this stage includes not only sexual intercourse, but also touching, cuddling, and masturbation. Sexual activity fulfills an older person's basic human need for physical closeness, warmth, and intimacy. Studies have shown that sexual behavior patterns of late adulthood correlate with those of earlier years. Some decline in sexual activity may be related to decreased opportunities or acceptance of the stereotype that older adults are sexless. Sexual difficulties are usually related to poor health, disease, medications, or other social problems.

Often young adults feel that sex is perfectly natural for them but have difficulty seeing their parents' sexuality as natural. Because of these negative attitudes, many older people feel guilty about their sexual needs and fear ridicule of their behavior. Some practices in health care facilities may further reinforce negative stereotyping. Very few institutions provide privacy and space for couples to be alone or have sex. In fact, some administrators in long-term care (LTC) settings go so far as to separate married residents from one another. Caring displays of affection allow people to feel good about themselves. Other benefits of sexual expression include physical exercise and improved circulation for the heart and lungs. For all these reasons, sexual expression is important and meaningful in the lives of older people. Nurses can foster a climate of support in which sexual expression is not suppressed but accepted as a natural part of life. Box 13.5 lists practices that promote sexual expression in older people.

The Inevitability of Death

Until a certain age healthy people usually do not think of the nearness of death. Death takes on different meanings for different people. Some face death with a sense of tranquility, whereas others fear it and feel that their time is running out. Older adults begin to face the reality of dying as their friends and loved ones die. Multiple losses are part of an older person's world. Losses serve to remind

---

BOX 13.5 Promoting Sexual Expression in Older People

- Allow for privacy.
- Be nonjudgmental.
- Maximize strengths and minimize weaknesses.
- Encourage attempts at grooming and the use of cosmetics.
- Suggest wearing clothing that enhances appearance.
- Avoid belittling or ridiculing older people's interest in the opposite sex.

---

people of their own mortality. Loss of a spouse or dear friend may cause loneliness and isolation. Community and religious affiliation and support groups can ease the pain and help with adjustment to loss. Spiritual awareness may become strengthened and help guide and support people through their losses. Death and dying are emotionally difficult issues for many people. Nurses themselves need to be comfortable when working with dying individuals. They must respect an individual's wishes, help the family of a dying person cope with the event, honor living wills, and so on. Although this is a sad time for many people, helping patients in a humane and compassionate manner can ease the process and perhaps make it more meaningful and growth producing for all involved.

Many older people nearing death attempt to resolve old conflicts between friends and family members. This helps them move forward with less guilt and unrest. Individuals should be encouraged to openly discuss their feelings about dying and burial plans. Wills designating property and possessions, living wills, and appointment of a health care proxy are needed for peace of mind. Refer to Chapter 14 for more on death and dying.

Cognitive Development

Older healthy people may retain their cognitive abilities well into late life. The Wechsler Adult

---

HELPFUL HINTS

Are You Prepared for Death?

1. Do you have a will?
2. Have you discussed your wishes with a loved one?
3. Have you discussed organ donation with a loved one?
4. Have you organized and gathered all of your important documents?

Intelligence Scale (WAIS), developed in 1955, continues to be used to assess adults' cognitive abilities. However, this test measures content that is not related to everyday cognitive tasks and therefore is not useful in determining older people's actual performance outside of the testing area. Tests that use material relevant to everyday functioning show that older people have no decline in intelligence with advancing age.

Many factors influence intelligence, including genetic inheritance, education, socioeconomic background, and state of health. Older individuals are generally less competitive and less interested in impressing others with their scores or performance. New material is learned more slowly as one ages. Attitudes toward learning new concepts are often different among those in this age group. An older person may be more reluctant to try new things and to learn. For example, children placed in front of a computer look at it as a challenge to master, whereas many older adults view it as a threat and fear its use. Old stereotypes and beliefs—such as "You can't teach an old dog new tricks"—can become self-fulfilling prophecies. Older individuals usually solve problems by using their life experiences rather than looking for new solutions.

Learning, perception, and cognition may be affected by normal age-related changes. Older people suffering from sensory losses have difficulty concentrating on more than one task at a time. They usually find it more difficult to focus and eliminate extraneous noise or interference. Reaction time slows down with aging, making it more difficult to process information at one's usual rate. Older adults can compensate for these changes and learn more efficiently when they set their own pace.

Memory shows slight changes with advancing age. Most older people remember what is heard better than what is read or seen. Research testing shows that older people are slower to retrieve stored information. Instead of attempting to remember, some elders say that they do not know. Recent, or short-term, memory stores a limited amount of information. Remote, or long-term, memory stores and encodes information in a meaningful mode. Older individuals show greater losses in short-term than in long-term memory. They often remember their wedding parties better than what they did an hour ago. The state of health and the amount of sensory losses have a great effect on memory. In fact, many individuals who appear to have suffered from marked cognitive losses actually may have profound uncorrected sensory deficits.

We do not know exactly why individuals experience memory changes as they age. We do know that we lose some nerve cells, and that there is a decrease in the activity in the hippocampus of the brain, causing a loss of some stored information. As we get older, steps can be taken to enhance memory. Regular exercise increases the amount of blood pumped to the brain and thereby enhances memory. Mental exercises may also help stimulate the brain and memory. Some people call these exercises "mental jogging." Forms of mental exercises can be varied and specific to each individual's particular likes.

Researchers are investigating whether HRT stimulates memory. The decision to use HRT is an individual decision that should first be discussed with one's physician.

Another measure that can help enhance memory is maintaining good dietary habits. It is important not to skip meals. Selecting high-quality foods helps to maintain optimal functioning. Individuals should include whole grains, fruits, and vegetables at each meal. These are good sources of both glucose and antioxidants, which are believed to stimulate brain functioning. Individuals should also try to avoid alcohol and drugs because of their adverse effects on the brain and memory.

Stress reduction and adequate sleep are also important to overall health and memory. Table 13.2 lists suggestions for improving mental functioning.

TABLE
13.2   Improving Mental Functioning

Risks for Mental Decline	Suggestions to Improve Mental Functioning
Family history of Alzheimer's disease	Maintain regular medical checkups.
History of untreated hypertension, heart disease, or diabetes	Follow medical regimen.
History of lead exposure	Avoid lead paint exposure.

Continued

TABLE
13.2   Improving Mental Functioning—cont'd

Risks for Mental Decline	Suggestions to Improve Mental Functioning
Smoking	Avoid smoking.
Illegal drug use	Refrain from drug usage.
Overindulgence in alcohol	Limit alcohol intake.
Lack of physical exercise	Remain active and exercise regularly.
Lack of social interaction	Stay socially active and involved.
High stress	Avoid stressful situations and practice stress-reduction techniques.
Lack of higher education	Remain intellectually involved. Enroll in classes, read, and do mental exercises.

The use of hearing aids, eyeglasses, and other assistive devices can enhance learning, promote independence, and boost self-esteem (Fig. 13.5). Older people suffering from chronic physical illnesses are easily fatigued, which further reduces their learning abilities. Healthy older adults may choose to return to school or college with successful outcomes. Those actively pursuing their educational goals find satisfaction and self-fulfillment.

Moral Development

The wisdom ascribed to older people since ancient times implies that their levels of moral reasoning have reached optimal points. In reality, however, the moral and ethical concerns of this age group are no different from those of any other age group. Moral beliefs are based on a lifetime of experiences and interactions with others. The older person's basic moral code may change as a result of illness or need. Disease or medication can interfere with a person's moral reasoning, which depends on intact cognitive skills.

Many older people have more time to devote to their spiritual needs. There is no evidence, however, that older people become more religious at this stage in their lives. Still, many find meaning in life based on their spiritual beliefs by accepting and following the teachings of a particular religion. Those who have strong beliefs may find peace and satisfaction in their lives.

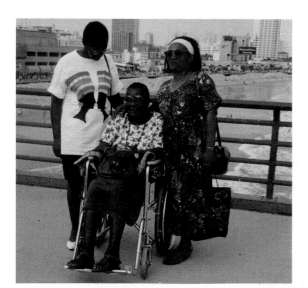

FIGURE 13.5 Assistive devices help maintain independence.

NUTRITION

Older adults are at an increased risk of inadequate diet and malnutrition, and the increasing numbers of older adults in society places more individuals at risk. Results of inadequate nutrition include the following: a decline in functional status, impaired muscle function, decreased muscle mass, immune dysfunction, anemia, reduced cognitive function, poor wound healing, and higher hospital admission rates and costs. Screening is vital in identifying problems and monitoring older clients. It is imperative that individuals with physical and cognitive decline be given special attention and care. Oral liquid high-energy supplements or enteral feeding should be considered in high-risk clients or in persons who are unable to meet their daily requirements.

Many factors affect an older person's nutritional status and eating habits. Nutritional status may be affected by a person's lifestyle, changes in body composition, and use of medications. Inflation and fixed incomes may prevent some older people from buying the foods necessary for adequate diets. Social situations (living alone or with others) and levels of education may also affect whether older individuals can adequately meet their nutritional needs or understand their dietary requirements. Weight maintenance is important for elderly people. Weight loss may reflect actual loss of muscle tissue.

Living alone often results in decreased appetite and less desire to prepare meals. Disabilities, sensory losses, and other age-related changes in various body systems may further complicate the older person's ability to shop for, prepare, eat, and enjoy food. Table 13.3 summarizes health implications of diet in elderly people. Other concerns for elderly people may include inadequate transportation to stores and fear of violence in the neighborhood. Title VII of the Older Americans Act offers nutritional programs for elderly people. Meals on Wheels is an example of a program used to provide homebound elders with nutritional meals.

TABLE
13.3   Dietary Implications for Older Adults

System	Physiological Changes	Dietary Suggestions
Cardiovascular system	Reduced elasticity of blood vessels Decreased cardiac output Decreased force of contraction	Reduce sodium intake. Lose weight if overweight.
Respiratory system	Lost elasticity Decreased maximum breathing capacity Decreased blood flow	Reduce caloric intake to prevent obesity.
Renal system	Decreased blood flow Decreased filtration, reduced numbers of nephrons	Drink plenty of fluids.
Neuromuscular system	Decreased responses Reduced physical strength and motor function	Maintain a well-balanced diet.
Nervous system	Reduced reaction time Decreased speed of nerve impulses	Maintain a well-balanced diet.
Sensory system	Appetite may be adversely affected by the loss of taste and smell.	Serve foods attractively and use fresh herbs and condiments to enhance flavor.
Endocrine system	Reduced blood levels of some hormones Decreased glucose tolerance	Reduce use of simple sugars.
Gastrointestinal system	Lost teeth Decreased taste, saliva, and digestive enzymes Decreased peristalsis	Use dentures. Use broth and juices to moisten foods. Eat small, frequent meals. Increase the amount of fiber. Maintain adequate fluid intake. Take vitamin C and adequate protein to aid healing.
Skin	Reduced subcutaneous fat Atrophied sweat glands Discolored, thin, wrinkled, and fragile skin	Drink plenty of water and maintain a well-balanced diet.

By old age, eating patterns are well-established habits largely fixed by culture, religion, and family structure that are difficult to change. If changes in diet are necessary, it is important that the nurse carefully review not only the individual's diet, but also all of the previously cited factors.

After age 21 the resting basal metabolic rate declines at a rate of 2% per decade, resulting in decreased caloric needs. Total caloric needs also depend on the individual's activity level. Between ages 51 and 75 most men should consume 2,000 to 2,300 calories per day, whereas most men ages 76 and older need 1,650 to 2,000 calories per day. Women between ages 51 and 75 usually need 1,600 to 1,800 calories per day, whereas women ages 76 and older need about 1,500 to 1,600 calories per day.

Carbohydrates should represent 60% of the older person's caloric intake. The best carbohydrates are those that are complex starches and sugars, such as whole-grain breads and cereals. These foods are digested over a long period and therefore are more satisfying to the appetite. Carbohydrates are also relatively inexpensive, tasty, and capable of being stored for long periods without refrigeration. A carbohydrate intake of 100 g daily is recommended for all adults. If intake goes below 50 g per day, there is a danger of developing *ketosis*, an accumulation of ketones when fats are improperly metabolized. Ketosis can lead to a disturbance in the acid–base balance.

Proteins should represent 12% to 13% of caloric intake. Because high-protein foods are more expensive, they may be missing from the older person's diet. A complete range of amino acids is found in eggs, meats, milk, fish, or poultry or in mixtures of rice, beans, cereals, nuts, and seeds. The protein needs of a healthy older adult differ greatly from those of an older ill person. For example, after surgery older individuals need greater amounts of protein to help the body build and repair tissues.

It is important to have some daily fat in the diet to help provide energy, transport fat-soluble vitamins, insulate and cushion the body, and make body compounds. However, it has been suggested that older adults need no more than 30% of their daily calories from fats. Diets restricted in cholesterol and high in unsaturated fats have been useful in minimizing the risk of cardiovascular disease.

Dietary fiber has multiple purposes. It helps to prevent constipation by increasing the bulk of the stool. It also helps to control weight because it satisfies hunger and gives the sensation of fullness without extra calories. Research shows that it may protect against colon and breast cancers. The recommended level of dietary fiber is 25 to 50 g per day. Foods such as whole grains, brown rice, unpeeled fruits and vegetables, legumes, nuts, and bran add fiber to the diet. Fluid intake should be increased to prevent the development of fecal impaction and possible intestinal obstruction.

Older people are often less aware of the sensation of thirst, may not be able to obtain fluids, or may avoid fluids to prevent nocturia (nighttime urination). These factors place older adults at greater risk for dehydration than young adults. Some elderly adults have conditions that further increase their need for fluids, such as diuretic therapy, fever, vomiting, and diarrhea. Normally, there should be a balance between water intake and output. Liquid intake should be sufficient enough to produce 1,000 mL of urine daily. Health care workers should be alert to the signs of dehydration, which include confusion; dry mouth and tongue; sunken eyes; dry, loose skin; urine-specific gravity greater than 1.030; and urine output of less than 500 mL per day.

Many older people take some type of vitamin supplement. Vitamin supplements that meet or are less than the recommended daily allowance levels are convenient, inexpensive means of providing some dietary needs. They should never be substituted for a balanced diet, however. It is also important that older people be cautioned against using excessive amounts of vitamins.

Moderate alcohol intake—one drink a day for women and two drinks a day for men—is associated with lower risks of coronary heart disease in some individuals.

Both physiological and psychological changes may have an impact on older persons developing poor nutrition. Undernutrition and overnutrition are potential problems for the older client. Several factors may contribute to these problems, including inadequate intake, problems with malabsorption, loss of nutrients, infection, and drug therapy.

Problems with malnutrition affect 40% to 60% of hospitalized older patients, and 40% to 80% of nursing home residents are at risk of developing malnutrition. The percentage of older home care clients is similar to that in the LTC setting. Caregivers in all settings and family caregivers must be alert to signs of malnutrition. Signs of malnutrition include weight loss, poor healing, cognitive impairment, visual disturbances, and muscle wasting. Undetected or untreated malnutrition may predispose the individual to pressure ulcers, infection, and other complications. Interventions to help identify nutritional problems in older institutionalized persons include making a referral to a dietitian as soon as a problem is suspected. A thorough review of the individual's medications will help identify any potential drug–nutrient interactions. Individuals complaining of a dry mouth may be advised to chew sugarless gum or suck on sugarless hard candies. Family members should be encouraged to bring in favorite foods, when allowed. Mealtimes should be a social time in an atmosphere that is conducive to one's appetite. The presence of family members, staff, or volunteers during mealtimes can help further stimulate appetite.

SLEEP AND REST

Older individuals need more rest and less sleep than do younger adults. Rest and sleep help to restore the body's energy reserve and prevent fatigue. However, the quality of sleep deteriorates during old age. The older person may take a longer time to fall asleep and may awaken more frequently during the night. It has been reported that 30% to 50% of elderly people have difficulty sleeping. Physical discomfort, anxiety, and nocturia are factors that cause these awakenings. The results of poor sleep are readily apparent the next day, causing poor performance, irritability, and exhaustion.

An assessment of sleep history can be useful in planning nursing interventions. Answers to questions about falling asleep and night waking can provide clues to sleep problems and tips on helping to promote better sleep habits. Nurses should follow individuals' prior sleep habits when caring for them in institutional settings. To make people comfortable before going to sleep, nurses can keep them warm and covered, suggest toileting, and provide a warm drink. Other measures that may help promote sleep include daytime naps, exercise in the early part of the day, and avoidance of stimulants (coffee, alcohol, and nicotine) and large or heavy meals before bedtime. Box 13.6 lists ideas for promoting sleep.

EXERCISE AND LEISURE

Lack of activity results in physical decline in older individuals. Research shows that more than 40% of older adults do not engage in exercise or physical activity. Less than one-third of this age group participate in moderate physical activity such as walking and gardening. Only 10% engage in any vigorous

---

B O X 13.6 | **Promoting Sleeping Among Older People**

- Meet the comfort needs of the individual (toileting, hygiene, and nutrition).
- Follow the person's normal sleep routine.
- Provide a quiet, relaxing environment.
- Maintain room temperature between 68°F and 72°F.

---

activity. Yet exercise has been recognized as a means to help maintain physical fitness across the life span. Regular exercise has been shown to slow the effects of the aging process, maximize the body systems' efficiencies, and decrease the incidence of coronary artery disease, hypertension, adult-onset diabetes, colon cancer, anxiety, and depression. Before beginning any exercise program, individuals need to consult their physician for medical clearance. Moderation is the key to all exercise programs. Box 13.7 lists the benefits of exercise.

SAFETY

Decreased auditory and visual acuity, gait changes, and neurological disorders increase an older person's risk of falling. Older people need to be taught safety practices, including getting up slowly and avoiding hot showers, which may make them dizzy. Normal circulatory and skin changes make their skin fragile and more prone to injury. Injuries to the skin heal more slowly.

Statistical studies show that, contrary to popular belief, elderly people are no more likely to be victims of crime than are younger adults. They are, however, often victims of purse snatching, thefts, and fraudulent schemes. Elderly persons may limit their activities out of fear that they are easy prey to

---

B O X 13.7 | **Benefits of Exercise**

Exercise should be habitual but not unduly strenuous. An example of beneficial exercise is sustained walking for 30 minutes per day. Regular exercise does the following:

- Reduces the risk for coronary heart disease
- Promotes cardiorespiratory fitness
- Builds muscle strength, endurance, and flexibility
- Is important for weight control
- Lowers blood pressure, blood lipids, and glucose tolerance
- Enhances well-being and helps reduce the risk of depression

criminals. This same fear that causes them to stay home may result in some feelings of social isolation and loneliness.

Abuse is defined as the willful infliction of physical or emotional pain or the deprivation of basic care necessary for survival or comfort. The exact number of cases of elder abuse is difficult to estimate, but studies indicate that it is increasing in a variety of settings. Abuse crosses all social, cultural, and socioeconomic boundaries. Most often abuse is related to caregivers' stress, unresolved family conflicts, or familial history of abuse. All forms of abuse are destructive and, at the very least, reduce an individual's self-esteem. Health care workers must be aware of elder abuse and understand that they are legally required to report acts of abuse that they have witnessed. The individual who fails to report an abusive act may be held responsible by the courts. Box 13.8 lists indicators of elder abuse.

HEALTH PROMOTION

The focus of health promotion is different for older adults than for younger people (Fig. 13.6). The emphasis is no longer solely prevention but also health maintenance. Exercise, diet modification, and healthy lifestyles can be useful in maximizing wellness and reducing risk factors in this age group. Health education and a positive attitude toward aging also help promote health during the later years. Lack of knowledge about health and health promotion and the devaluation of old age can prevent older people from seeking proper health care services. Older adults use many health services, as they often have many complex conditions that require professional expertise to meet their specific needs. Many programs need to target minorities and underserved populations. Issues directed at the health of older adults include helping them to coordinate care and manage their own care, establishing

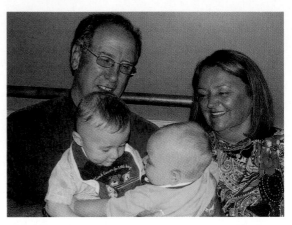

FIGURE 13.6 Family interactions may promote health.

quality measures, and determining the minimum level of training for people who care for older adults.

Health screening and maintenance include tests to detect for abnormalities and illnesses at early stages. All older adults need annual physical examinations. Health examinations should include an assessment of diet, activity level, medication usage (prescribed and over the counter), smoking, and alcohol intake. Vision and hearing tests should also be conducted annually. Immunizations are important at this time because there is a decrease in the immune response. Vaccinations against tetanus, pneumonia, and influenza are important. Pneumococcal pneumonia is three times more common in people 65 and older. The U.S. Department of Health and Human Services recommends that persons 65 and older receive the influenza vaccine each year and a pneumococcal vaccination at least once after age 65. Women are slightly more likely to receive the vaccines than men.

Elderly people are more likely to suffer from at least one chronic condition, and many have multiple conditions. Common chronic conditions include hypertension, arthritis, heart disease, cancer, diabetes, and sinusitis.

The leading causes of death among elderly people are heart disease, cancer, stroke, arteriosclerosis, diabetes, lung disease, and cirrhosis of the liver. Breast cancer is a concern after age 50. Early diagnosis of breast cancer has proved to be effective in increasing survival rates. Mortality rates have been reduced by 25% to 35% in women ages 50 to 59 with proper mammography screening.

Older people are particularly susceptible to ultraviolet rays because of their normal age-related skin changes. Brief periods of sunlight may precipitate photosensitive reactions in older adults who

B O X
13.8   Indicators of Elder Abuse

- Evidence of substance abuse
- Social isolation
- Lack of support systems
- Financial problems
- Marital difficulties
- Outward aggression
- Previous psychiatric history, neglect, or mistreatment

are taking certain medications. Older clients should be taught measures that promote healthy skin, including adequate fluid intake and avoidance of skin and perfume products that contain alcohol. They should be instructed to use an emollient after bathing to help keep the skin soft and moist.

Older individuals use a wide range of services in an ever-changing health care arena. For acute or serious illnesses, they usually require inpatient hospitalization. LTC facilities provide elderly residents with skilled nursing services and rehabilitation as needed. With increasing numbers of older patients being discharged from hospitals after brief stays, the level of acuity in LTC facilities has increased dramatically. Box 13.9 lists factors to consider when selecting a nursing home. Nurses practicing in these settings now need to expand their understanding and knowledge of the more acutely ill elderly resident.

Other older individuals have opted for community-based services such as home care. The typical older home care client has multiple complex health care problems, challenging the skills of home care nurses. Today's home care nurse, in addition to possessing excellent clinical skills, must be a self-directed member of a multidisciplinary team. Assisted living is another type of community-based living arrangement. Assisted living is usually an apartment or condominium complex that provides supportive services to its residents. The aim is to assist the individual who wants to maintain his or her independence. The types of services that are included are those that assist persons with their activities of daily living in a homelike setting. This type of living arrangement is costly and appeals to individuals with upper-middle and upper incomes.

Hospice services provide support and nursing care in the home and inpatient settings to older people with terminal illnesses. Mental health services are offered in both the community and hospital settings. These services provide health care and help individuals to maintain psychological well-being. A variety of outpatient services are available to older adults, including senior centers, day care, and respite care for clients with Alzheimer's disease. Older people who are homebound can benefit from homemaker services and visiting nursing care.

There are a number of special health concerns and health-related issues for elderly people, including dementia, depression, and suicide. Government programs are available to assist and protect older people.

Special Health Concerns

Delirium
Delirium is an acute response in brain functioning. It manifests itself as an acute impairment in cognition and attention. Delirium can occur at any age, but it is common in older persons. Symptoms may vary in patients, but classic symptoms include disorientation, emotional lability, hallucinations, and delusions. Possible causes of delirium may be *systemic* (resulting from acute conditions that interfere with the brain's metabolic processes), *mechanical* (referring to a cause such as blockage or obstruction), or *psychosocial–environmental* (referring to external nonphysical causes that diminish personal meaning). Symptoms of delirium develop over several hours or days. There is usually a disturbance in the sleep–wake cycle and disturbances in psychomotor behavior including restlessness, hyperactivity or decreased activity, and emotional lability.

Dementia
Contrary to what was once thought, dementia is not inevitable or part of the normal aging process. Dementia refers to a loss of cognitive abilities. The symptoms of dementia—memory loss, disorientation, and confusion—may be caused by more than 70 different diseases. Alzheimer's disease is the leading cause of dementia and cognitive impairment affecting the older age group. There are other similar but treatable forms of dementia also characterized by loss of memory, disorientation, and poor social functioning. Among people 65 to 80, the incidence of dementia is 5% to 10%; for those

BOX 13.9 Factors to Consider in Selecting a Nursing Home

Costs: daily rate, insurance accepted, services available
Administration: ownership, accessibility of medical services
Philosophy of care: staff selection, accessibility of staff, approach to residents
Other services: speech therapy, physical therapy, social services, occupational therapy

HELPFUL HINTS

Determining Onset of Delirium
Ask the following two questions:
1. How long has this been going on?
2. How abruptly did it start?

older than 80, it is 20% to 40%. Of these cases, 10% to 20% are caused by drug toxicity. The age-related physiological changes affecting the liver and kidneys increase the incidence of drug toxicity. Drug metabolism and excretion slow with aging. A routine part of a complete geriatric physical examination should include an assessment of cognitive functioning. Many older individuals in early stages of dementia go undiagnosed because their social skills and behavior can obscure other losses. A mini-mental state examination (MMSE), or an abbreviated, portable examination, may be used to easily determine cognitive functioning. These examinations test memory, judgment, abstract thinking, attention, and calculation abilities. Care must be taken to provide an atmosphere that is quiet and conducive to producing valid test results. Baseline cognitive functioning is important to properly manage the care of the older individual. Refer to Box 13.10 for factors that distinguish dementia from delirium.

Depression and Suicide

Multiple losses, disease, and medication may lead to depression in the older age group. Again, stereotypical beliefs about older people often prevent families and health professionals from properly identifying depression in elderly persons. Symptoms include hopelessness and profound sadness. The use of support services may help cushion the many losses that are experienced at this age. Proper diagnosis and treatment of disease may help prevent depression in some cases. In chronic conditions with debilitation and unrelenting pain, depression is common. Some cases of depression are related to the medications that are prescribed for older people. *Polypharmacy*, or the use of multiple medications, can create pseudodepression. Reducing or eliminating the medication may help reverse the symptoms. Once it is diagnosed, depression often responds favorably to medication and other treatment modalities.

Untreated depression may lead to suicide. The incidence of suicide in elderly persons is rapidly increasing. Family members and caregivers must be alert to sudden changes in mood or other possible warning signs of suicide. See Chapter 10 for information on these signs.

Health Care Services

Social Security

The Social Security Act was established in 1935 as part of President Roosevelt's New Deal. The original intent of Social Security was to supplement income after retirement. The system is comprehensive and jointly administered by the state and federal governments. Funding for Social Security benefits comes from payroll taxes deducted from both employer and employee. At retirement, workers receive benefits equal to their contributions over their working years.

In 1939 the Social Security Act was strengthened to provide millions of older Americans with assistance and as a means toward a better standard of living. Benefits were recalculated based on average earnings over a shorter period rather than over a lifetime. Another amendment in 1950 provided benefits to surviving spouses and dependents. It later included government employees and self-employed workers, who were originally excluded. In 1957 disability insurance was set up to provide funds to workers older than age 50 who became disabled on the job. In 1960 this was expanded further to remove the age barrier and offer benefits to any disabled worker.

The Social Security Administration has tried to keep benefits at a level equal to inflation and rising health care costs. At this time benefit levels have increased faster than earning levels; therefore, the Social Security Administration has projected that at the present rate, funds may be depleted by the year 2015. This is the time when the baby boomers will become eligible for pensions.

Medicare and Medicaid

In the past, Medicare and Medicaid were the two programs that provided universal health care

---

BOX 13.10 Factors That Distinguish Dementia from Delirium

Dementia

- Gradual onset, cannot be dated
- Chronic, progressive over years
- Generally irreversible
- Disorientation later in illness
- Stable day-to-day
- Day/night reversal in a disturbed sleep–wake cycle
- Psychomotor changes late in disease

Delirium

- Abrupt, precise onset
- Acute illness precedes
- Usually reversible with prompt treatment
- Disorientation early
- Clouded, altered consciousness
- Disturbed sleep–wake cycle
- Marked psychomotor changes, either hypoactivity or hyperactivity

coverage to the older population. Today the Medicare and Medicaid plans have been rolled into the Affordable Care Act (ACA). The ACA is discussed further in Chapter 1.

Medicare is one of the most expensive federal programs. It is divided into four parts: Parts A through D. Part A is financed by mandatory contributions from both employer and employee and functions in a similar fashion to hospital insurance. Part B is a voluntary supplemental medical insurance financed by premiums and general revenues. Premiums are about $104.90 per month, and the deductible is $147.00 per year. Part B coverage pays for doctor fees and other services. Recipients must be 65 years of age or older or disabled and entitled to Social Security benefits.

Part C is the Medicare Advantage Plan, which is composed of a variety of health plans such as health maintenance organizations (HMOs) and preferred provider organizations (PPOs). Part D is the prescription drug program. It lowers the cost of prescription drugs for recipients. Individuals must be aware of the entry dates required for Part D; penalties are imposed for late enrollment. Private insurance companies now offer Medigap programs that cover charges not covered by Medicare, such as deductibles and copayments.

Medicaid comes under Title XIX of the Social Security Act and was first introduced in 1965. Today, Medicaid has been included in the ACA with the goal of reducing the number of uninsured. In 2010 the ACA expanded the minimum Medicaid eligibility to all individuals with incomes at or below 133% of the federal poverty level. States have the right to create their own basic health plan for uninsured individuals. Medicaid is still the main source of financing for long-term care.

Rights of Elderly People

In 1987 the federal Older Americans Act was passed. This act is designed to protect institutionalized elderly people by means of ombudsman programs. The ombudsman acts as a representative and spokesperson for older clients, making certain that their rights are protected.

In 1990 Congress passed the Patient Self-Determination Act, which was intended to ensure that patients' wishes would be followed if they were unable to speak for themselves. This is accomplished by using one of two types of advance directives: the living will and the health care proxy. Living wills are written when individuals are still competent and able to determine the type of future treatment they desire. The health care proxy, or durable power of attorney, designates someone to make decisions in the event that the person is unable to do so. See Appendix C for sample living will and health care proxy forms.

Do Not Resuscitate (DNR) orders can be written by a physician at a patient's or family's request. This document legally protects both doctors and health care workers in the event of a patient's sudden death. It is imperative that nurses become familiar with the laws in their states because states have varying laws regarding living wills, DNR orders, and other such advance directives.

Elderly persons have the right to look forward to successful aging. Successful aging can be defined as the ability to enjoy health of the mind and body through one's later years. A part of successful aging is the desire to live independently while remaining socially active and involved with family and friends. Although good health is not possible for all older individuals, optimism and a positive outlook may enhance an individual's ability to adapt to and cope with age-related changes.

SUMMARY

1. Old age is divided into three periods: young old (65 to 74 years), old (75 to 90 years), and very old (90 years and older).

2. Elderly people are the fastest-growing segment of the population in this country. Life expectancy is longer for women than for men. The most accurate predictor of life expectancy is the life span of one's biological parents.

3. Several theories attempt to explain aging. Biological theories include the clockwork, free-radical, wear-and-tear, immune-system-failure, and autoimmune theories.

4. Several psychosocial theories attempt to explain how aging affects socialization and life satisfaction. These include the disengagement, activity, and continuity-developmental theories.

5. Many physical changes occur as a part of the normal aging process.

6. Psychosocial tasks for old age include accepting and adjusting to changing body image, family roles, work and leisure patterns, and sexuality, and facing the inevitability of death.

7. According to Erikson, an older individual who has accomplished the first seven developmental tasks can now set out to achieve the task of ego integrity. People who lack ego integrity develop helplessness and despair.

8. Older people use the process of reminiscing, or life review, to help give meaning to their life and reinforce their feelings of worth.

9. Elderly people usually retain their cognitive abilities until late in life. Memory shows slight changes with advancing age. Older people tend to show greater losses in short-term than in long-term memory.

10. Moral beliefs develop from a lifetime of experiences and interactions with others. Many elders find peace and satisfaction through spirituality and religion.

11. Good nutrition has been shown to prevent late-life diseases and improve a person's response to treatment.

12. Older individuals need more rest and less sleep than do younger adults. Rest and sleep help to restore the body's energy reserve and prevent fatigue.

13. Exercise has been recognized as a means of maintaining physical fitness across the life span.

14. Older people are more likely to suffer from at least one chronic condition; many have multiple conditions.

15. The leading causes of death among elderly people are heart disease, cancer, stroke, arteriosclerosis, diabetes, lung disease, and cirrhosis of the liver.

16. The focus of health promotion and health maintenance is exercise, diet modification, and a healthy lifestyle.

17. Accidents can be prevented by recognizing the increased risk factors unique to this age group. Changes in sensory perceptions and gait and neurological disorders may increase the older person's risk for falls.

18. Crime toward and abuse of elderly people cross all social, cultural, and economic boundaries.

19. Social Security, Medicare, and Medicaid are programs that provide assistance to older people.

20. Depression and suicide among elderly persons may result from multiple losses, diseases, and medication usage.

CRITICAL THINKING

Alice Thompson, an 80-year-old woman, lives with her daughter and son-in-law. She is beginning her second week as a day-care client in an LTC facility. She has been very quiet and withdrawn since her arrival. Today she responds to your interaction by stating, "My daughter is not human." She asks you to promise to tell her daughter that she wants her Social Security check back.

1. What would be your first verbal response to this client?
2. Outline a planned intervention for Alice and her family.
3. Describe the function of life review.

MULTIPLE-CHOICE QUESTIONS

1. The majority of older Americans live in:
   a. Chronic LTC facilities
   b. Acute rehabilitation facilities
   c. Hospitals as patients
   d. Their own homes alone or with their families

2. The psychological theories of aging serve to explain:
   a. Physical changes of aging
   b. A person's life satisfaction
   c. Life expectancy
   d. Life span

3. Older people are at increased risk for falling because of:
   a. An accumulation of cerumen
   b. Postmenopausal symptoms
   c. A shift in the center of gravity
   d. Marked decrease in height

4. Falls in the older adult may contribute to: (Select all that apply)
   a. Permanent loss of function
   b. Sedentary behavior
   c. Poor quality of life
   d. Prolonged institutional care

5. As the older person loses adipose tissue:
   a. Muscle weight increases
   b. Memory loss increases
   c. Temperature control is difficult
   d. The biological clock speeds up

6. The characteristic hearing loss of old age means that the nurse must communicate in:
   a. Low, moderate tones
   b. High-frequency tones
   c. A soft whisper
   d. A loud shout

7. The following retirement phase is characterized by a feeling of euphoria:
   a. Remote
   b. Reorientation
   c. Stability
   d. Honeymoon

8. Which of the following statements about aging is correct?
   a. As individuals age, they are always ill.
   b. Most elderly are in nursing homes.
   c. Older people can learn new things.
   d. All older people become senile.

9. Dementia seen in the older adult:
   a. Is always irreversible
   b. Is a natural outcome of aging
   c. Is a symptom of an underlying disorder
   d. Is caused by Alzheimer's disease

10. Which of the following symptoms is characteristic of delirium?
    a. Onset over weeks
    b. Irreversible
    c. Chronic and progressive
    d. May result from acute illness

11. Older adults need a diet consisting of adequate proteins, carbohydrates, fats, fiber, and fluids. Following surgery the older adult requires greater amounts of _____ to help build and repair tissues.
    a. Carbohydrates
    b. Proteins
    c. Fats
    d. Fluids

12. Marital conflict, substance abuse, and financial difficulties may be contributing factors to:
    a. Unwanted pregnancy
    b. Family violence
    c. Disengagement
    d. Ageism

13. The _____ theory of aging suggests that one should remain involved in activities as long as possible.
    a. Disengagement
    b. Clockwork
    c. Wear-and-tear
    d. Activity

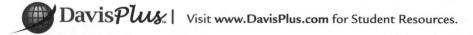 **DavisPlus** | Visit **www.DavisPlus.com** for Student Resources.

Student Activity

Visit a cemetery and examine your feelings about dying.

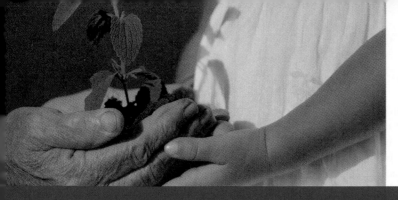

Chapter Outline

Learning Objectives

At the end of this chapter, you should be able to:

- Define key terms related to death and dying.
- Describe Kübler-Ross's stages of death and dying.
- List different types of losses.
- Describe the development of a concept of death.
- Contrast cultural aspects of death.
- Name signs of approaching death.
- Describe ethical concerns regarding end-of-life issues.

DEATH AS A PART OF LIFE

The journey of life can be predictable in stages for various ages but unpredictable in overall length. Death is the inevitable fate of all living creatures. The concept of death may give meaning and purpose to life. Death and loss are very personal issues, and individual responses to it vary. Loss is an encounter that one faces during the course of his or her life. Loss challenges the person's priorities and importance of relationships. A significant loss may influence the need for change and adaptation. Coping is a complex process that involves an individual's self-identity. How an individual copes depends on his or her manner of dealing with previous losses. The person's coping mechanism will in turn affect how that individual overcomes future losses in his or her lifetime. Ideally, a loss will result in a greater appreciation of life and its fragility.

Death can occur at any age. Sudden, unexpected death at any age creates unique issues in addition to those normally surrounding death. The loss of a loved one of any age is traumatic. Grief is the feeling tone or the outward expression in response to a loss. Typically, individuals experience grief in response to a death. The grief reaction to loss is a painful process. Some researchers refer to what is called anticipatory grief. Anticipatory grief is a reaction to an expected loss, such as in terminal illness. Family members become aware that their loved one is dying and they experience a sense of loss before the death occurs. Anticipatory grief may permit family members to express feelings, complete unfinished business with the dying person, and begin dealing with the inevitable loss. Grief responses may be considered adaptive or healthy in that they run over a predictable course of time and they are self-limiting and result in a healthy resolution. Maladaptive grief responses usually exhibit an exaggerated, lengthy, unpredictable course that results in unresolved conflicts. No individual should deny or ignore his or her need for emotional support during the grieving process. Professional help is available and recommended to ease the pain and suffering associated with loss. Mourning is the natural process that one goes through following a major loss. Mourning is personal and facilitates adjustment to the loss. The course of mourning may be short or long, ranging from months to years. The outcome is resumption of normal life. Individual grief varies in intensity. Some individuals experience anger, guilt, anxiety, depression, preoccupation with thoughts, and somatic complaints. Others may experience insomnia. Grief is considered a healthy, normal response of a person to a loss. A delayed, prolonged grief period beyond the usual length of time can indicate pathological reactions and require interventions. Bereavement is a state of having sustained a loss.

Grief encompasses many reactions, including emotional, cognitive, and restorative responses. Emotional responses to grief include numbness, sadness, crying, loneliness, anxiety, and depression. Individuals may overeat or undereat, or become hyperactive or socially withdrawn. Many individuals experience a variety of somatic responses including dry mouth, tightness in the throat, and abdominal complaints that may lead to weakness and fatigue. The typical cognitive responses to grief and loss are usually denial, disbelief, and anger. Dreams and thoughts of the deceased are common during the grieving process. Restorative responses follow after a period of contemplation and resolution. Individuals describe having thoughts of the past, with their associated feelings of pleasure. They once again develop an interest in activities. At this stage new relationships may develop. New roles are tried and bring about new priorities and goals.

THEORIES OF LOSS AND GRIEF

Elisabeth Kübler-Ross's Stages

Elisabeth Kübler-Ross was the first physician to identify five distinct stages of death and dying that patients and their families go through. The patient and the family may go through the stages in any order and not necessarily at the same time. The order of these five stages of dying is based on a person's individuality, cultural influences, and length of illness.

Stage 1: Denial
Denial occurs when the patient or family member believes that the doctor has made a mistake in the diagnosis and that death will not occur. Denial may occur in cases of unexpected death with the surviving family and friends left in shock and disbelief. Denial allows individuals time to deal with the full implication of the prognosis or the death.

Stage 2: Anger
Anger occurs when the individual internalizes the truth of the impending death. This anger may be

turned inward or displaced by the person and family toward the physician, nurse, or even God. The health care worker must be able to interact in a supportive manner when anger is directed toward him or her. The family can also direct anger toward their dying loved one, blaming the dying person for leaving. Children may feel abandoned by their loss and may blame themselves for the death of a loved one.

Stage 3: Bargaining

When the patient or family member knows that death is inevitable, he or she may try to get more time by striking a bargain with God. Usually the bargain is for a few extra months or one more year to see a task through.

Stage 4: Depression

Depression is a feeling of sadness or loneliness experienced when the person knows that he or she cannot change the outcome. The person is often withdrawn and quiet.

Stage 5: Acceptance

Acceptance is ownership of the inevitability of death by the patient or family. Accepting individuals are able to work through unresolved feelings and problems together. All personal business is put in order. Final good-byes are said.

John Bowlby's Stages of Separation

John Bowlby also studied reactions to attachment and loss. Bowlby studied the child's reaction to separation from his or her mother, and noted similarities between this reaction and patterns of adult grief. In Bowlby's description, the initial reaction by the child to separation is *Protest*. In this stage the child is upset and crying and reacting to the loss. This stage of protest can be seen in the adult's first response to a significant loss. Bowlby described stage two as *Despair*. Children are quiet, sad, and subdued. They show little interest in their environment and often refuse food and lose weight. These are similar to characteristics of individuals after losing a loved one. The final stage is *Detachment*. During this stage the child appears disinterested in the mother when she returns. The child's remote responses indicate his or her attempt to reorganize and resign to the loss.

Bowlby developed a theory of mourning using his theory of attachment as a foundation and backdrop. In the first of his four phases of mourning, the individual passes through a numbing stage. This serves as a protective mechanism, allowing the individual time to mobilize his or her strength to deal with the loss. Following this phase is a painful stage in which the individual faces the magnitude of the loss. During this stage the person feel a tremendous longing for the deceased. The third phase is one of disorganization and despair. Often individuals feel anger over their loss and search for answers to why this has happened to them. Last, persons having experienced a significant loss will need to reorganize, adapt to new roles, and revise priorities. This reorganization stage is the final stage and requires support and encouragement from friends and family.

TYPES OF LOSSES

Some losses are predictable and universal, whereas others are unexpected. Losses may occur at all stages of development. Many losses are classified as *physical losses* in that they are readily evident and visible. Death of a spouse, parent, child, or other close person represents this type of loss. Other losses are less apparent to the outside world, and they are known as *symbolic losses*. These losses may be the loss of work or status or change in roles such as in divorce or desertion. All losses create a grief response.

Loss of a Spouse

Loss of a spouse is considered a loss of great magnitude. The surviving spouse must deal with loneliness and changing roles. Studies have shown that there is great risk of death of the remaining husband or wife, especially in the first two years after the loss. Some researchers have noted a difference in the way men and women react to becoming a widow or widower. Men seem to react to the loss of their wife by feeling alone and believing they have lost a part of themselves. Women, however, react with feelings of being abandoned, deserted, and left to carry on by themselves. The age of the surviving spouse plays an important part in the way the person reacts to and deals with the loss. For men, widowhood often occurs late in life, whereas women often experience it at a much younger age. Age may influence the person's adjustment to his or her new role.

Loss of a Parent

Loss of a parent at any age is difficult. For children the meaning of this loss depends on their stage of development chronologically, developmentally, and cognitively. Children should be encouraged to openly express their fears, worries, and feelings. Young children may be better able to act out their feelings during play sessions. They need to be reassured that they will be loved and taken care of and that they are not alone. Older children need to feel loved, supported, and accepted. Questions should be answered honestly at their level of comprehension. Loss of a parent during the adult years may be somewhat anticipated and natural but nonetheless very difficult to bear. Parents are the individual's source of unconditional love and support. The death of a parent ends this support and brings the need for a change in roles. The adult child may now be needed to look after the surviving parent. Families should seek out support groups for added support and comfort at these difficult times.

Loss of a Child

Loss of a child is thought to be one of the most difficult losses to comprehend and accept. We naturally think that our children will outlive us in a long and healthy life. When a child dies either from an accident or because of an illness, parents and family members are left with insurmountable feelings of despair, disbelief, and anger. Often parents will express a need to blame someone or something when death is the result of an accident. Casting blame in a way helps the person gain some control over the senseless loss.

Loss of an Unborn Child

Another significant kind of loss is the death of an unborn child. Parents and their families experience significant trauma and grief following a fetal death or stillbirth. Regardless of how long the pregnancy lasted, there is an enormous sense of loss and disappointment. When the death occurs close to term, it is important for staff to allow the parents the opportunity to see and possibly hold their child. The parents first should be told what to expect in terms of the child's appearance, color, and temperature. The baby can be wrapped in warm blankets and brought to the parents. Nursing staff should be sensitive to whether the parents would like to be alone with their baby or prefer the staff to stay with them while they say their good-byes. Parents have said that even seeing an infant's deformity was not as bad as what they had imagined. Some parents who experienced a loss during childbirth later expressed that they believed that maybe their child had really

survived. Allowing them to see and hold their baby may help them begin the grieving process.

Loss of a Sibling

The death of a sibling causes great pain and sorrow at any age and stage. When the death is a child, other siblings find it hard to bear and sometimes blame themselves. Surviving children have to learn to deal with their parents' reactions and mourning as well as their own grief. Death of an adult sibling creates a void and a break in the family chain. Whether the death is a result of illness, accident, or a disaster, survivors try to make some sense of it. There is an effort to attempt to put the loss into perspective that can be understood and eventually accepted. With the loss of a loved one, there is an inevitable family reorganization and adjustment.

Facing One's Own Death

Facing one's death occurs in terminal illness. Regardless of what the person has been told, he or she is aware of impending death. Age, religion, culture, support of family and friends, and personal beliefs affect the way a person accepts death. Having family and close friends near helps decrease the loneliness that otherwise might occur.

Older individuals think about the inevitability of death, and some make necessary preparations. Allowing persons to discuss their wishes for their funeral, burial, and disposition of their possessions gives control and comfort to the individuals involved. Families and friends should encourage open communication and discussion of end-of-life concerns and preferences.

DEVELOPMENT OF A CONCEPT OF DEATH

Children's understanding of death is related to their age and developmental and cognitive stage. The infant has no concept of death. Gradually, young toddlers become aware of themselves as separate persons apart from their mother. Toddlers' main concern is separation anxiety. Death to them means "less alive." By preschool, children are concerned with getting hurt and the pain related to injuries or illness. This age group expresses fear about going to the doctor and getting shots or having pain. They frequently ask, "Is it going to hurt?" By age 5 or 6 years, children seem concerned about punishment for wrongdoings. They have seen death portrayed on television and in the movies, and some have already experienced loss in their family. They have a vivid imagination and often dream about or become frightened by what they have seen or believe to be true or possible. School-aged children have the capacity to understand the finality of death (Fig. 14.1). They often associate death with an accident, illness, or old age. Children living in violence-prone areas may be introduced to death at an early age. With the ever-increasing number of guns, drugs, and gangs, some children see shootings, stabbings, and violence as everyday occurrences.

Adolescent teens see death as final and understand rituals and customs. Death is seen as a distant possibility for adolescents because they believe they are invincible and hearty. When death happens to a friend or person of their age, the teen is shocked and angry. Death is a deterrent to achieving goals. Teens usually struggle with finding the meaning of life and their purpose in society. Adults view death according to their perspective on life.

In early adulthood, individuals are determining their goals and aspirations. Their focus is placed on starting a family, raising children, and advancing their education and career. Planning for the future, although distant, begins during this stage. Concerns about their own mortality surface periodically when someone their age dies suddenly or someone becomes gravely ill.

Middle-aged adults focus on physical changes and losses that they begin to experience. These losses challenge the middle-aged adult to think about his or her own mortality. The death of a parent forces the surviving child to reevaluate his or her priorities and values. Death and losses create the need for change and adaptation. The outcome may eventually be positive in that the person develops a keen appreciation for and satisfaction with life.

Older adults may realize that they will die in the near future and prepare by talking about death and their final wishes and by completing their life review. In doing so, individuals can move on with a sense of peace and comfort.

CULTURAL AND RELIGIOUS DIFFERENCES

Culture, as defined in Chapter 2, refers to all the learned patterns of behavior that are passed on through generations. Religion is a formal system of beliefs and practices. Cultural patterns or traits and religion largely direct individuals through key life events including birth, marriage, and death. These rituals help persons to know what to do at specific times and events. This guidance also helps families respond and function at the time of death and loss of a loved one. Health care professionals can better meet the needs of patients and their families by increasing their knowledge and understanding of people from different cultures. Greater knowledge will lead to an improved quality of health care.

Christianity is a broad term that encompasses several religions, including Catholicism, Protestantism, and Eastern Orthodoxy, among others. The U.S. population also includes persons of numerous

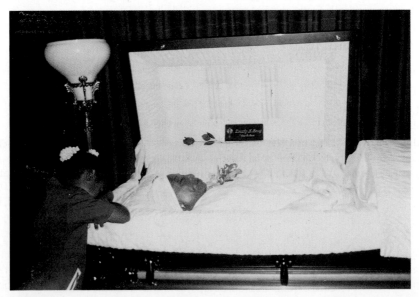

FIGURE 14.1 Loss is painful at all stages.

non-Christian religious faiths. The following sections list beliefs and traditions from some of these religions and their denominations as they relate to death and dying. This information is further summarized in Table 14.1.

Catholicism

Catholics believe in death, burial, resurrection, and an eternal future for body and soul. Priests, nuns, or church members administer rituals to the sick and dying. These prayer rituals continue through death and mourning and for several days after. The purposes of these rituals are to provide absolution for the soul and to console family members and help them cope with separation in the company of family and friends. The dying person must first make a confession to help the soul qualify for departure. Next, the person receives the Holy Eucharist to prepare for the passage to eternal joy. Last, the sacrament of the anointing of the sick is administered to those who are gravely ill or dying or undergoing major surgery. The purpose is for recovery or spiritual strength. This may be repeated as often as necessary. At the time of death the deceased body is treated with dignity and reverence. The body is cleansed and prepared for viewing, eulogizing, and burial. Church

teachings require a special service (Mass of the Resurrection) where Christ's life is remembered and related to the deceased. This is followed by entombment in a Catholic cemetery, where the body returns to the earth. Cremation is acceptable but must be quickly followed by entombment of the ashes or burial at sea. The ashes cannot be scattered or kept in the home. Mourning continues after burial through nonreligious services such as wakes.

Protestantism

The Protestant religion is divided into several denominations and is similar to the Catholic religion in that Protestants believe in laying the body to rest in the hope for resurrection and eternal life. In some of these denominations death is not natural but a punishment for one's sins. In others, at the time of death the spirit and body separate and go to judgment. In this instance one's life experiences determine whether one goes to heaven or to hell. Prayer vigils by clergy or members of the congregation are kept during illness and death. At the time of death the body is treated with reverence. Cleansing is necessary to prepare the body for viewing, funeral service, burial, or cremation. The last viewing of the body occurs before the funeral service is performed

TABLE

14.1   Religious Beliefs and Practices Related to Death and Dying

Religion	Beliefs and Practices Related to Death and Dying
Catholicism	Priest offers the anointing of the sick.
Protestantism	Prayer vigils by clergy or members of the congregation are kept during illness and death. Some give last rites.
Jehovah's Witnesses	At death the soul is believed to die. Last rites are not given.
Christian Science	Visit from the Christian Science reader. No last rites are performed and autopsies are forbidden.
Seventh-Day Adventist	No specific practices related to death. Person treated with dignity.
Eastern Orthodox	Last rites are given to raise hope and courage and offer peace to the sick and dying.
Hinduism	Visit by priest, family cleanses body after death, and cremation is accepted.
Buddhism	At death the body is left undisturbed for 8 hours. The body is cleansed, then dressed in new clothing and jewelry. Cremation usually takes place within 7 days after death.
Islam	At death family members wash the body; the eyes are closed, and the body is wrapped in a clean white sheet. Prayer continues to the burial.
Judaism	Presence of rabbi desired; autopsy and cremation are forbidden.

(Fig. 14.2). After the funeral service, the casket is closed and mourners may pray at the burial site or throw earth or flowers on the coffin. A ceremonial feast after the burial is a tradition for many of these denominations and may take place in the home of the deceased, a family members' residence, a church hall, or a restaurant, where family and friends come together to share memories and anecdotes about the deceased's life.

Jehovah's Witnesses

Jehovah's Witnesses believe that God and his son will keep one free of sickness and disease and that the dead will reunite here on earth under more peaceful, righteous conditions. This denomination interprets the Bible as the true readings from God and takes from these readings the return of Christ's reign on earth. This return is anticipated after the final battle on earth. This final battle is called The Armageddon, which is believed to be imminent. At the time of death Jehovah's Witnesses do not believe in last rites or sacraments. At death the soul is believed to die. Grief is accepted, and it is believed that God is near to those who are broken or crushed.

Christian Science

Christian Science believes in the power of prayer and counsel for ill persons. Members of this denomination believe in the birth of Christ, the crucifixion, the resurrection of the body, and the ascension. In this divine science the universe, including man, is spiritual, harmonious, and eternal. God is life. Sin, sickness, and death can be overcome by understanding and applying God's divine teachings. Healing is possible through the power of prayer. Death is not seen as a spiritual reality but as a changed state.

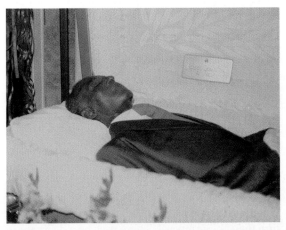

FIGURE 14.2 Customs and rituals surrounding death vary.

Christian Scientists believe that there is no death in God. This oneness with God and reliance on spiritual healing make it unlikely that patients who are terminally ill will seek medical intervention or means to prolong life. At the time of death there are no last rites performed, and autopsies are forbidden.

Seventh-Day Adventists

Followers of the Seventh-Day Adventist denomination believe in a Christian life of love and unity with Christ as the head of the church. One must first repent and live in faith and obedience to God's commandments, and one's name will be written in the good book of life. Health is important to the holiness of one's body. Belief in the purity of the human body leads many followers to become vegetarians. The seventh day of Yah, the Sabbath, is a day of spiritual rest. This begins Friday sundown and continues until Saturday sundown. Judgment of the dead is ongoing, with the belief that one will reap what one sows. Followers live an orderly life as they await the second coming of Christ. Medical treatment and other support are accepted.

Eastern Orthodoxy

The Orthodox Church dates back to the time of the apostles, when the Christian message was first carried to Greece. Orthodoxy is the predominant form of worship today in Greece, Russia, and parts of Western Europe and Asia. Followers see God as the creator with ultimate power over life and death. They believe in the unity of body and soul. In early times, physicians practiced medicine in addition to a healing ministry. Church clergy may marry and offer communion to infants. Redemption is obtained through baptism and the sacraments. Members of the church take part in various rituals of fasting and feast to commemorate the saints. The sacrament of Holy Unction is offered to the sick and dying for the ultimate pardon in the face of death.

Hinduism

The Hindu religion believes death is a natural part of living and the cyclic reincarnation of one's soul. The ultimate goal is to transcend the need for reincarnation. Many rituals are directed to help the soul transcend and eliminate the need for rebirth. Rebirth is based on past thoughts and actions. At death the body is washed, dressed, adorned, and made ready for cremation. Prayers and chanting go on as the body is carried to the cremation site and continue for several days to satisfy the deceased soul and ensure its voyage to the other world. Hindu teachings state that the soul is released to the heavens on the 11th day after death and that it reaches its destination and is joined with its ancestors on the 12th day. Special offerings are necessary on these two days to help the departed soul. Cremation releases the soul from its earlier existence, and at burial there is a call for the ashes to be thrown in the Ganges, the holy river in India, or to be placed in a nearby flowing river or ocean. The chief mourner is usually the one to light the pyre.

Buddhism

The Buddhist religion has a deep belief in impermanence, meaning life is concurrent with dying. One must accept impermanence to prepare for and reach the ultimate state of transcendence or rebirth. To transcend, one must accumulate merits through one's daily selfless acts. Dying is a gradual process where there is a separation of the two factors of human life—consciousness and warmth. In death, consciousness separates and the body becomes cold; at that time, the person begins a journey to the beginning of a new life. Professionals or voluntary groups conduct rituals; the objective of these rituals is elevation of one's soul and gaining merits toward the new life. Rituals that elevate one's soul include chanting, prostration, lighting of candles, and consumption of food and drinks. Rituals that promote merit include contributions to worthwhile causes.

The dying person must be in a comfortable environment. Chanting can be done in person or via a recording. After death the body is left undisturbed for 8 hours until it is cold. After this period the body is cleansed and dressed in new clothing and jewelry. Cremation usually takes place within 7 days after death. At the deceased's home, an altar is set up to represent the consciousness, with the deceased's picture and name written on a sheet of paper. There are offerings of food, incense, and candles that will burn for 49 days. During this period friends will show their respect and support.

Islam

According to Islam, death is seen as a departure from this world to eternal life. At the time of death the family provides physical and spiritual comfort. The dying person, aided by family members, must recite verses from the holy Quran as a reminder of God's mercy and forgiveness. The Muslim's last word must be the declaration of faith to Allah. At death, family members wash the body, the eyes are closed, and the body is wrapped in a clean white sheet. Prayer continues into the burial, which is usually quick to prevent the need for embalming. Autopsy can be performed only if necessary. The objective is to make certain that there is as little disturbance of the body as possible. Men usually accompany the body at the graveside, where the deceased is laid in the grave on the right side. The mourning period for families is usually 3 days, but for the spouse mourning can be extended from 10 days to 4 months.

Judaism

Jewish law is known as Torah. The degree to which one practices the customs and rituals depends on one's following: orthodox, conservative, or reform. According to Torah, Friday sunset to Saturday sunset is to be celebrated as the Sabbath, a day of rest. Orthodox Jews strictly observe the Sabbath by not using any appliances or turning on or off light switches. Some Jews will eat only kosher foods that have been prepared under strict guidelines. These guidelines include the method of slaughtering the animals and the separation of dairy and meat. Included in these dietary restrictions is the avoidance of shellfish and pork. During the Passover holiday, leavened bread is omitted from the diet. Jewish laws advocate that everything must be done to prolong life. Strict observers believe that the dying person should never be left alone. The presence of a rabbi is desired. Following the death of an immediate family member, family members cut a garment or black ribbon and wear it, symbolizing that the person has been torn away from one's heart. Autopsy and cremation are forbidden by the Orthodox. Close observers hold the funeral the day after death. At the gravesite, family members may place some earth into the grave, symbolizing the finality of the death. They also say a mourner's prayer known as the Mourner's Kaddish. Mourning begins with the funeral and lasts for 7 days. This period is known as *shivah*. Mourning continues for 30 days.

SIGNS OF APPROACHING DEATH

No one can accurately predict the time of death. There are, however, signs that an individual is weakening and near death. Some persons begin to withdraw from what is going on around them. They turn their focus inward. There may be a decrease in senses, although hearing is said to remain until death. Some are quiet and still, whereas others are restless and agitated. Breathing patterns change. Respiratory rates may become irregular with periods of apnea, referred to as **Cheyne-Stokes respirations.** Vital signs change, with blood pressure dropping and pulse slowing down. Bowel and bladder control weakens. The person's level of consciousness changes, making him or her less alert and aware. As death approaches there may be a loss of heat, producing a cool sensation to the body. Spiritual needs may take on new importance. Family and friends may be a real source of comfort to the dying person even if there is little acknowledgment of their presence. Family members need assistance and support in dealing with the approaching death of a loved one. Refer to Box 14.1 for help in communicating with family members. Individuals suffering a significant loss can be assisted by following the recommendations listed in Box 14.2.

END-OF-LIFE ISSUES

An **advance directive** is a legal document that states the person's wishes for medical treatment in the event that he or she cannot make these decisions. Health care facilities must inform individuals of their right to have this legal protection on admission. In 1991 the federal government passed the **Patient Self-Determination Act** (PSDA). According to this law a patient has the right to have

---

BOX 14.1   Help in Communicating With Family Members

Remember:
Ask open-ended questions.
Be nonjudgmental.

Ask:
What are your concerns?

Determine:
What is important for them at this time?

Always:
Ensure privacy.

Attempt to:
Determine level of knowledge.
Support and acknowledge feelings.

Don't:
Use clichés, such as "He is better off."

BOX 14.2   Ways to Survive a Loss

- **Accept** the help of people—surround yourself with family and friends. Join support groups to share with others who have had similar losses.
- **Be open** with feelings. Do not keep feelings and emotions bottled up. Express your feelings.
- **Do not** neglect your health. Be aware of changes in mood and sleeping and eating patterns.
- **Avoid** major life changes. Postpone making decisions related to moving, remarrying, or changing jobs. Attempt to adjust to loss before making major changes.
- **Be good** to yourself. Plan pleasant activities and recognize that it is OK to feel happy.
- **Seek** professional help if needed.

---

advance directives in place. Failure of an institution to inform a person of this right will result in withholding reimbursement of funding to the institution.

A **living will** is a form of advance directive that states the wishes of a person regarding life-sustaining treatment in case of serious illness. This legal document is available throughout the United States. Each state may have slight differences in format or content. Some individuals decide to use a document called a **durable power of attorney for health care** to appoint someone to make their wishes known and carry out some decisions regarding their medical care in the event that they can no longer express themselves. On admission to a health care facility, patients are asked if they wish to sign a **Do Not Resuscitate** (DNR) order. This order should guide health care workers with regard to the wishes of patients should they go into cardiac or respiratory arrest. See Appendix C for a sample living will and health care proxy forms.

Ethical decisions often surface and present challenges for patients and families. Frequently, surviving family members are asked to consider donating the organs of their recently deceased relative. Health care professionals must use extreme tact and care in approaching family members with such a request. The decision ultimately rests with the family and may represent the patient's wishes, if known, or surviving family members' beliefs. At no time should the family be pressured or judged for their decisions.

Several of the following concepts are controversial and evoke many reactions because they touch on culture, religion, and ethical values. **Euthanasia** (or assisted suicide), known as "mercy killing" in the past, refers to the deliberate ending of one's life and the withholding of treatment. Assisted suicide is currently legal in the states of Oregon, Washington, and Vermont but is illegal throughout the rest of the United States. This ethical issue continues to be actively debated. **Right to die** proponents believe that persons have the right to refuse medical treatment even though it may result in death. Health care professionals who support the right to die are not doing so to cause death but because they do not wish to prolong life in every case. **Palliative care** is another form of helping to relieve the suffering of the terminally ill. Although this process may shorten the individual's life, it is said not to be the intention of this care method. **Hospice care** provides care for the terminally ill in the comfort of their home or in a hospice designated unit. Hospice emphasizes comfort rather than curative measures. The dying process is viewed as a natural process with the emphasis on meeting physical, psychological, spiritual, and family needs. Hospice care is provided by a number of different disciplines, including nursing, social work, physical therapy, and clergy if desired. The patient determines his or her needs in each of these areas. Following the death, hospice offers bereavement counseling for family members for 13 months. During this period, family may receive individual or group counseling at no cost. Hospice care is now covered under the Affordable Care Act. Box 14.3 lists the requirements for hospice care.

B O X
14.3   Requirements for Hospice Care

- Less than 6 months life expectancy
- Available primary caregiver
- Patient elects hospice care
- Physician supports hospice care
- Established palliative care plan

Each individual has the right to be fully informed of his or her condition and the benefits and risks of all of the possible treatments. Families should plan for opportunities to openly discuss a person's concerns and wishes. Each individual and his or her family then must make the decision that best suits their needs. As heartbreaking as terminal illness is, it is awful for everyone concerned to fight over treatment options instead of offering comfort and support to each other.

H E L P F U L   H I N T S

Do not underestimate the importance of giving of one's self.
Remain with the dying person.
Silence can be comforting when all is said and done.
Your presence can say that you care.

SUMMARY

1. Death is the inevitable fate of all living creatures.

2. Death and loss are personal issues.

3. Loss is an encounter that one faces during the course of one's life.

4. Death can occur at any age.

5. Grief is the feeling tone or outward expression in response to a loss.

6. Mourning is the natural process that one goes through following a major loss.

7. Bereavement is a state of having sustained a loss.

8. Grief encompasses emotional, cognitive, and restorative responses.

9. Emotional responses to grief include numbness, sadness, crying, loneliness, anxiety, and depression.

10. Elisabeth Kübler-Ross first identified the five stages of loss and dying.

11. John Bowlby studied children and their reactions to loss and separation, and these reactions may be similar to adult grief patterns.

12. The concept of death varies with the age and stage of development.

13. Culture and religion serve to guide and direct individuals and families through a loss.

14. Many physical and social changes are witnessed before death.

15. Advance directives legally state the person's wishes in the event that he or she cannot make health care decisions.

16. A living will is a form of an advance directive that spells out the individual's wishes for life-sustaining treatment.

17. A durable power of attorney for health care may be used to give another person the power to carry out one's wishes in the event of illness.

18. A Do Not Resuscitate (DNR) order is a legal form that directs caregivers in the event of cardiac or respiratory arrest.

19. Euthanasia refers to the deliberate ending of one's treatment or life.

20. Palliative care is an approach to care that helps relieve suffering in the terminally ill.

21. Hospice care uses many disciplines to provide comfort and a peaceful death in the home or in a hospice unit.

CRITICAL THINKING

Exercise #1

Seven-year-old Timothy has just found out that his grandfather has died. His parents and immediate family are all very sad and busy making arrangements. Timothy was very close to his grandfather and spent time with him after school. Later that day his parents are uncertain if Timothy should be present at the funeral.

1. How should Timothy's parents handle their child's response to his grandfather's death?
2. Should Timothy be present at the funeral? Explain your answer.

Exercise #2

List five suggestions that help to bring solace and peace to family members of a dying loved one:

1.
2.
3.
4.
5.

Exercise #3

An 85-year old Chinese woman has been admitted to your long-term care facility. After 3 weeks, the nurse notes that she rarely touches the food on her tray and relies on her family for food from home. She doesn't participate or socialize with other residents despite their attempts to get to know her. The nurse also notices that she refuses to drink her bedside water. How would you interpret her behavior and what changes would you institute?

MULTIPLE-CHOICE QUESTIONS

1. The feeling tone or emotional reaction to a death is known as:
   a. Bereavement
   b. Grief
   c. Mourning
   d. Loss

2. According to Kübler-Ross, the last stage of dying is:
   a. Denial
   b. Anger
   c. Bargaining
   d. Acceptance

3. Which of the following age groups has a concept of death's finality?
   a. Toddlers
   b. Preschool
   c. Infants
   d. School age

4. Which one of the following groups does not believe in autopsy?
   a. Roman Catholic
   b. Islam
   c. Protestant
   d. Orthodox Judaism

5. Which of the following may be seen as a sign of approaching death?
   a. Rapid pulse
   b. Loss of hearing
   c. Irregular breathing with periods of apnea
   d. Anxiety

6. The focus of hospice care is on:
   a. Curative measures
   b. Experimental treatment
   c. Drug trial and error
   d. Promoting comfort

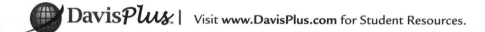 **DavisPlus** | Visit **www.DavisPlus.com** for Student Resources.

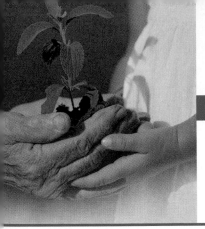

Community Help Services

Abuse Hotline
(800) 604-2923
Affordable Care Act (ACA)
Healthcare.gov

Alcoholics Anonymous
www.aa.org

American Association of Retired Persons (AARP)
www.aarp.org

American Heart Association
www.americanheart.org

Child Help USA Inc.
(800) 4-A-CHILD
www.childhelp.org

Meals on Wheels Foundation
www.meals-on-wheels.org

National Adoption Center
www.adopt.org

National Committee for the Prevention of Elder Abuse
www.preventelderabuse.org

National Council on Alcoholism and Drug Dependence
www.ncadd.org

National Domestic Violence Hotline
www.ndvh.org

National Institute on Aging
www.nia.org

Planned Parenthood Federation of America
www.plannedparenthood.org

Prevent Child Abuse NY and **1-800 Children**
www.preventchildabuseny.org

U.S. Centers for Disease Control and Prevention
CDC.gov

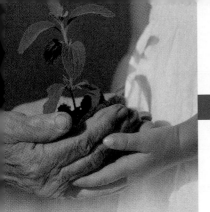

Recommendations for Health Promotion

Figure 1. Recommended immunization schedule for persons aged 0 through 18 years – United States, 2014.

(FOR THOSE WHO FALL BEHIND OR START LATE, SEE THE CATCH-UP SCHEDULE [FIGURE 2]).

These recommendations must be read with the footnotes that follow. For those who fall behind or start late, provide catch-up vaccination at the earliest opportunity as indicated by the green bars in Figure 1. To determine minimum intervals between doses, see the catch-up schedule (Figure 2). School entry and adolescent vaccine age groups are in bold.

Vaccine	Birth	1 mo	2 mos	4 mos	6 mos	9 mos	12 mos	15 mos	18 mos	19–23 mos	2–3 yrs	4–6 yrs	7–10 yrs	11–12 yrs	13–15 yrs	16–18 yrs
Hepatitis B[1] (HepB)	1st dose	←——2nd dose——→			3rd dose											
Rotavirus[2] (RV) RV1 (2-dose series); RV5 (3-dose series)			1st dose	2nd dose	See footnote 2											
Diphtheria, tetanus, & acellular pertussis[3] (DTaP: <7 yrs)			1st dose	2nd dose	3rd dose		←——4th dose——→					5th dose				
Tetanus, diphtheria, & acellular pertussis[4] (Tdap: ≥7 yrs)														(Tdap)		
Haemophilus influenzae type b[5] (Hib)			1st dose	2nd dose	See footnote 5		←—3rd or 4th dose, See footnote 5—→									
Pneumococcal conjugate[6] (PCV13)			1st dose	2nd dose	3rd dose		←——4th dose——→									
Pneumococcal polysaccharide[6] (PPSV23)																
Inactivated poliovirus[7] (IPV) (<18 yrs)			1st dose	2nd dose	←——3rd dose——→							4th dose				
Influenza[8] (IIV; LAIV) 2 doses for some: See footnote 8					Annual vaccination (IIV only)							Annual vaccination (IIV or LAIV)				
Measles, mumps, rubella[9] (MMR)							←—1st dose—→					2nd dose				
Varicella[10] (VAR)							←—1st dose—→					2nd dose				
Hepatitis A[11] (HepA)							←——2-dose series, See footnote 11——→									
Human papillomavirus[12] (HPV2: females only; HPV4: males and females)														(3-dose series)		
Meningococcal[13] (Hib-MenCY ≥ 6 weeks; MenACWY-D ≥9 mos; MenACWY-CRM ≥ 2 mos)							See footnote 13							1st dose		Booster

Legend:
- Range of recommended ages for all children
- Range of recommended ages for catch-up immunization
- Range of recommended ages for certain high-risk groups
- Range of recommended ages during which catch-up is encouraged and for certain high-risk groups
- Not routinely recommended

This schedule includes recommendations in effect as of January 1, 2014. Any dose not administered at the recommended age should be administered at a subsequent visit, when indicated and feasible. The use of a combination vaccine generally is preferred over separate injections of its equivalent component vaccines. Vaccination providers should consult the relevant Advisory Committee on Immunization Practices (ACIP) statement for detailed recommendations, available online at http://www.cdc.gov/vaccines/hcp/acip-recs/index.html. Clinically significant adverse events that follow vaccination should be reported to the Vaccine Adverse Event Reporting System (VAERS) online (http://www.vaers.hhs.gov) or by telephone (800-822-7967). Suspected cases of vaccine-preventable diseases should be reported to the state or local health department. Additional information, including precautions and contraindications for vaccination, is available from CDC online (http://www.cdc.gov/vaccines/recs/vac-admin/contraindications.htm) or by telephone (800-CDC-INFO [800-232-4636]).

This schedule is approved by the Advisory Committee on Immunization Practices (http://www.cdc.gov/vaccines/acip), the American Academy of Pediatrics (http://www.aap.org), the American Academy of Family Physicians (http://www.aafp.org), and the American College of Obstetricians and Gynecologists (http://www.acog.org).

NOTE: The above recommendations must be read along with the footnotes of this schedule.

FIGURE 2. Catch-up immunization schedule for persons aged 4 months through 18 years who start late or who are more than 1 month behind —United States, 2014.

The figure below provides catch-up schedules and minimum intervals between doses for children whose vaccinations have been delayed. A vaccine series does not need to be restarted, regardless of the time that has elapsed between doses. Use the section appropriate for the child's age. Always use this table in conjunction with Figure 1 and the footnotes that follow.

Vaccine	Minimum Age for Dose 1	Minimum Interval Between Doses			
		Dose 1 to dose 2	Dose 2 to dose 3	Dose 3 to dose 4	Dose 4 to dose 5
Persons aged 4 months through 6 years					
Hepatitis B[1]	Birth	4 weeks	8 weeks and at least 16 weeks after first dose; minimum age for the final dose is 24 weeks		
Rotavirus[2]	6 weeks	4 weeks	4 weeks[2]		
Diphtheria, tetanus, & acellular pertussis[3]	6 weeks	4 weeks	4 weeks	6 months	6 months[3]
Haemophilus influenzae type b[5]	6 weeks	4 weeks if first dose administered at younger than age 12 months 8 weeks (as final dose) if first dose administered at age 12 through 14 months No further doses needed if first dose administered at age 15 months or older	4 weeks[5] if current age is younger than 12 months and first dose administered at < 7 months old 8 weeks (as final dose)[5] if current age is younger than 12 months and first dose administered between 7 through 11 months (regardless of Hib vaccine [PRP-T or PRP-OMP] used for first dose); OR if current age is 12 through 59 months and first dose administered at younger than age 12 months; OR first 2 doses were PRP-OMP and administered at younger than 12 months. No further doses needed if previous dose administered at age 15 months or older	8 weeks (as final dose) This dose only necessary for children aged 12 through 59 months who received 3 (PRP-T) doses before age 12 months and started the primary series before age 7 months	
Pneumococcal[6]	6 weeks	4 weeks if first dose administered at younger than age 12 months 8 weeks (as final dose for healthy children) if first dose administered at age 12 months or older No further doses needed for healthy children if first dose administered at age 24 months or older	4 weeks if current age is younger than 12 months 8 weeks (as final dose for healthy children) if current age is 12 months or older No further doses needed for healthy children if previous dose administered at age 24 months or older	8 weeks (as final dose) This dose only necessary for children aged 12 through 59 months who received 3 doses before age 12 months or for children at high risk who received 3 doses at any age	
Inactivated poliovirus[7]	6 weeks	4 weeks[7]	4 weeks[7]	6 months[7] minimum age 4 years for final dose	
Meningococcal[13]	6 weeks	8 weeks[13]	See footnote 13	See footnote 13	
Measles, mumps, rubella[9]	12 months	4 weeks			
Varicella[10]	12 months	3 months			
Hepatitis A[11]	12 months	6 months			
Persons aged 7 through 18 years					
Tetanus, diphtheria; tetanus, diphtheria, & acellular pertussis[4]	7 years[4]	4 weeks	4 weeks if first dose of DTaP/DT administered at younger than age 12 months 6 months if first dose of DTaP/DT administered at age 12 months or older or older and no further doses needed for catch-up	6 months if first dose of DTaP/DT administered at younger than age 12 months	
Human papillomavirus[12]	9 years	Routine dosing intervals are recommended[12]			
Hepatitis A[11]	12 months	6 months			
Hepatitis B[1]	Birth	4 weeks	8 weeks (and at least 16 weeks after first dose)		
Inactivated poliovirus[7]	6 weeks	4 weeks	4 weeks[7]	6 months[7]	
Meningococcal[13]	6 weeks	8 weeks[13]	See footnote 13		
Measles, mumps, rubella[9]	12 months	4 weeks			
Varicella[10]	12 months	3 months if person is younger than age 13 years 4 weeks if person is aged 13 years or older			

NOTE: The above recommendations must be read along with the footnotes of this schedule.

Footnotes — Recommended immunization schedule for persons aged 0 through 18 years—United States, 2014

For further guidance on the use of the vaccines mentioned below, see: http://www.cdc.gov/vaccines/hcp/acip-recs/index.html.
For vaccine recommendations for persons 19 years of age and older, see the adult immunization schedule.

Additional information

- For contraindications and precautions to use of a vaccine and for additional information regarding that vaccine, vaccination providers should consult the relevant ACIP statement available online at http://www.cdc.gov/vaccines/hcp/acip-recs/index.html.
- For purposes of calculating intervals between doses, 4 weeks = 28 days. Intervals of 4 months or greater are determined by calendar months.
- Vaccine doses administered ≤4 days before the minimum interval are considered valid. Doses of any vaccine administered ≥5 days earlier than the minimum interval or minimum age should not be counted as valid doses and should be repeated as age-appropriate. The repeat dose should be spaced after the invalid dose by the recommended minimum interval. For further details, see MMWR, General Recommendations on Immunization and Reports / Vol. 60 / No. 2; Table 1. Recommended and minimum ages and intervals between vaccine doses available online at http://www.cdc.gov/mmwr/pdf/rr/rr6002.pdf.
- Information on travel vaccine requirements and recommendations is available at http://wwwnc.cdc.gov/travel/destinations/list.
- For vaccination of persons with primary and secondary immunodeficiencies, see Table 13, "Vaccination of persons with primary and secondary immunodeficiencies," in General Recommendations on Immunization (ACIP), available at http://www.cdc.gov/mmwr/pdf/rr/rr6002.pdf; and American Academy of Pediatrics. Immunization in Special Clinical Circumstances, in Pickering LK, Baker CJ, Kimberlin DW, Long SS eds. Red Book: 2012 report of the Committee on Infectious Diseases. 29th ed. Elk Grove Village, IL: American Academy of Pediatrics.

1. Hepatitis B (HepB) vaccine. (Minimum age: birth)

Routine vaccination:

At birth:

- Administer monovalent HepB vaccine to all newborns before hospital discharge.
- For infants born to hepatitis B surface antigen (HBsAg)-positive mothers, administer HepB vaccine and 0.5 mL of hepatitis B immune globulin (HBIG) within 12 hours of birth. These infants should be tested for HBsAg and antibody to HBsAg (anti-HBs) 1 to 2 months after completion of the HepB series, at age 9 through 18 months (preferably at the next well-child visit).
- If mother's HBsAg status is unknown, within 12 hours of birth administer HepB vaccine regardless of birth weight. For infants weighing less than 2,000 grams, administer HBIG in addition to HepB vaccine within 12 hours of birth. Determine mother's HBsAg status as soon as possible and, if mother is HBsAg-positive, also administer HBIG for infants weighing 2,000 grams or more as soon as possible, but no later than age 7 days.

Doses following the birth dose:

- The second dose should be administered at age 1 or 2 months. Monovalent HepB vaccine should be used for doses administered before age 6 weeks.
- Infants who did not receive a birth dose should receive 3 doses of a HepB-containing vaccine on a schedule of 0, 1 to 2 months, and 6 months starting as soon as feasible. See Figure 2.
- Administer the second dose 1 to 2 months after the first dose (minimum interval of 4 weeks), administer the third dose at least 8 weeks after the second dose AND at least 16 weeks after the first dose. The final (third or fourth) dose in the HepB vaccine series should be administered no earlier than age 24 weeks.
- Administration of a total of 4 doses of HepB vaccine is permitted when a combination vaccine containing HepB is administered after the birth dose.

Catch-up vaccination:

- Unvaccinated persons should complete a 3-dose series.
- A 2-dose series (doses separated by at least 4 months) of adult formulation Recombivax HB is licensed for use in children aged 11 through 15 years.
- For other catch-up guidance, see Figure 2.

2. Rotavirus (RV) vaccines. (Minimum age: 6 weeks for both RV1 [Rotarix] and RV5 [RotaTeq])

Routine vaccination:

Administer a series of RV vaccine to all infants as follows:

1. If Rotarix is used, administer a 2-dose series at 2 and 4 months of age.
2. If RotaTeq is used, administer a 3-dose series at ages 2, 4, and 6 months.
3. If any dose in the series was RotaTeq or vaccine product is unknown for any dose in the series, a total of 3 doses of RV vaccine should be administered.

Catch-up vaccination:

- The maximum age for the first dose in the series is 14 weeks, 6 days; vaccination should not be initiated for infants aged 15 weeks, 0 days or older.
- The maximum age for the final dose in the series is 8 months, 0 days.
- For other catch-up guidance, see Figure 2.

3. Diphtheria and tetanus toxoids and acellular pertussis (DTaP) vaccine. (Minimum age: 6 weeks.

Exception: DTaP-IPV [Kinrix]: 4 years)

Routine vaccination:

- Administer a 5-dose series of DTaP vaccine at ages 2, 4, 6, 15 through 18 months, and 4 through 6 years. The fourth dose may be administered as early as age 12 months, provided at least 6 months have elapsed since the third dose.

Catch-up vaccination:

- The fifth dose of DTaP vaccine is not necessary if the fourth dose was administered at age 4 years or older.
- For other catch-up guidance, see Figure 2.

4. Tetanus and diphtheria toxoids and acellular pertussis (Tdap) vaccine. (Minimum age: 10 years for Boostrix, 11 years for Adacel)

Routine vaccination:

- Administer 1 dose of Tdap vaccine to all adolescents aged 11 through 12 years.
- Tdap may be administered regardless of the interval since the last tetanus and diphtheria toxoid-containing vaccine.
- Administer 1 dose of Tdap vaccine to pregnant adolescents during each pregnancy (preferred during 27 through 36 weeks gestation) regardless of time since prior Td or Tdap vaccination.

Catch-up vaccination:

- Persons aged 7 years and older who are not fully immunized with DTaP vaccine should receive Tdap vaccine as 1 (preferably the first) dose in the catch-up series; if additional doses are needed, use Td vaccine. For children 7 through 10 years who receive a dose of Tdap as part of the catch-up series, an adolescent Tdap vaccine dose at age 11 through 12 years should NOT be administered. Td should be administered instead 10 years after the Tdap dose.
- Persons aged 11 through 18 years who have not received Tdap vaccine should receive a dose followed by tetanus and diphtheria toxoids (Td) booster doses every 10 years thereafter.

Inadvertent doses of DTaP vaccine:

- If administered inadvertently to a child aged 7 through 10 years may count as part of the catch-up series. This dose may count as the adolescent Tdap dose, or the child can later receive a Tdap booster dose at age 11 through 12 years.
- If administered inadvertently to an adolescent aged 11 through 18 years, the dose should be counted as the adolescent Tdap booster.
- For other catch-up guidance, see Figure 2.

5. Haemophilus influenzae type b (Hib) conjugate vaccine. (Minimum age: 6 weeks for PRP-T [ACTHIB, DTaP-IPV/Hib (Pentacel) and Hib-MenCY (MenHibrix)], PRP-OMP [PedvaxHIB or COMVAX], 12 months for PRP-T [Hiberix])

Routine vaccination:

- Administer a 2- or 3-dose Hib vaccine primary series and a booster dose (dose 3 or 4 depending on vaccine used in primary series) at age 12 through 15 months to complete a full Hib vaccine series.
- The primary series with ActHIB, MenHibrix, or Pentacel consists of 3 doses and should be administered at 2, 4, and 6 months of age. The primary series with PedvaxHib or COMVAX consists of 2 doses and should be administered at 2 and 4 months of age; a dose at age 6 months is not indicated.
- One booster dose (dose 3 or 4 depending on vaccine used in primary series) of any Hib vaccine should be administered at age 12 through 15 months. An exception is Hiberix vaccine. Hiberix should only be used for the booster (final) dose in children aged 12 months through 4 years who have received at least 1 prior dose of Hib-containing vaccine.

For further guidance on the use of the vaccines mentioned below, see: http://www.cdc.gov/vaccines/hcp/acip-recs/index.html.

5. Haemophilus influenzae type b (Hib) conjugate vaccine (cont'd)

- For recommendations on the use of MenHibrix in patients at increased risk for meningococcal disease, please refer to the meningococcal vaccine footnotes and also to MMWR March 22, 2013; 62(RR02):1-22, available at http://www.cdc.gov/mmwr/pdf/rr/rr6202.pdf.

Catch-up vaccination:

- If dose 1 was administered at ages 12 through 14 months, administer a second (final) dose at least 8 weeks after dose 1, regardless of Hib vaccine used in the primary series.
- If the first 2 doses were PRP-OMP (PedvaxHIB or COMVAX), and were administered at age 11 months or younger, the third (and final) dose should be administered at age 12 through 15 months and at least 8 weeks after the second dose.
- If the first dose was administered at age 7 through 11 months, administer the second dose at least 4 weeks later and a third (and final) dose at age 12 through 15 months or 8 weeks after second dose, whichever is later, regardless of Hib vaccine used for first dose.
- If first dose is administered at younger than 12 months of age and second dose is given between 12 through 14 months of age, a third (and final) dose should be given 8 weeks later.
- For unvaccinated children aged 15 months or older, administer only 1 dose.
- For other catch-up guidance, see Figure 2. For catch-up guidance related to MenHibrix, please see the meningococcal vaccine footnotes and also MMWR March 22, 2013; 62(RR02):1-22, available at http://www.cdc.gov/mmwr/pdf/rr/rr6202.pdf.

Vaccination of persons with high-risk conditions:

- Children aged 12 through 59 months who are at increased risk for Hib disease, including chemotherapy recipients and those with anatomic or functional asplenia (including sickle cell disease), human immunodeficiency virus (HIV) infection, immunoglobulin deficiency, or early component complement deficiency, who have received either no doses or only 1 dose of Hib vaccine before 12 months of age, should receive 2 additional doses of Hib vaccine 8 weeks apart; children who received 2 or more doses of Hib vaccine before 12 months of age should receive 1 additional dose.
- For patients younger than 5 years of age undergoing chemotherapy or radiation treatment who received a Hib vaccine dose(s) within 14 days of starting therapy or during therapy, repeat the dose(s) at least 3 months following therapy completion.
- Recipients of hematopoietic stem cell transplant (HSCT) should be revaccinated with a 3-dose regimen of Hib vaccine starting 6 to 12 months after successful transplant, regardless of vaccination history; doses should be administered at least 4 weeks apart.
- A single dose of any Hib-containing vaccine should be administered to unimmunized* children and adolescents 15 months of age and older undergoing an elective splenectomy; if possible, vaccine should be administered at least 14 days before procedure.
- Hib vaccine is not routinely recommended for patients 5 years or older. However, 1 dose of Hib vaccine should be administered to unimmunized* persons aged 5 years or older who have anatomic or functional asplenia (including sickle cell disease) and unvaccinated persons 5 through 18 years of age with human immunodeficiency virus (HIV) infection.

Patients who have not received a primary series and booster dose or at least 1 dose of Hib vaccine after 14 months of age are considered unimmunized.

6. Pneumococcal vaccines. (Minimum age: 6 weeks for PCV13, 2 years for PPSV23)

Routine vaccination with PCV13:

- Administer a 4-dose series of PCV13 vaccine at ages 2, 4, and 6 months and at age 12 through 15 months.
- For children aged 14 through 59 months who have received an age-appropriate series of 7-valent PCV (PCV7), administer a single supplemental dose of 13-valent PCV (PCV13).

Catch-up vaccination with PCV13:

- Administer 1 dose of PCV13 to all healthy children aged 24 through 59 months who are not completely vaccinated for their age.
- For other catch-up guidance, see Figure 2.

Vaccination of persons with high-risk conditions with PCV13 and PPSV23:

- All recommended PCV13 doses should be administered prior to PPSV23 vaccination if possible.
- For children 2 through 5 years of age with any of the following conditions: chronic heart disease (particularly cyanotic congenital heart disease and cardiac failure); chronic lung disease (including asthma if treated with high-dose oral corticosteroid therapy); diabetes mellitus; cerebrospinal fluid leak; cochlear implant; sickle cell disease; anatomic or functional asplenia; HIV infection; chronic renal failure; nephrotic syndrome; diseases associated with treatment with immunosuppressive drugs or radiation therapy, including malignant neoplasms, leukemias, lymphomas, and Hodgkin disease; solid organ transplantation; or congenital immunodeficiency:
  1. Administer 1 dose of PCV13 if 3 doses of PCV (PCV7 and/or PCV13) were received previously.
  2. Administer 2 doses of PCV13 at least 8 weeks apart if fewer than 3 doses of PCV (PCV7 and/or PCV13) were received previously.

6. Pneumococcal vaccines (cont'd)

  3. Administer 1 supplemental dose of PCV13 if 4 doses of PCV7 or other age-appropriate complete PCV7 series was received previously.
  4. The minimum interval between doses of PPSV23 at least 8 weeks.
  5. For children with no history of PPSV23 vaccination, administer PPSV23 at least 8 weeks after the most recent dose of PCV13.

- For children aged 6 through 18 years who have cerebrospinal fluid leak; cochlear implant; sickle cell disease and other hemoglobinopathies; anatomic or functional asplenia; congenital or acquired immunodeficiencies; HIV infection; chronic renal failure; nephrotic syndrome; diseases associated with treatment with immunosuppressive drugs or radiation therapy, including malignant neoplasms, leukemias, lymphomas, and Hodgkin disease; generalized malignancy; solid organ transplantation; or multiple myeloma:
  1. If neither PCV13 nor PPSV23 has been received previously, administer 1 dose of PCV13 now and 1 dose of PPSV23 at least 8 weeks later.
  2. If PCV13 has been received previously but PPSV23 has not, administer 1 dose of PPSV23 at least 8 weeks after the most recent dose of PCV13.
  3. If PPSV23 has been received but PCV13 has not, administer 1 dose of PCV13 at least 8 weeks after the most recent dose of PPSV23.
- For children aged 6 through 18 years with chronic heart disease (particularly cyanotic congenital heart disease and cardiac failure), diabetes mellitus, alcoholism, or chronic liver disease, who have not received PPSV23, administer 1 dose of PPSV23. If PCV13 has been received previously, then PPSV23 should be administered at least 8 weeks after any prior PCV13 dose.
- A single revaccination with PPSV23 should be administered 5 years after the first dose to children with sickle cell disease or other hemoglobinopathies; anatomic or functional asplenia; congenital or acquired immunodeficiencies; HIV infection; chronic renal failure; nephrotic syndrome; diseases associated with treatment with immunosuppressive drugs or radiation therapy, including malignant neoplasms, leukemias, lymphomas, and Hodgkin disease; generalized malignancy; solid organ transplantation; or multiple myeloma.

7. Inactivated poliovirus vaccine (IPV). (Minimum age: 6 weeks)

Routine vaccination:

- Administer a 4-dose series of IPV at ages 2, 4, 6 through 18 months, and 4 through 6 years. The final dose in the series should be administered on or after the fourth birthday and at least 6 months after the previous dose.

Catch-up vaccination:

- In the first 6 months of life, minimum age and minimum intervals are only recommended if the person is at risk for imminent exposure to circulating poliovirus (i.e., travel to a polio-endemic region or during an outbreak).
- If 4 or more doses are administered before age 4 years, an additional dose should be administered at age 4 through 6 years and at least 6 months after the previous dose.
- A fourth dose is not necessary if the third dose was administered at age 4 years or older and at least 6 months after the previous dose.
- If both OPV and IPV were administered as part of a series, a total of 4 doses should be administered, regardless of the child's current age. IPV is not routinely recommended for U.S. residents aged 18 years or older.
- For other catch-up guidance, see Figure 2.

8. Influenza vaccines. (Minimum age: 6 months for inactivated influenza vaccine [IIV], 2 years for live, attenuated influenza vaccine [LAIV])

Routine vaccination:

- Administer influenza vaccine annually to all children beginning at age 6 months. For most healthy, nonpregnant persons aged 2 through 49 years, either LAIV or IIV may be used. However, LAIV should NOT be administered to some persons, including 1) those with asthma, 2) children 2 through 4 years who had wheezing in the past 12 months, or 3) those who have any other underlying medical conditions that predispose them to influenza complications. For all other contraindications to use of LAIV, see MMWR 2013;62 (No. RR-7):1-43, available at http://www.cdc.gov/mmwr/pdf/rr/rr6207.pdf.

For children aged 6 months through 8 years:

- For the 2013–14 season, administer 2 doses (separated by at least 4 weeks) to children who are receiving influenza vaccine for the first time. Some children in this age group who have been vaccinated previously will also need 2 doses. For additional guidance, follow dosing guidelines in the 2013-14 ACIP influenza vaccine recommendations, MMWR 2013; 62 (No. RR-7):1-43, available at http://www.cdc.gov/mmwr/pdf/rr/rr6207.pdf.
- For the 2014–15 season, follow dosing guidelines in the 2014 ACIP influenza vaccine recommendations.

For persons aged 9 years and older:

- Administer 1 dose.

For further guidance on the use of the vaccines mentioned below, see: http://www.cdc.gov/vaccines/hcp/acip-recs/index.html.

9. **Measles, mumps, and rubella (MMR) vaccine. (Minimum age: 12 months for routine vaccination)**

   Routine vaccination:
   - Administer a 2-dose series of MMR vaccine at ages 12 through 15 months and 4 through 6 years. The second dose may be administered before age 4 years, provided at least 4 weeks have elapsed since the first dose.
   - Administer 1 dose of MMR vaccine to infants aged 6 through 11 months before departure from the United States for international travel. These children should be revaccinated with 2 doses of MMR vaccine, the first at age 12 through 15 months (12 months if the child remains in an area where disease risk is high), and the second dose at least 4 weeks later.
   - Administer 2 doses of MMR vaccine to children aged 12 months and older before departure from the United States for international travel. The first dose should be administered on or after age 12 months and the second dose at least 4 weeks later.

   Catch-up vaccination:
   - Ensure that all school-aged children and adolescents have had 2 doses of MMR vaccine; the minimum interval between the 2 doses is 4 weeks.

10. **Varicella (VAR) vaccine. (Minimum age: 12 months)**

    Routine vaccination:
    - Administer a 2-dose series of VAR vaccine at ages 12 through 15 months and 4 through 6 years. The second dose may be administered before age 4 years, provided at least 3 months have elapsed since the first dose. If the second dose was administered at least 4 weeks after the first dose, it can be accepted as valid.

    Catch-up vaccination:
    - Ensure that all persons aged 7 through 18 years without evidence of immunity (see MMWR 2007; 56 [No. RR-4], available at http://www.cdc.gov/mmwr/pdf/rr/rr5604.pdf) have 2 doses of varicella vaccine. For children aged 7 through 12 years, the recommended minimum interval between doses is 3 months (if the second dose was administered at least 4 weeks after the first dose, it can be accepted as valid); for persons aged 13 years and older, the minimum interval between doses is 4 weeks.

11. **Hepatitis A (HepA) vaccine. (Minimum age: 12 months)**

    Routine vaccination:
    - Initiate the 2-dose HepA vaccine series at 12 through 23 months; separate the 2 doses by 6 to 18 months.
    - Children who have received 1 dose of HepA vaccine before age 24 months should receive a second dose 6 to 18 months after the first dose.
    - For any person aged 2 years and older who has not already received the HepA vaccine series, 2 doses of HepA vaccine separated by 6 to 18 months may be administered if immunity against hepatitis A virus infection is desired.

    Catch-up vaccination:
    - The minimum interval between the two doses is 6 months.

    Special populations:
    - Administer 2 doses of HepA vaccine at least 6 months apart to previously unvaccinated persons who live in areas where vaccination programs target older children, or who are at increased risk for infection. This includes persons traveling to or working in countries that have high or intermediate endemicity of infection; men having sex with men; users of injection and non-injection illicit drugs; persons who work with HAV-infected primates or with HAV in a research laboratory; persons with clotting-factor disorders; persons with chronic liver disease; and persons who anticipate close, personal contact (e.g., household or regular babysitting) with an international adoptee during the first 60 days after arrival in the United States from a country with high or intermediate endemicity. The first dose should be administered as soon as the adoption is planned, ideally 2 or more weeks before the arrival of the adoptee.

12. **Human papillomavirus (HPV) vaccines. (Minimum age: 9 years for HPV2 [Cervarix] and HPV4 [Gardasil])**

    Routine vaccination:
    - Administer a 3-dose series of HPV vaccine on a schedule of 0, 1-2, and 6 months to all adolescents aged 11 through 12 years. Either HPV4 or HPV2 may be used for females, and only HPV4 may be used for males.
    - The vaccine series may be started at age 9 years.
    - Administer the second dose 1 to 2 months after the first dose (minimum interval of 4 weeks), administer the third dose 24 weeks after the first dose and 16 weeks after the second dose (minimum interval of 12 weeks).

    Catch-up vaccination:
    - Administer the vaccine series to females (either HPV2 or HPV4) and males (HPV4) at age 13 through 18 years if not previously vaccinated.
    - Use recommended routine dosing intervals (see above) for vaccine series catch-up.

13. **Meningococcal conjugate vaccines. (Minimum age: 6 weeks for Hib-MenCY [MenHibrix], 9 months for MenACWY-D [Menactra], 2 months for MenACWY-CRM [Menveo])**

    Routine vaccination:
    - Administer a single dose of Menactra or Menveo vaccine at age 11 through 12 years, with a booster dose at age 16 years.
    - Adolescents aged 11 through 18 years with human immunodeficiency virus (HIV) infection should receive a 2-dose primary series of Menactra or Menveo with at least 8 weeks between doses.
    - For children aged 2 months through 18 years with high-risk conditions, see below.

    Catch-up vaccination:
    - Administer Menactra or Menveo vaccine at age 13 through 18 years if not previously vaccinated.
    - If the first dose is administered at age 13 through 15 years, a booster dose should be administered at age 16 through 18 years with a minimum interval of at least 8 weeks between doses.
    - If the first dose is administered at age 16 years or older, a booster dose is not needed.
    - For other catch-up guidance, see Figure 2.

    Vaccination of persons with high-risk conditions and other persons at increased risk of disease:

    Children with anatomic or functional asplenia (including sickle cell disease):
    1. For children younger than 19 months of age, administer a 4-dose infant series of MenHibrix or Menveo at 2, 4, 6, and 12 through 15 months of age.
    2. For children aged 19 through 23 months who have not completed a series of MenHibrix or Menveo, administer 2 primary doses of Menveo at least 3 months apart.
    3. For children aged 24 months and older who have not received a complete series of MenHibrix or Menveo or Menactra, administer 2 primary doses of either Menactra or Menveo at least 2 months apart. If Menactra is administered to a child with asplenia (including sickle cell disease), do not administer Menactra until 2 years of age and at least 4 weeks after the completion of all PCV13 doses.

    Children with persistent complement component deficiency:
    1. For children younger than 19 months of age, administer a 4-dose infant series of either MenHibrix or Menveo at 2, 4, 6, and 12 through 15 months of age.
    2. For children 7 through 23 months who have not initiated vaccination, two options exist depending on age and vaccine brand:
       a. For children who initiate vaccination with Menveo at 7 months through 23 months of age, a 2-dose series should be administered with the second dose after 12 months of age and at least 3 months after the first dose.
       b. For children who initiate vaccination with Menactra at 9 months through 23 months of age, a 2-dose series of Menactra should be administered at least 3 months apart.
       c. For children aged 24 months and older who have not received a complete series of MenHibrix, Menveo, or Menactra, administer 2 primary doses of either Menactra or Menveo at least 2 months apart.

    - For children who travel to or reside in countries in which meningococcal disease is hyperendemic or epidemic, including countries in the African meningitis belt or the Hajj, administer an age-appropriate formulation and series of Menactra or Menveo for protection against serogroups A and W meningococcal disease. Prior receipt of MenHibrix is not sufficient for children traveling to the meningitis belt or the Hajj because it does not contain serogroups A or W.
    - For persons at risk during a community outbreak attributable to a vaccine serogroup, administer or complete an age- and formulation-appropriate series of MenHibrix, Menactra, or Menveo.
    - For booster doses among persons with high-risk conditions, refer to MMWR 2013; 62(RR02);1-22, available at http://www.cdc.gov/mmwr/preview/mmwrhtml/rr6202a1.htm.

    Catch-up recommendations for persons with high-risk conditions:
    1. If MenHibrix is administered to achieve protection against meningococcal disease, a complete age-appropriate series of MenHibrix should be administered.
    2. If the first dose of MenHibrix is given at or after 12 months of age, a total of 2 doses should be given at least 8 weeks apart to ensure protection against serogroups C and Y meningococcal disease.
    3. If the first dose of vaccination with Menveo at 7 months through 9 months of age, a 2-dose series should be administered with the second dose after 12 months of age and at least 3 months after the first dose.
    4. For other catch-up recommendations for these persons, refer to MMWR 2013;62(RR02);1-22, available at http://www.cdc.gov/mmwr/preview/mmwrhtml/rr6202a1.htm.

    For complete information on use of meningococcal vaccines, including guidance related to vaccination of persons at increased risk of infection, see MMWR March 22, 2013; 62(RR02);1-22, available at http://www.cdc.gov/mmwr/pdf/rr/rr6202.pdf.

Recommended Adult Immunization Schedule—United States - 2014

Note: These recommendations must be read with the footnotes that follow containing number of doses, intervals between doses, and other important information.

Figure 1. Recommended adult immunization schedule, by vaccine and age group[1]

VACCINE ▼ AGE GROUP ►	19-21 years	22-26 years	27-49 years	50-59 years	60-64 years	≥ 65 years
Influenza [2,*]	1 dose annually					
Tetanus, diphtheria, pertussis (Td/Tdap) [3,*]	Substitute 1-time dose of Tdap for Td booster; then boost with Td every 10 yrs					
Varicella [4,*]	2 doses					
Human papillomavirus (HPV) Female [5,*]	3 doses					
Human papillomavirus (HPV) Male [5,*]	3 doses					
Zoster [6]					1 dose	
Measles, mumps, rubella (MMR) [7,*]	1 or 2 doses					
Pneumococcal 13-valent conjugate (PCV13) [8,*]	1 dose					
Pneumococcal polysaccharide (PPSV23) [9,10]	1 or 2 doses					1 dose
Meningococcal [11,*]	1 or more doses					
Hepatitis A [12,*]	2 doses					
Hepatitis B [13,*]	3 doses					
Haemophilus influenzae type b (Hib) [14,*]	1 or 3 doses					

*Covered by the Vaccine Injury Compensation Program

For all persons in this category who meet the age requirements and who lack documentation of vaccination or have no evidence of previous infection; zoster vaccine recommended regardless of prior episode of zoster

Recommended if some other risk factor is present (e.g., on the basis of medical, occupational, lifestyle, or other indication)

No recommendation

Report all clinically significant postvaccination reactions to the Vaccine Adverse Event Reporting System (VAERS). Reporting forms and instructions on filing a VAERS report are available at www.vaers.hhs.gov or by telephone, 800-822-7967.

Information on how to file a Vaccine Injury Compensation Program claim is available at www.hrsa.gov/vaccinecompensation or by telephone, 800-338-2382. To file a claim for vaccine injury, contact the U.S. Court of Federal Claims, 717 Madison Place, N.W., Washington, D.C. 20005; telephone, 202-357-6400.

Additional information about the vaccines in this schedule, extent of available data, and contraindications for vaccination is also available at www.cdc.gov/vaccines or from the CDC-INFO Contact Center at 800-CDC-INFO (800-232-4636) in English and Spanish, 8:00 a.m. - 8:00 p.m. Eastern Time, Monday - Friday, excluding holidays.

Use of trade names and commercial sources is for identification only and does not imply endorsement by the U.S. Department of Health and Human Services.

The recommendations in this schedule were approved by the Centers for Disease Control and Prevention's (CDC) Advisory Committee on Immunization Practices (ACIP), the American Academy of Family Physicians (AAFP), the American College of Physicians (ACP), American College of Obstetricians and Gynecologists (ACOG) and American College of Nurse-Midwives (ACNM).

Figure 2. Vaccines that might be indicated for adults based on medical and other indications[1]

VACCINE ▼ INDICATION ►	Pregnancy	Immuno-compromising conditions (excluding human immunodeficiency virus [HIV])[4,6,7,8,15]	HIV infection CD4+ T lymphocyte count [4,6,7,8,15] < 200 cells/µL	HIV infection CD4+ T lymphocyte count ≥ 200 cells/µL	Men who have sex with men (MSM)	Kidney failure, end-stage renal disease, receipt of hemodialysis	Heart disease, chronic lung disease, chronic alcoholism	Asplenia (including elective splenectomy and persistent complement component deficiencies)[8,14]	Chronic liver disease	Diabetes	Healthcare personnel
Influenza [2,*]	1 dose IIV annually				1 dose IIV or LAIV annually	1 dose IIV annually					1 dose IIV or LAIV annually
Tetanus, diphtheria, pertussis (Td/Tdap) [3,*]	1 dose Tdap each pregnancy	Substitute 1-time dose of Tdap for Td booster; then boost with Td every 10 yrs									
Varicella [4,*]	Contraindicated			2 doses							
Human papillomavirus (HPV) Female [5,*]	3 doses through age 26 yrs				3 doses through age 26 yrs						
Human papillomavirus (HPV) Male [5,*]	3 doses through age 26 yrs				3 doses through age 21 yrs						
Zoster [6]	Contraindicated			1 dose							
Measles, mumps, rubella (MMR) [7,*]	Contraindicated			1 or 2 doses							
Pneumococcal 13-valent conjugate (PCV13) [8,*]	1 dose										
Pneumococcal polysaccharide (PPSV23) [9,10]	1 or 2 doses										
Meningococcal [11,*]	1 or more doses										
Hepatitis A [12,*]	2 doses										
Hepatitis B [13,*]	3 doses										
Haemophilus influenzae type b (Hib) [14,*]	post-HSCT recipients only	1 or 3 doses									

*Covered by the Vaccine Injury Compensation Program

For all persons in this category who meet the age requirements and who lack documentation of vaccination or have no evidence of previous infection; zoster vaccine recommended regardless of prior episode of zoster

Recommended if some other risk factor is present (e.g., on the basis of medical, occupational, lifestyle, or other indications)

No recommendation

CDC
U.S. Department of Health and Human Services
Centers for Disease Control and Prevention

These schedules indicate the recommended age groups and medical indications for which administration of currently licensed vaccines is commonly indicated for adults ages 19 years and older, as of February 1, 2014. For all vaccines being recommended on the Adult Immunization Schedule: a vaccine series does not need to be restarted, regardless of the time that has elapsed between doses. Licensed combination vaccines may be used whenever any components of the combination are indicated and when the vaccine's other components are not contraindicated. For detailed recommendations on all vaccines, including those used primarily for travelers or that are issued during the year, consult the manufacturers' package inserts and the complete statements from the Advisory Committee on Immunization Practices (www.cdc.gov/vaccines/hcp/acip-recs/index.html). Use of trade names and commercial sources is for identification only and does not imply endorsement by the U.S. Department of Health and Human Services.

Footnotes
Recommended Immunization Schedule for Adults Aged 19 Years or Older: United States, 2014

1. **Additional information**
   - Additional guidance for the use of the vaccines described in this supplement is available at www.cdc.gov/vaccines/hcp/acip-recs/index.html.
   - Information on vaccination recommendations when vaccination status is unknown and other general immunization information can be found in the General Recommendations on Immunization at www.cdc.gov/mmwr/preview/mmwrhtml/rr6002a1.htm.
   - Information on travel vaccine requirements and recommendations (e.g., for hepatitis A and B, meningococcal, and other vaccines) is available at http://wwwnc.cdc.gov/travel/destinations/list.
   - Additional information and resources regarding vaccination of pregnant women can be found at http://www.cdc.gov/vaccines/adults/rec-vac/pregnant.html.

2. **Influenza vaccination**
   - Annual vaccination against influenza is recommended for all persons aged 6 months or older.
   - Persons aged 6 months or older, including pregnant women and persons with hives-only allergy to eggs, can receive the inactivated influenza vaccine (IIV). An age-appropriate IIV formulation should be used.
   - Adults aged 18 to 49 years can receive the recombinant influenza vaccine (RIV) (FluBlok). RIV does not contain any egg protein.
   - Healthy, nonpregnant persons aged 2 to 49 years without high-risk medical conditions can receive either intranasally administered live, attenuated influenza vaccine (LAIV) (FluMist), or IIV. Health care personnel who care for severely immunocompromised persons (i.e., those who require care in a protected environment) should receive IIV or RIV rather than LAIV.
   - The intramuscularly or intradermally administered IIV are options for adults aged 18 to 64 years.
   - Adults aged 65 years or older can receive the standard-dose IIV or the high-dose IIV (Fluzone High-Dose).

3. **Tetanus, diphtheria, and acellular pertussis (Td/Tdap) vaccination**
   - Administer 1 dose of Tdap vaccine to pregnant women during each pregnancy (preferred during 27 to 36 weeks' gestation) regardless of interval since prior Td or Tdap vaccination.
   - Persons aged 11 years or older who have not received Tdap vaccine or for whom vaccine status is unknown should receive a dose of Tdap followed by tetanus and diphtheria toxoids (Td) booster doses every 10 years thereafter. Tdap can be administered regardless of interval since the most recent tetanus or diphtheria-toxoid containing vaccine.
   - Adults with an unknown or incomplete history of completing a 3-dose primary vaccination series with Td-containing vaccines should begin or complete a primary vaccination series including a Tdap dose.
   - For unvaccinated adults, administer the first 2 doses at least 4 weeks apart and the third dose 6 to 12 months after the second.
   - For incompletely vaccinated (i.e., less than 3 doses) adults, administer remaining doses.
   - Refer to the ACIP statement for recommendations for administering Td/Tdap as prophylaxis in wound management (see footnote 1).

4. **Varicella vaccination**
   - All adults without evidence of immunity to varicella (as defined below) should receive 2 doses of single-antigen varicella vaccine or a second dose if they have received only 1 dose.
   - Vaccination should be emphasized for those who have close contact with persons at high risk for severe disease (e.g., health care personnel and family contacts of persons with immunocompromising conditions) or are at high risk for exposure or transmission (e.g., teachers; child care employees; residents and staff members of institutional settings, including correctional institutions; college students; military personnel; adolescents and adults living in households with children; nonpregnant women of childbearing age; and international travelers).
   - Pregnant women should be assessed for evidence of varicella immunity. Women who do not have evidence of immunity should receive the first dose of varicella vaccine upon completion or termination of pregnancy and before discharge from the health care facility. The second dose should be administered 4 to 8 weeks after the first dose.
   - Evidence of immunity to varicella in adults includes any of the following:
     — documentation of 2 doses of varicella vaccine at least 4 weeks apart;
     — U.S.-born before 1980, except health care personnel and pregnant women;
     — history of varicella based on diagnosis or verification of varicella disease by a health care provider;
     — history of herpes zoster based on diagnosis or verification of herpes zoster disease by a health care provider; or
     — laboratory evidence of immunity or laboratory confirmation of disease.

5. **Human papillomavirus (HPV) vaccination**
   - Two vaccines are licensed for use in females, bivalent HPV vaccine (HPV2) and quadrivalent HPV vaccine (HPV4), and one HPV vaccine for use in males (HPV4).
   - For females, either HPV4 or HPV2 is recommended in a 3-dose series for routine vaccination at age 11 or 12 years and for those aged 13 through 26 years, if not previously vaccinated.
   - For males, HPV4 is recommended in a 3-dose series for routine vaccination at age 11 or 12 years and for those aged 13 through 21 years, if not previously vaccinated. Males aged 22 through 26 years may be vaccinated.

5. **Human papillomavirus (HPV) vaccination (cont'd)**
   - HPV4 is recommended for men who have sex with men through age 26 years for those who did not get any or all doses when they were younger.
   - Vaccination is recommended for immunocompromised persons (including those with HIV infection) through age 26 years for those who did not get any or all doses when they were younger.
   - A complete series for either HPV4 or HPV2 consists of 3 doses. The second dose should be administered 4 to 8 weeks (minimum interval of 4 weeks) after the first dose; the third dose should be administered 24 weeks after the first dose and 16 weeks after the second dose (minimum interval of at least 12 weeks).
   - HPV vaccines are not recommended for use in pregnant women. However, pregnancy testing is not needed before vaccination. If a woman is found to be pregnant after initiating the vaccination series, no intervention is needed; the remainder of the 3-dose series should be delayed until completion of pregnancy.

6. **Zoster vaccination**
   - A single dose of zoster vaccine is recommended for adults aged 60 years or older regardless of whether they report a prior episode of herpes zoster. Although the vaccine is licensed by the U.S. Food and Drug Administration for use among and can be administered to persons aged 50 years or older, ACIP recommends that vaccination begin at age 60 years.
   - Persons aged 60 years or older with chronic medical conditions may be vaccinated unless their condition constitutes a contraindication, such as pregnancy or severe immunodeficiency.

7. **Measles, mumps, rubella (MMR) vaccination**
   - Adults born before 1957 are generally considered immune to measles and mumps. All adults born in 1957 or later should have documentation of 1 or more doses of MMR vaccine unless they have a medical contraindication to the vaccine or laboratory evidence of immunity to each of the three diseases. Documentation of provider-diagnosed disease is not considered acceptable evidence of immunity for measles, mumps, or rubella.
   Measles component:
   - A routine second dose of MMR vaccine, administered a minimum of 28 days after the first dose, is recommended for adults who:
     — are students in postsecondary educational institutions;
     — work in a health care facility; or
     — plan to travel internationally.
   - Persons who received inactivated (killed) measles vaccine or measles vaccine of unknown type during 1963–1967 should be revaccinated with 2 doses of MMR vaccine.
   Mumps component:
   - A routine second dose of MMR vaccine, administered a minimum of 28 days after the first dose, is recommended for adults who:
     — are students in a postsecondary educational institution;
     — work in a health care facility; or
     — plan to travel internationally.
   - Persons vaccinated before 1979 with either killed mumps vaccine or mumps vaccine of unknown type who are at high risk for mumps infection (e.g., persons who are working in a health care facility) should be considered for revaccination with 2 doses of MMR vaccine.
   Rubella component:
   - For women of childbearing age, regardless of birth year, rubella immunity should be determined. If there is no evidence of immunity, women who are not pregnant should be vaccinated. Pregnant women who do not have evidence of immunity should receive MMR vaccine upon completion or termination of pregnancy and before discharge from the health care facility.
   Health care personnel born before 1957:
   - For unvaccinated health care personnel born before 1957 who lack laboratory evidence of measles, mumps, and/or rubella immunity or laboratory confirmation of disease, health care facilities should consider vaccinating personnel with 2 doses of MMR vaccine at the appropriate interval for measles and mumps or 1 dose of MMR vaccine for rubella.

8. **Pneumococcal conjugate (PCV13) vaccination**
   - Adults aged 19 years or older with immunocompromising conditions (including chronic renal failure and nephrotic syndrome), functional or anatomic asplenia, cerebrospinal fluid leaks, or cochlear implants who have not previously received PCV13 or PPSV23 should receive a single dose of PCV13 followed by a dose of PPSV23 at least 8 weeks later.
   - Adults aged 19 years or older with the aforementioned conditions who have previously received 1 or more doses of PPSV23 should receive a dose of PCV13 one or more years after the last PPSV23 dose was received. For adults who require additional doses of PPSV23, the first such dose should be given no sooner than 8 weeks after PCV13 and at least 5 years after the most recent dose of PPSV23.
   - When indicated, PCV13 should be administered to patients who are uncertain of their vaccination status history and have no record of previous vaccination.
   - Although PCV13 is licensed by the U.S. Food and Drug Administration for use among and can be administered to persons aged 50 years or older, ACIP recommends PCV13 for adults aged 19 years or older with the specific medical conditions noted above.

9. Pneumococcal polysaccharide (PPSV23) vaccination

- When PCV13 is also indicated, PCV13 should be given first (see footnote 8).
- Vaccinate all persons with the following indications:
  - all adults aged 65 years or older;
  - adults younger than 65 years with chronic lung disease (including chronic obstructive pulmonary disease, emphysema, and asthma), chronic cardiovascular diseases, diabetes mellitus, chronic renal failure, nephrotic syndrome, chronic liver disease (including cirrhosis), alcoholism, cochlear implants, cerebrospinal fluid leaks, immunocompromising conditions, and functional or anatomic asplenia (e.g., sickle cell disease and other hemoglobinopathies, congenital or acquired asplenia, splenic dysfunction, or splenectomy [if elective splenectomy is planned, vaccinate at least 2 weeks before surgery]);
  - residents of nursing homes or long-term care facilities; and
  - adults who smoke cigarettes.
- Persons with immunocompromising conditions and other selected conditions are recommended to receive PCV13 and PPSV23 vaccines. See footnote 8 for information on timing of PCV13 and PPSV23 vaccinations.
- Persons with asymptomatic or symptomatic HIV infection should be vaccinated as soon as possible after their diagnosis.
- When cancer chemotherapy or other immunosuppressive therapy is being considered, the interval between vaccination and initiation of immunosuppressive therapy should be at least 2 weeks. Vaccination during chemotherapy or radiation therapy should be avoided.
- Routine use of PPSV23 vaccine is not recommended for American Indians/Alaska Natives or other persons younger than 65 years unless they have underlying medical conditions that are PPSV23 indications. However, public health authorities may consider recommending PPSV23 for American Indians/Alaska Natives who are living in areas where the risk for invasive pneumococcal disease is increased.
- When indicated, PPSV23 vaccine should be administered to patients who are uncertain of their vaccination status and have no record of vaccination.

10. Revaccination with PPSV23

- One-time revaccination 5 years after the first dose of PPSV23 is recommended for persons aged 19 through 64 years with chronic renal failure or nephrotic syndrome, functional or anatomic asplenia (e.g., sickle cell disease or splenectomy), or immunocompromising conditions.
- Persons who received 1 or 2 doses of PPSV23 before age 65 years for any indication should receive another dose of the vaccine at age 65 years or later if at least 5 years have passed since their previous dose.
- No further doses of PPSV23 are needed for persons vaccinated with PPSV23 at or after age 65 years.

11. Meningococcal vaccination

- Administer 2 doses of quadrivalent meningococcal conjugate vaccine (MenACWY [Menactra, Menveo]) at least 2 months apart to adults of all ages with functional asplenia or persistent complement component deficiencies. HIV infection is not an indication for routine vaccination with MenACWY. If an HIV-infected person of any age is vaccinated, 2 doses of MenACWY should be administered at least 2 months apart.
- Administer a single dose of meningococcal vaccine to microbiologists routinely exposed to isolates of *Neisseria meningitidis*, military recruits, persons at risk during an outbreak attributable to a vaccine serogroup, and persons who travel to or live in countries in which meningococcal disease is hyperendemic or epidemic.
- First-year college students up through age 21 years who are living in residence halls should be vaccinated if they have not received a dose on or after their 16th birthday.
- MenACWY is preferred for adults with any of the preceding indications who are aged 55 years or younger as well as for adults aged 56 years or older who a) were vaccinated previously with MenACWY and are recommended for revaccination, or b) for whom multiple doses are anticipated. Meningococcal polysaccharide vaccine (MPSV4 [Menomune]) is preferred for adults aged 56 years or older who have not received MenACWY previously and who require a single dose only (e.g., travelers).
- Revaccination with MenACWY every 5 years is recommended for adults previously vaccinated with MenACWY or MPSV4 who remain at increased risk for infection (e.g., adults with anatomic or functional asplenia, persistent complement component deficiencies, or microbiologists).

12. Hepatitis A vaccination

- Vaccinate any person seeking protection from hepatitis A virus (HAV) infection and persons with any of the following indications:
  - men who have sex with men and persons who use injection or non-injection illicit drugs;
  - persons working with HAV-infected primates or with HAV in a research laboratory setting;
  - persons with chronic liver disease and persons who receive clotting factor concentrates;
  - persons traveling to or working in countries that have high or intermediate endemicity of hepatitis A; and

12. Hepatitis A vaccination (cont'd)

  - unvaccinated persons who anticipate close personal contact (e.g., household or regular babysitting) with an international adoptee during the first 60 days after arrival in the United States from a country with high or intermediate endemicity. (See footnote 1 for more information on travel recommendations.) The first dose of the 2-dose hepatitis A vaccine series should be administered as soon as adoption is planned, ideally 2 or more weeks before the arrival of the adoptee.
- Single-antigen vaccine formulations should be administered in a 2-dose schedule at either 0 and 6 to 12 months (Havrix), or 0 and 6 to 18 months (Vaqta). If the combined hepatitis A and hepatitis B vaccine (Twinrix) is used, administer 3 doses at 0, 1, and 6 months; alternatively, a 4-dose schedule may be used, administered on days 0, 7, and 21 to 30 followed by a booster dose at month 12.

13. Hepatitis B vaccination

- Vaccinate persons with any of the following indications and any person seeking protection from hepatitis B virus (HBV) infection:
  - sexually active persons who are not in a long-term, mutually monogamous relationship (e.g., persons with more than 1 sex partner during the previous 6 months); persons seeking evaluation or treatment for a sexually transmitted disease (STD); current or recent injection drug users; and men who have sex with men;
  - health care personnel and public safety workers who are potentially exposed to blood or other infectious body fluids;
  - persons with diabetes who are younger than age 60 years as soon as feasible after diagnosis; persons with diabetes who are age 60 years or older at the discretion of the treating clinician based on the likelihood of acquiring HBV infection, including the risk posed by an increased need for assisted blood glucose monitoring in long-term care facilities, the likelihood of experiencing chronic sequelae if infected with HBV, and the likelihood of immune response to vaccination;
  - persons with end-stage renal disease, including patients receiving hemodialysis, persons with HIV infection, and persons with chronic liver disease;
  - household contacts and sex partners of hepatitis B surface antigen–positive persons, clients and staff members of institutions for persons with developmental disabilities, and international travelers to countries with high or intermediate prevalence of chronic HBV infection; and
  - all adults in the following settings: STD treatment facilities, HIV testing and treatment facilities, facilities providing drug abuse treatment and prevention services, health care settings targeting services to injection drug users or men who have sex with men, correctional facilities, end-stage renal disease programs and facilities for chronic hemodialysis patients, and institutions and nonresidential day care facilities for persons with developmental disabilities.
- Administer missing doses to complete a 3-dose series of hepatitis B vaccine to those persons not vaccinated or not completely vaccinated. The second dose should be administered 1 month after the first dose; the third dose should be given at least 2 months after the second dose (and at least 4 months after the first dose). If the combined hepatitis A and hepatitis B vaccine (Twinrix) is used, give 3 doses at 0, 1, and 6 months; alternatively, a 4-dose Twinrix schedule, administered on days 0, 7, and 21 to 30 followed by a booster dose at month 12 may be used.
- Adult patients receiving hemodialysis or with other immunocompromising conditions should receive 1 dose of 40 mcg/mL (Recombivax HB) administered on a 3-dose schedule at 0, 1, and 6 months or 2 doses of 20 mcg/mL (Engerix-B) administered simultaneously on a 4-dose schedule at 0, 1, 2, and 6 months.

14. *Haemophilus influenzae* type b (Hib) vaccination

- One dose of Hib vaccine should be administered to persons who have functional or anatomic asplenia or sickle cell disease or are undergoing elective splenectomy if they have not previously received Hib vaccine. Hib vaccination 14 or more days before splenectomy is suggested.
- Recipients of a hematopoietic stem cell transplant should be vaccinated with a 3-dose regimen 6 to 12 months after a successful transplant, regardless of vaccination history; at least 4 weeks should separate doses.
- Hib vaccine is not recommended for adults with HIV infection since their risk for Hib infection is low.

15. Immunocompromising conditions

- Inactivated vaccines generally are acceptable (e.g., pneumococcal, meningococcal, and inactivated influenza vaccine) and live vaccines generally are avoided in persons with immune deficiencies or immunocompromising conditions. Information on specific conditions is available at http://www.cdc.gov/vaccines/hcp/acip-recs/index.html.

TABLE. Contraindications and precautions to commonly used vaccines in adults: United States, 2014 [1][*][†]		
Vaccine	**Contraindications**	**Precautions**
Influenza, inactivated vaccine (IIV)[2]	Severe allergic reaction (e.g., anaphylaxis) after previous dose of any IIV or LAIV or to a vaccine component, including egg protein.	Moderate or severe acute illness with or without fever. History of Guillain-Barré Syndrome within 6 weeks of previous influenza vaccination. Persons who experience only hives with exposure to eggs may receive RIV (if age 18-49 years) or, with additional safety precautions, IIV.[2]
Influenza, recombinant (RIV)	Severe allergic reaction (e.g., anaphylaxis) after previous dose of RIV or to a vaccine component. RIV does not contain any egg protein.[2]	Moderate or severe acute illness with or without fever. History of Guillain-Barré Syndrome within 6 weeks of previous influenza vaccination.
Influenza, live attenuated (LAIV)[2,3]	Severe allergic reaction (e.g., anaphylaxis) after previous dose of any IIV or LAIV or to a vaccine component, including egg protein. Conditions for which the Advisory Committee on Immunization Practices (ACIP) recommends against use, but which are not contraindications in vaccine package insert: immune suppression, certain chronic medical conditions (such as asthma, diabetes, heart or kidney disease). and pregnancy.[2,3]	Moderate or severe acute illness with or without fever. History of Guillain-Barré Syndrome within 6 weeks of previous influenza vaccination. Receipt of specific antivirals (i.e., amantadine, rimantadine, zanamivir, or oseltamivir) within 48 hours before vaccination. Avoid use of these antiviral drugs for 14 days after vaccination.
Tetanus, diphtheria, pertussis (Tdap); tetanus, diphtheria (Td)	Severe allergic reaction (e.g., anaphylaxis) after a previous dose or to a vaccine component. For pertussis-containing vaccines: encephalopathy (e.g., coma, decreased level of consciousness, or prolonged seizures) not attributable to another identifiable cause within 7 days of administration of a previous dose of Tdap or diphtheria and tetanus toxoids and pertussis (DTP) or diphtheria and tetanus toxoids and acellular pertussis (DTaP) vaccine.	Moderate or severe acute illness with or without fever. Guillain-Barré Syndrome within 6 weeks after a previous dose of tetanus toxoid–containing vaccine. History of Arthus-type hypersensitivity reactions after a previous dose of tetanus or diphtheria toxoid–containing vaccine; defer vaccination until at least 10 years have elapsed since the last tetanus toxoid-containing vaccine. For pertussis-containing vaccines: progressive or unstable neurologic disorder, uncontrolled seizures, or progressive encephalopathy until a treatment regimen has been established and the condition has stabilized.
Varicella[3]	Severe allergic reaction (e.g., anaphylaxis) after a previous dose or to a vaccine component. Known severe immunodeficiency (e.g., from hematologic and solid tumors, receipt of chemotherapy, congenital immunodeficiency, or long-term immunosuppressive therapy[4] or patients with human immunodeficiency virus (HIV) infection who are severely immunocompromised). Pregnancy.	Recent (within 11 months) receipt of antibody-containing blood product (specific interval depends on product).[5] Moderate or severe acute illness with or without fever. Receipt of specific antivirals (i.e., acyclovir, famciclovir, or valacyclovir) 24 hours before vaccination; avoid use of these antiviral drugs for 14 days after vaccination.
Human papillomavirus (HPV)	Severe allergic reaction (e.g., anaphylaxis) after a previous dose or to a vaccine component.	Moderate or severe acute illness with or without fever. Pregnancy.
Zoster[3]	Severe allergic reaction (e.g., anaphylaxis) to a vaccine component. Known severe immunodeficiency (e.g., from hematologic and solid tumors, receipt of chemotherapy, or long-term immunosuppressive therapy[4] or patients with HIV infection who are severely immunocompromised). Pregnancy.	Moderate or severe acute illness with or without fever. Receipt of specific antivirals (i.e., acyclovir, famciclovir, or valacyclovir) 24 hours before vaccination; avoid use of these antiviral drugs for 14 days after vaccination.
Measles, mumps, rubella (MMR)[3]	Severe allergic reaction (e.g., anaphylaxis) after a previous dose or to a vaccine component. Known severe immunodeficiency (e.g., from hematologic and solid tumors, receipt of chemotherapy, congenital immunodeficiency, or long-term immunosuppressive therapy[4] or patients with HIV infection who are severely immunocompromised). Pregnancy.	Moderate or severe acute illness with or without fever. Recent (within 11 months) receipt of antibody-containing blood product (specific interval depends on product).[5] History of thrombocytopenia or thrombocytopenic purpura. Need for tuberculin skin testing.[6]
Pneumococcal conjugate (PCV13)	Severe allergic reaction (e.g., anaphylaxis) after a previous dose or to a vaccine component, including to any vaccine containing diphtheria toxoid.	Moderate or severe acute illness with or without fever.
Pneumococcal polysaccharide (PPSV23)	Severe allergic reaction (e.g., anaphylaxis) after a previous dose or to a vaccine component.	Moderate or severe acute illness with or without fever.
Meningococcal, conjugate, (MenACWY); meningococcal, polysaccharide (MPSV4)	Severe allergic reaction (e.g., anaphylaxis) after a previous dose or to a vaccine component.	Moderate or severe acute illness with or without fever.
Hepatitis A (HepA)	Severe allergic reaction (e.g., anaphylaxis) after a previous dose or to a vaccine component.	Moderate or severe acute illness with or without fever.
Hepatitis B (HepB)	Severe allergic reaction (e.g., anaphylaxis) after a previous dose or to a vaccine component.	Moderate or severe acute illness with or without fever.
Haemophilus influenzae Type b (Hib)	Severe allergic reaction (e.g., anaphylaxis) after a previous dose or to a vaccine component.	Moderate or severe acute illness with or without fever.

1. Vaccine package inserts and the full ACIP recommendations for these vaccines should be consulted for additional information on vaccine-related contraindications and precautions and for more information on vaccine excipients. Events or conditions listed as precautions should be reviewed carefully. Benefits of and risks for administering a specific vaccine to a person under these circumstances should be considered. If the risk from the vaccine is believed to outweigh the benefit, the vaccine should not be administered. If the benefit of vaccination is believed to outweigh the risk, the vaccine should be administered. A contraindication is a condition in a recipient that increases the chance of a serious adverse reaction. Therefore, a vaccine should not be administered when a contraindication is present.

2. For more information on use of influenza vaccines among persons with egg allergies and a complete list of conditions that CDC considers to be reasons to avoid receiving LAIV, see CDC. Prevention and control of seasonal influenza with vaccines: recommendations of the Advisory Committee on Immunization Practices (ACIP) — United States, 2013–14. *MMWR* 2013;62(RR07):1-43. Available at http://www.cdc.gov/mmwr/preview/mmwrhtml/rr6207a1.htm.

3. LAIV, MMR, varicella, or zoster vaccines can be administered on the same day. If not administered on the same day, live vaccines should be separated by at least 28 days.

4. Immunosuppressive steroid dose is considered to be ≥2 weeks of daily receipt of 20 mg of prednisone or the equivalent. Vaccination should be deferred for at least 1 month after discontinuation of such therapy. Providers should consult ACIP recommendations for complete information on the use of specific live vaccines among persons on immune-suppressing medications or with immune suppression because of other reasons.

5. Vaccine should be deferred for the appropriate interval if replacement immune globulin products are being administered. See CDC. General recommendations on immunization: recommendations of the Advisory Committee on Immunization Practices (ACIP). *MMWR* 2011;60(No. RR-2). Available at www.cdc.gov/vaccines/hcp/acip-recs/index.html.

6. Measles vaccination might suppress tuberculin reactivity temporarily. Measles-containing vaccine may be administered on the same day as tuberculin skin testing. If testing cannot be performed until after the day of MMR vaccination, the test should be postponed for at least 4 weeks after the vaccination. If an urgent need exists to skin test, do so with the understanding that reactivity might be reduced by the vaccine.

* Adapted from CDC. Table 6. Contraindications and precautions to commonly used vaccines. General recommendations on immunization: recommendations of the Advisory Committee on Immunization Practices. *MMWR* 2011;60(No. RR-2):40–41 and from Atkinson W, Wolfe S, Hamborsky J, eds. Appendix A. Epidemiology and prevention of vaccine preventable diseases. 12th ed. Washington, DC: Public Health Foundation, 2011. Available at www.cdc.gov/vaccines/pubs/pinkbook/index.html.
† Regarding latex allergy, consult the package insert for any vaccine administered.

U.S. Department of Health and Human Services
Centers for Disease and Prevention

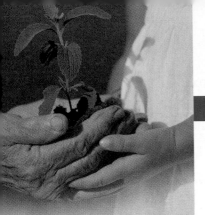

Sample of Living Will and Health Care Proxy

New York Health Care Proxy

PRINT YOUR NAME

PRINT NAME, HOME ADDRESS AND TELEPHONE NUMBER OF YOUR AGENT

(1) I, _____ , hereby appoint:

(name)

_____

(name, home address and telephone number of agent)

_____

as my health care agent to make any and all health care decisions for me, except to the extent that I state otherwise. My agent does know my wishes regarding artificial nutrition and hydration.

This Health Care Proxy shall take effect in the event I become unable to make my own health care decisions.

ADD PERSONAL INSTRUCTIONS (IF ANY)

(2) Optional instructions: I direct my agent to make health care decisions in accord with my wishes and limitations as stated below, or as he or she otherwise knows.

PRINT NAME, HOME ADDRESS AND TELEPHONE NUMBER OF YOUR ALTERNATE AGENT

(3) Name of substitute or fill-in agent if the person I appoint above is unable, unwilling or unavailable to act as my health care agent.

_____

(name, home address and telephone number of agent)

_____

ORGAN DONATION (OPTIONAL)

(4) Donation of Organs at Death: Upon my death:

[ ] I **do not** wish to donate my organs, tissues or parts.
[ ] I **do** wish to be an organ donor and upon my death I wish to donate:
[ ] (a) Any needed organs, tissues, or parts;

OR

[ ] (b) The following organs, tissues, or parts:

_____

_____

[ ] (c) My gift is for the following purposes:
   (put a line through any of the following you do not want)

   (i) Transplant   (ii) Therapy   (iii) Research   (iv) Education

ENTER A DURATION OR A CONDITION (IF ANY)

(5) Unless I revoke it, this proxy shall remain in effect indefinitely, or until the date or condition I have stated below. This proxy shall expire (specific date or conditions, if desired):_____

_____

(6) Signature _____ Date _____

Address _____

SIGN AND DATE THE DOCUMENT AND PRINT YOUR ADDRESS

WITNESSING PROCEDURE

Statement by Witnesses (must be 18 or older)

I declare that the person who signed this document appeared to execute the proxy willingly and free from duress. He or she signed (or asked another to sign for him or her) this document in my presence. I am not the person appointed as proxy by this document.

Witness 1_____

Address _____

Witness 2_____

Address _____

Courtesy of Caring Connections
1700 Diagonal Road, Suite 625, Alexandria, VA 22314
www. caringinfo.org, 800/658-8898

New York Living Will

INSTRUCTIONS

This Living Will has been prepared to conform to the law in the State of New York, as set forth in the case In re Westchester County Medical Center, 72 N.Y.2d 517 (1988). In that case the Court established the need for "clear and convincing" evidence of a patient's wishes and stated that the "ideal situation is one in which the patient's wishes were expressed in some form of writing, perhaps a 'living will.'"

PRINT YOUR NAME

I, _____ , being of sound mind, make this statement as a directive to be followed if I become permanently unable to participate in decisions regarding my medical care. These instructions reflect my firm and settled commitment to decline medical treatment under the circumstances indicated below:

I direct my attending physician to withhold or withdraw treatment that merely prolongs my dying, if I should be in an **incurable or irreversible mental or physical condition with no reasonable expectation of recovery,** including but not limited to: (a) **a terminal condition;** (b) a **permanently unconscious condition;** or (c) **a minimally conscious condition in which I am permanently unable to make decisions or express my wishes.**

I direct that my treatment be limited to measures to keep me comfortable and to relieve pain, including any pain that might occur by withholding or withdrawing treatment.

While I understand that I am not legally required to be specific about future treatments **if I am in the condition(s) described above I feel especially strongly about the following forms of treatment:**

**CROSS OUT
ANY STATEMENTS
THAT DO NOT
REFLECT YOUR
WISHES**

I do not want cardiac resuscitation.
I do not want mechanical respiration.
I do not want artificial nutrition and hydration.
I do not want antibiotics.

However, **I do want** maximum pain relief, even if it may hasten my death.

**ADD PERSONAL
INSTRUCTIONS
(IF ANY)**

Other directions:

**SIGN AND DATE
THE DOCUMENT AND
PRINT YOUR ADDRESS**

These directions express my legal right to refuse treatment, under the law of New York. I intend my instructions to be carried out, unless I have rescinded them in a new writing or by clearly indicating that I have changed my mind.

Signature _____ Date _____

Address _____

**WITNESSING
PROCEDURE**

I declare that the person who signed this document appeared to execute the living will willingly and free from duress. He or she signed (or asked another to sign for him or her) this document in my presence.

**YOUR WITNESSES
MUST SIGN AND PRINT
THEIR ADDRESSES**

Witness 1 _____

Address _____

Witness 2 _____

Address _____

Courtesy of Caring Connections
1700 Diagonal Road, Suite 625, Alexandria, VA 22314
www. caringinfo.org, 800/658-8898

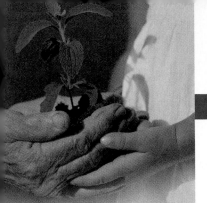

Answers to Multiple-Choice Questions

Chapter 1
1. b
2. d
3. b
4. c
5. a
6. b
7. c
8. c
9. b
10. d
11. d
12. b, c, d

Chapter 2
1. c
2. a
3. a
4. d
5. c
6. d
7. c
8. c
9. d
10. b, c

Chapter 3
1. d
2. a
3. a
4. d
5. c
6. d
7. c

8. c
9. d
10. b
11. True

Chapter 4
1. c
2. a
3. c
4. c
5. c
6. b
7. d
8. d
9. b
10. a

Chapter 5
1. c
2. c
3. b
4. d
5. c
6. a
7. c
8. b
9. c
10. d
11. b

Chapter 6
1. c
2. b, c
3. c
4. a

5. c
6. c
7. b
8. a
9. a
10. d
11. c
12. d
13. a
14. b

Chapter 7
1. b
2. c
3. b
4. d
5. b
6. b
7. c
8. d
9. b
10. d
11. d
12. c
13. d
14. c

Chapter 8
1. a, b, c
2. b, c
3. c
4. c
5. b
6. b

7. d
8. b
9. c
10. d
11. b
12. c

Chapter 9

1. c
2. d
3. c
4. b
5. b
6. b
7. c
8. c
9. d
10. b

Chapter 10

1. c
2. b
3. c
4. d
5. b
6. b

7. c
8. c
9. c
10. c
11. b
12. d

Chapter 11

1. d
2. c
3. c
4. b
5. b
6. b
7. a
8. a
9. d

Chapter 12

1. b
2. d
3. c
4. d
5. d
6. c
7. c
8. b

9. HDL high density lipoprotein
10. d

Chapter 13

1. d
2. b
3. c
4. a, b, c, d
5. c
6. a
7. d
8. b
9. c
10. d
11. b
12. b
13. d

Chapter 14

1. b
2. d
3. d
4. d
5. c
6. d

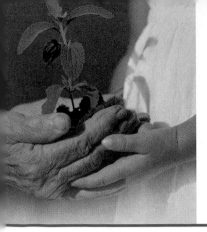

Glossary

acrocyanosis a bluish discoloration of the newborn's hands and feet as a result of poor peripheral circulation.

activity theory the aging theory that suggests that individuals remain active and engaged throughout their later years.

acuity sharpness or clearness.

adducted referring to movement of the extremities toward the center of the body.

adenohypophysis the anterior lobe of the pituitary gland.

adolescence a transitional period beginning with sexual maturity and ending with growth cessation and movement toward emotional maturity.

advance directive a legal document that states the person's wishes for medical treatment in the event that he or she cannot make these decisions.

aerobic exercise exercise that works the large body muscles and elevates the cardiac output and metabolic rate.

ageism discrimination against older persons.

aging normal, inevitable, progressive process that produces irreversible changes over an extended period.

ambivalence an emotional state of having conflicting, opposite feelings, such as love and hate for a person or object.

amblyopia known as "lazy eye," a condition seen in early childhood caused by weaker muscles in one eye that, if not corrected, may lead to blindness.

anorexia nervosa an eating disorder that is characterized by willful starvation and severe weight loss.

anticipatory grief a reaction to an expected loss such as in terminal illness.

antioxidants agents that prevent the formation of free radicals and may affect the aging process.

anxiety the response to a stressful situation.

apathy a lack of interest in one's surroundings.

Apgar score an assessment scale used to indicate an overall picture of the newborn's status.

apnea absence of respirations.

apocrine glands sweat glands in the axillae and pubic region.

atrophy wasting away.

autoimmune theory a theory of aging that suggests that aging is related to the body's weakening immune system, which fails to recognize its own tissues and may destroy itself.

autonomy independence and a sense of self.

basal metabolic rate the amount of energy that an individual uses at rest.

beliefs truths held by a culture.

benign prostatic hypertrophy a benign enlargement of the prostate gland that causes difficulty voiding, diminished urine stream, dribbling, and frequency.

bereavement a state of having sustained a loss.

bias a prejudice or a negative belief about someone or something.

blastocyst the developing mass of cells at the point of implantation of a fertilized egg.

bottle-mouth syndrome dental caries caused by sugar in the milk or juice; it usually occurs when bottles are given at nighttime.

bulimia an eating disorder characterized by a series of binges followed by purging or self-induced vomiting.

carcinogens cancer-producing agents such as cigarettes, radiation, etc.

cataract a cloudy formation on the lens of the eye.

cephalocaudal a directional term that refers to growth and development that begins at the head and progresses downward toward the feet.

cerumen wax buildup found in the ear.

cervix the lower "neck" portion of the uterus.

Cheyne-Stokes respirations irregular respiratory rates with periods of apnea.

cholesterol a component of many foods in our diet. It is an essential component of cells in the brain, nerves, blood, and hormones.

chromosomes substances that carry the genes that transmit inherited characteristics.

circumcision surgical removal of the foreskin performed for hygienic or religious reasons.

cleft palate incomplete congenital formation and nonunion of the hard palate.

climacteric change of life.

clockwork theory a theory of aging suggesting that connective-tissue cells have an internal clock that determines length of life.

coitus another term for sexual intercourse.

colostrum precursor of breast milk, present as early as the seventh month of fetal life.

communication an interaction between two or more persons.

compatibility a sympathetic, comfortable feeling tone in a relationship.

compensation a mental mechanism that allows the person to make up for deficiencies in one area by excelling in another.

conception union of the female ovum and the male sperm cell; also called fertilization.

congruence an agreement between the verbal and nonverbal language.

conscience a person's internal system of values, similar to the superego.

continuity-developmental theory an aging theory that suggests that aging should be viewed as part of the life cycle, not as a separate terminal stage.

conversion a mental mechanism that converts unconscious feelings and anxiety into physical symptoms that have no underlying organic basis for the complaints.

cooperative/associative play a play style typical of preschool children in which they begin to take turns and share in a cooperative manner.

culture all of the learned patterns of behavior passed down through generations.

deciduous teeth "baby" or primary teeth, which usually appear at about 6 to 7 months of age.

defense mechanisms also known as mental mechanisms, techniques used at all stages of the life cycle to help individuals cope with the threat of anxiety.

delirium an acute response in brain functioning that manifests itself as an acute impairment in cognition and attention.

demographics the study of a group of people including the size of the group, changes within the group, and information about where the group lives.

denial the mental mechanism whereby the individual is unable to recognize the event or emotions surrounding an occurrence. These events are so painful they are pushed out of consciousness.

dental caries tooth decay.

depression prolonged feelings of profound sadness and unworthiness.

dermis the inner layer of the skin directly below the epidermis.

development the progressive acquisition of skills and the capacity to function.

dilation widening or expansion of an opening.

disease prevention divided into three levels: primary, secondary, and tertiary. Aimed at disease prevention, includes proper education, nutrition, exercise, and immunization. Early diagnosis and treatment help prevent permanent disability. When permanent disability arises, the aim is to maximize the level of functioning.

disengagement theory a theory of aging that suggests that older persons and society gradually withdraw from one another to assist the transfer of power from the old to the young.

displacement a mental mechanism that transfers emotions associated with a person or object to another, less threatening person or object.

Do Not Resuscitate order (DNR) an order that guides health care workers with regard to the wishes of patients should the patient go into cardiac or respiratory arrest.

dominant genes those genes that are more capable of expressing their traits than are other genes.

durable power of attorney for health care the appointing of someone to make one's wishes known and carry out some decisions regarding one's medical care in the event that one can no longer express oneself.

dysfunctional family a family that is unable to offer its members a stable structure.

dyspareunia pain or discomfort during intercourse.

dysphagia difficulty swallowing.

effacement shortening and thinning of the cervix.

ego the executive of the mind. It relates most closely to reality.

ego integrity a period of self-satisfaction that occurs during old age.

egocentricity self-centered thought or actions.

ejaculation the release of sperm and semen.

Electra complex a young girl's sexual attraction toward her father and unconscious wish to replace her mother.

embryo the developing organism. Called this until the end of the eighth week.

emotions expressed feeling tones that influence a person's behavior.

empowerment a form of self-responsibility that demands that people take charge of their own decision making.

empty-nest syndrome a term used to define the reaction to having grown children leave the home.

engrossment the process of neonatal–father bonding.

enuresis bed-wetting after the age when urinary control has been established.

epiphyseal cartilage the center for ossification and growth at the end of long bones.

equilibrium a balance or a state of homeostasis.

estrogen hormone produced by the ovary.

ethnicity stable cultural patterns shared by a group of families with the same historical roots.

eustachian tube the structure that connects the pharynx to the middle ear.

euthanasia known as mercy killing in the past, now refers to the deliberate ending of one's life as well as the withholding of treatment.

family two or more people who have chosen to live together and share their interests, roles, and resources.

feedback the response to a message.

fertilization the union of the female ovum and male sperm cell; also called conception.

fetus the developing organism. Called this from the eighth week until birth.

fibrocystic breast disease benign cystic growths found in breast tissue.

fight-or-flight response a state of readiness to attack or flee caused by a perceived threat.

folkways the customs within the culture that determine how we greet one another.

fontanels commonly called soft spots. Spaces found between the infant's cranial bones where the sutures cross.

free-radical theory a theory of aging that states that highly unstable molecules contribute to the aging process.

free radicals highly unstable chemical substances produced by metabolism.

functional family a family that fosters the growth and development of its members.

general adaptation syndrome (GAS) a response to stress that was described by Hans Selye.

generativity Erikson's task for middle-aged adults. It involves individuals' desires to serve the larger community and have positive influences on their children.

genes found on strands of deoxyribonucleic acid (DNA) within the cell nucleus.

gerontology the study of the normal aging process.

gingivitis an inflammation of the gums characterized by swelling, redness, and bleeding.

glaucoma a disease of the eye characterized by increased intraocular pressure.

gonads the male and female sex glands.

grief the feeling tone or the outward expression in response to a loss.

growth an increase in physical size.

health a state of complete physical, mental, and social well-being, not merely the absence of disease or infirmity.

health promotion health care directed toward increasing one's optimum level of wellness.

health restoration that which begins once the disease process is stabilized.

heredity all characteristics that are transmitted through the genes and determined at the time of fertilization.

holistic including not only physical aspects of health but also psychological, social, cognitive, and environmental influences.

homeostasis a balance.

hormone replacement therapy (HRT) giving estrogen during menopause to treat symptoms.

hospice care a health care organization, under Medicare and Medicaid and other third-party insurers, that provides care to terminally ill persons in the comfort of their homes.

hot flashes sensations caused by vasodilatation of the capillaries that produces a rush of blood to the skin surface.

hypertension high blood pressure.

id the body's basic, primitive urges.

identification a mental mechanism in which one takes on the personality traits of another person, usually one held in high esteem.

immune-system-failure theory a theory of aging that suggests that it results when the immune system is unable to perform its function.

industry Erikson's task for the school-age child. At this stage children are productive and focus on the real world and their roles in it.

infant mortality rate the number of infant deaths before the first birthday per 1,000 live births.

initiative Erikson's task for the preschool child demonstrated by pretend, exploration, and trying on of new roles.

insomnia inability to sleep.

integumentary system skin and related structures.

intimacy a feeling of warmth, love, and affection.

introspection a form of self-reflection. It may serve as a tool that permits sharing of our innermost thoughts.

involution the return of the uterus to its nonpregnant state.

karyotype the individual chromosomal pattern of a person.

keratosis skin thickening.

kyphosis curvature of the thoracic spine.

lacrimal ducts tear ducts.

lanugo soft, fine, downy hair covering newborns.

larynx the voice box that houses the vocal cords.

latency the period described by Freud when school-age children's sexual energies are relatively dormant.

laws written policies supported and enforced by the government.

libido sex drive.

life expectancy the average number of years a person is likely to live.

life span the maximum number of years that a species is capable of surviving.

lifestyle a person's habits and usual practices common to daily living.

lipofuscin a pigmented metabolic waste product that has been found in greater amounts in various organs of the aged body.

living will a form of advance directive that states the wishes of a person for life-sustaining treatment in case of serious illness.

lordosis an exaggerated lumbar curvature seen in the toddler period.

loss an encounter that one faces during the course of one's life.

lumen the opening or diameter of a vessel.

maladaptive grief responses to loss that usually exhibit an exaggerated, lengthy, unpredictable course that results in unresolved conflicts.

malnutrition poor dietary practice that results from the lack of essential nutrients or from failure to eat available foods.

malocclusion a malposition or imperfect contact between the upper and lower teeth.

mammography breast x-ray for diagnostic screening.

Mantoux skin test an intracutaneous test for tuberculosis.

maturation the unfolding of skills or potential regardless of practice or training.

meconium the first newborn stool, usually green–black in color and odorless.

melanocytes pigmented skin cells.

menarche the onset of menses (first menstrual period).

menopause the cessation of menses, usually between 45 and 55 years of age.

message the expression of thoughts and feelings in words, symbols, and body language.

method the way a message is conveyed.

milia small clusters of pearly white spots found mostly on the infant's nose, chin, and forehead. They result from nonfunctioning or clogged sebaceous glands.

molding an elongation or overriding of the cranial bones that occurs during passage through the birth canal.

mongolian spot a bluish-black, flat, irregularly pigmented area found in the lumbosacral region in darker pigmented infants.

mores moral issues that are strongly believed by a culture.

morula the mass of cells following fertilization that resembles a mulberry.

mourning the natural process that one goes through following a major loss.

negativistic behavior negative, rebellious behavior exhibited by toddlers that is caused by frustration or a conflict of wills.

neonate the newborn or the first 4 weeks of extrauterine life.

nephrons the functional, working units found in the kidneys.

neurons also known as nerve cells.

nonverbal communication communication using body language.

normal physiological weight loss a loss of 5% to 10% of birth weight occurring in the early neonatal period with a regain in approximately 10 days.

norms socially accepted rules and behavior that guide human behavior and interactions within a culture.

nurturance the provision of love, care, and attention to each family member.

nystagmus unequal eye movements (crossing) owing to immature ciliary muscles.

obesity the state of having 20% to 30% excess weight.

occult blood hidden or invisible blood.

Oedipus complex a young boy's sexual attraction for his mother and unconscious wish to replace his father.

old the period between age 75 and age 90.

omnipotence sense of unlimited power or authority.

opacity a clouding of the lens of the eye.

ossification the hardening process whereby bone tissue gradually replaces the soft cartilage tissue.

osteoporosis a disorder characterized by decreased bone mass resulting from the loss of minerals from the bones.

ova the plural form of ovum; female sex cells.

ovaries the female sex glands or gonads.

ovulation the rupture and release of the ovum.

ovum the female sex cell.

palliative care a form of helping to relieve the suffering of terminally ill persons.

Papanicolaou test a common screening test used to detect cancer of the cervix.

parallel play a play style typical of toddlers whereby they play alongside each other but do not really interact or share.

Patient Self-Determination Act (PSDA) the law that requires that a patient has the right to have advance directives in place. Failure of an institution to inform a person of this right will result in withholding reimbursement of funding to the institution.

penis the male sex organ.

peristalsis wavelike muscular movement in the gastrointestinal tract.

personality the unique behavior patterns that distinguish one person from another.

physiological jaundice a yellowish tinge to the skin of the newborn seen in the first 48 to 72 hours after birth.

placenta a flattened circular mass of tissue attached to the inner uterine wall. This organ has several functions: to produce hormones, transport nutrients and wastes, and protect the unborn from harmful substances.

preadolescence (or puberty) a time of rapid growth ending with reproductive maturation.

presbycusis an impairment of high-frequency hearing associated with advancing age.

presbyopia the decreased ability to see objects clearly at close distance. It occurs with advancing age.

primary sex characteristics the growth and maturation of the sex glands.

procreation the ability to reproduce.

progesterone a female sex hormone.

projection a mental mechanism referred to as the blaming mechanism; in projection the individual rejects unacceptable thoughts or feelings and attributes them to another person.

proximity nearness in location.

proximodistal a directional term that refers to growth and development that progresses from the center of the body toward the extremities.

pruritus a term used to describe itching.

pseudomenstruation a slight blood-tinged vaginal discharge that may appear shortly after birth. It is thought to be related to the maternal hormones and disappears without any treatment.

puberty the period following childhood and before adolescence in which the body prepares for the changes necessary for reproduction.

race a group of people sharing certain characteristics including skin color, hair texture, facial shape, and/or body size or shape.

rationalization a mental mechanism used to justify or excuse undesirable actions or feelings. It is a face-saving technique that may or may not deal with the truth.

reaction formation a mental mechanism that keeps unacceptable feelings or thoughts out of one's awareness and replaces them with opposite feelings or thoughts.

reaction time the speed at which a person responds to a stimulus.

receiver the person to whom a message is sent.

recessive genes genes for inherited traits that can only be transmitted if they exist in pairs.

reciprocity moral feelings of concern for what is fair to others, as described by Kohlberg.

regression a return to an earlier stage of development during stressful periods.

religion a specific system of beliefs and worship.

reminiscence a process of remembering and discussing key life events.

residual volume the amount of air left in the lungs after forceful exhalation.

resistance exercise weight lifting that builds muscle mass.

respectability emphasizes role modeling and valuing.

ritualistic behavior repetitive behavior, habits, or routines that serve to lower anxiety.

sanctions the social remedies for violating any of the norms.

saturated fats fats that come from animals. Found in meats and dairy products.

school phobia an intense fear of going to school.

scoliosis abnormal lateral curvature of the spine.

scrotum a sac that holds the testes.

secondary sex characteristics all the changes that play no direct role in reproduction, such as the appearance of pubic, axillary, and facial hair; an increase in activity of the sebaceous and apocrine glands; breast development; and widening of the pelvic and hip bones.

sender the person who delivers a message.

senescence the symptoms or changes associated with normal aging.

senile lentigo common, flat, discolored "age spots" found on the skin.

separation anxiety anxiety brought on by stress when the young child is separated from family by school, hospitalization, or family death.

sexuality a broad term that includes anatomy; gender roles; relationships; and a person's thoughts, feelings, and attitudes about sex.

sexually transmitted diseases (STDs) diseases that are transmitted through sexual intercourse.

sibling rivalry jealousy of siblings that causes feelings of insecurity.

social communication communication that is used every day and is light and superficial.

socialization the process of having the individual adapt to social customs.

socializing agent an agent that helps to instill beliefs, values, and mores in a child. The family is the first socializing agent for a child.

somatic pertaining to the body.

sperm the male sex cell.

stagnation the lack of generativity, characterized by having feelings of self-absorption and general dissatisfaction with life.

stress anything that upsets psychological or physiological balance.

sublimation a mental mechanism in which the individual channels or redirects unacceptable impulses into socially acceptable outlets.

sun protection factor (SPF) the amount of time a person can stay exposed to sunlight without burning.

superego the part of the mind that dictates right from wrong and is similar to the conscience.

suppression the mental mechanism whereby one consciously puts out of awareness one's distressing feelings.

sutures thick bands of cartilage that separate the infant's skull bones.

symbols expressed as language, gestures, or objects. A culture uses symbols to communicate with its members.

team play an advanced style of play typical of older children that requires the ability to follow rules and regulations. Team play may be competitive in nature.

teratogens chemical or physical substances that can adversely affect the unborn.

testes the male gonads.

testosterone the male sex hormone produced by the interstitial cells of the testes.

therapeutic communication communication that is purposeful and goal directed.

tinnitus ringing in the ears.

transcultural nursing a view of nursing as caring for one world with many cultures.

umbilical cord the connecting link between the fetus and the placenta.

undoing a mental mechanism in which the individual acts in a manner that symbolically cancels a previous unacceptable thought or action.

unsaturated fats fats that are usually liquid at room temperature and are derived from plant sources.

values deeply embedded feelings that determine what is considered good or bad, right or wrong.

verbal communication transmission of attitudes, thoughts, and feelings using spoken or written words.

vernix caseosa a white, cheeselike, protective covering found on the neonate's skin.

very old the period of age 90 and older.

vital capacity the ability of the lungs to move air in and out.

weaning the gradual substitution of the cup for the breast or bottle.

wear-and-tear theory theory suggesting that after repeated injury, cells wear out and cease to function, hastening the aging process.

wellness a relative state of health.

xerostomia a reduction in saliva and resultant drying of the mouth.

young old the period from ages 65 to 74.

zygote a fertilized ovum.

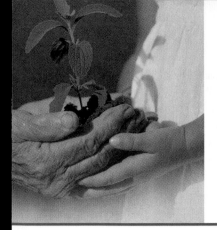

Index

Note: Illustrations are indicated by *(f);* tables by *(t);* boxes by *(b).*